ITI Treatment Guide
Volume 14

France Lambert
Adam Hamilton

International Team for Implantology

Immediate Implant Placement and Loading

Single or Multiple Teeth Requiring Replacement

EDITORS
Daniel Wismeijer
Stephen Barter
Nikolaos Donos

QUINTESSENCE PUBLISHING

Berlin | Chicago | Tokyo
Barcelona | London | Milan | Mexico City | Paris | Prague | Seoul | Warsaw
Beijing | Istanbul | Sao Paulo | Zagreb

The German National Library has listed this publication in the German National Bibliography. Detailed bibliographical data are available at https://dnb.ddb.de.

A CIP record for this book is available from the British Library.
ISBN 978-1-78698-127-1

QUINTESSENCE PUBLISHING DEUTSCHLAND

Ifenpfad 2–4
12107 Berlin
Germany
www.quintessence-publishing.com

Quintessence Publishing Co Ltd
Grafton Road, New Malden
Surrey KT3 3AB
United Kingdom
www.quintessence-publishing.com

Illustrations:	Ute Drewes, Basel (CH), www.drewes.ch
Copyediting:	Triacom Dental, Barendorf (DE), www.triacom.com
Layout | Production:	Janina Kuhn, Berlin (DE)
Printer:	Grafički zavod Hrvatske Mičevečka ulica 7 HR-10000 Zagreb, Croatia www.gzh.hr

Printed in Croatia
ISBN: 978-1-78698-127-1

The materials offered in the ITI Treatment Guide are for educational purposes only and intended as a step-by-step guide to the treatment of a particular case and patient situation. These recommendations are based on the conclusions of the ITI Consensus Conferences and, as such, are in line with the ITI treatment philosophy. These recommendations, nevertheless, represent the opinions of the authors. Neither the ITI nor the authors, editors, or publishers make any representation or warranty for the completeness or accuracy of the published materials and as a consequence do not accept any liability for damages (including, without limitation, direct, indirect, special, consequential, or incidental damages or loss of profits) caused by the use of the information contained in the ITI Treatment Guide. The information contained in the ITI Treatment Guide cannot replace an individual assessment by a clinician and its use for the treatment of patients is therefore the sole responsibility of the clinician.

The inclusion of or reference to a particular product, method, technique or material relating to such products, methods, or techniques in the ITI Treatment Guide does not represent a recommendation or an endorsement of the values, features, or claims made by its respective manufacturers.

Some of the manufacturer and product names referred to in this publication may be registered trademarks or proprietary names, even though specific reference to this fact is not made. Therefore, the appearance of a name without designation as proprietary is not to be construed as a representation by the publisher that it is in the public domain.

The tooth identification system used in this ITI Treatment Guide is that of the FDI World Dental Federation.

The ITI Mission is …

"… to serve the dental profession by providing a growing global network for life-long learning in implant dentistry through comprehensive quality education and innovative research to the benefit of the patient."

Acknowledgement

The authors would like to express their gratitude to Dr. Kati Benthaus for her excellent support in the preparation and coordination of this Treatment Guide. We would also like to thank Ms. Ute Drewes for the professional illustrations, Ms. Janina Kuhn (Quintessence Publishing) for the typesetting, Ms. Änne Kappeler (Quintessence Publishing) for the coordination of the production workflow, and Mr. Per N. Döhler (Triacom Dental) for the language editing. We also acknowledge Institut Straumann AG, the corporate partner of the ITI, for its continuing support.

Preface

The advantages of immediate implant placement and loading protocols are well documented and can be considered a desirable treatment approach if certain conditions are fulfilled.

A considerable body of literature supporting the use of immediate implant placement and loading protocols in partially edentulous patients has accumulated over the last two decades. However, a number of factors and procedures such as type of surgery, alveolar ridge preservation, and type of graft, among others, can make the clinical decisions involved challenging.

Referring to evidence-based methods, this volume of the ITI Treatment Guide series aims to provide a comprehensive overview of immediate implant placement and loading protocols for replacement of single or multiple teeth requiring extraction. It highlights the importance of patient and site selection in combination with comprehensive treatment planning and provides the reader with a risk-assessment table to aid in decision-making. The reader will also find a description of all key aspects of both surgical and loading procedures, providing clinical protocols for predictable treatment outcomes.

Step-by-step clinical cases performed by experts in the field underline the importance of careful patient selection in order to achieve successful outcomes, while also reducing patient treatment time. Overall, Volume 14 of the ITI Treatment Guide series will inform and support clinicians when faced with challenging cases of single and multiple tooth replacement.

D. Wismeijer S. Barter N. Donos

Editors and Authors

EDITORS

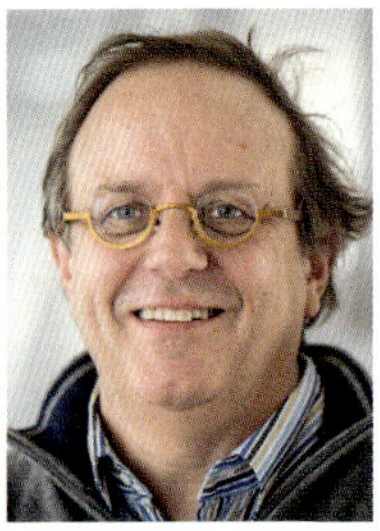

Daniel Wismeijer, Professor, DMD, PhD
Referral Practice for Oral Implantology and Prosthetic Dentistry
De Veluwezoom
p/a Zutphensestraatweg 26
6955 AH Ellecom
The Netherlands
Email: danwismeijer@gmail.com

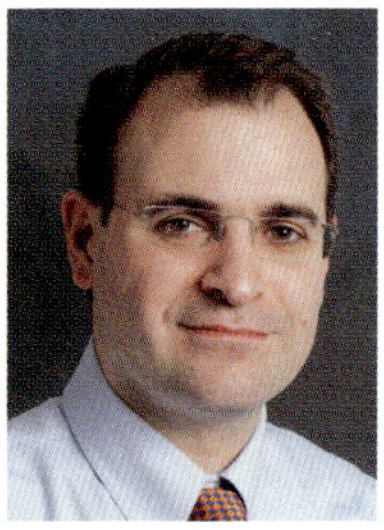

Nikolaos Donos, DDS, MS, FHEA, FDSRC, PhD
Director of Research
Professor and Chair of Periodontology and Implant Dentistry
Head of Clinical Research
Centre for Oral Clinical Research
Institute of Dentistry
Barts and The London School of Medicine and Dentistry
Turner Street
London E1 2AD
United Kingdom
Email: n.donos@qmul.ac.uk

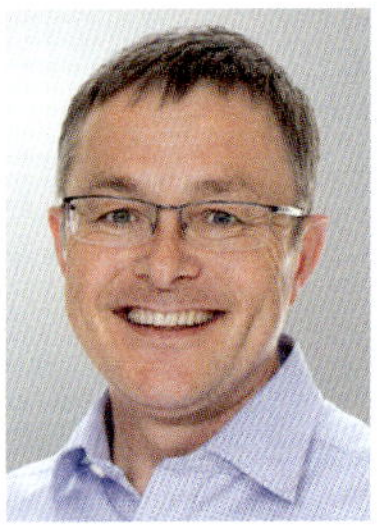

Stephen Barter, BDS, MSurgDent, RCS
Specialist in Oral Surgery
Honorary Senior Clinical Lecturer / Consultant Oral Surgeon
Centre for Oral Clinical Research
Institute of Dentistry
Barts and The London School of Medicine and Dentistry
Turner Street
London E1 2AD
United Kingdom
Email: s.barter@gmx.com

AUTHORS

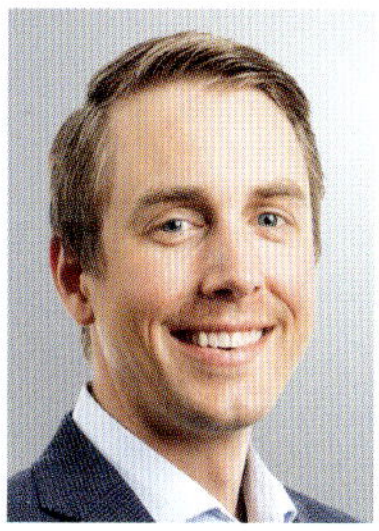

Adam Hamilton, BDSc, DCD, FRACDS
Discipline Lead in Prosthodontics and Graduate Program Convenor
Division of Oral Restorative and Rehabilitative Sciences
University of Western Australia
17 Monash Avenue
Nedlands, WA 6009
Australia
Email: adam.hamilton2@uwa.edu.au

Division of Regenerative and Implant Sciences
Department of Restorative Dentistry and Biomaterial Sciences
Harvard School of Dental Medicine
188 Longwood Avenue
Boston, MA 02118
United States of America
Email: adam_hamilton@hsdm.harvard.edu

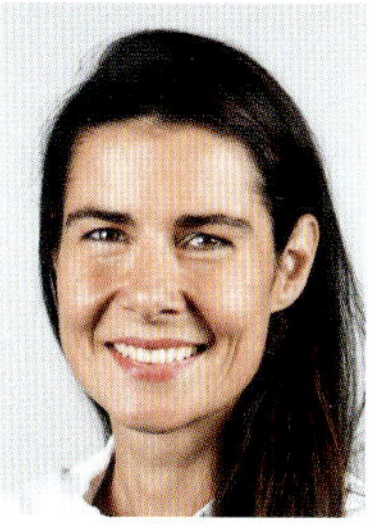

France Lambert, DDS, MSc, PhD
Professor and Head, Department of Periodontology, Oro-dental and Implant Surgery
Vice-director, Dental Biomaterial Research Unit
CHU of Liège
University of Liège
Domaine Universitaire du Sart Tilman B35
4000 Liège
Belgium
Email: france.lambert@chuliege.be

Contributors

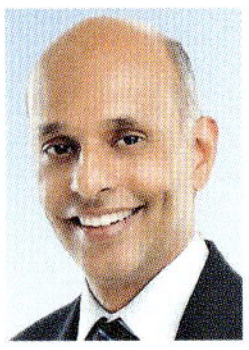

Mauricio G. Araújo, DDS, MSc, PhD
Professor, Head of Periodontics and Implant Dentistry Research Unit
Department of Dentistry
State University of Maringá
Av. Mandacaru 1550
87080-000 Maringá
Brazil
Email: odomar@hotmail.com

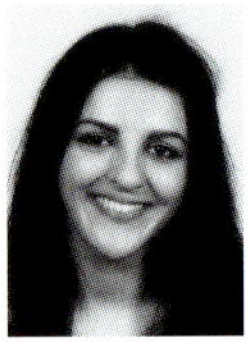

Miljana Baćević, DDS, PhD
Centre for Oral Clinical Research
Institute of Dentistry
Barts and The London School of Medicine and Dentistry
Turner Street
London E1 2AD
United Kingdom
Email: miljanabacevic@gmail.com

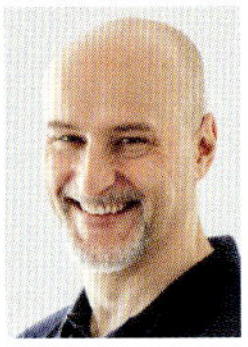

Thomas Borer, Dr med dent
Oral Surgery and Prosthetics
Private Clinic Basel Switzerland
Missionsstrasse 1
4055 Basel
Switzerland
Email: info@praxis-moser-borer.ch

Senior Doctor
Kantonsspital Aarau Switzerland
Haus 2a, Tellstrasse 25
5001 Aarau
Switzerland
Email: thomas.borer@ksa.ch

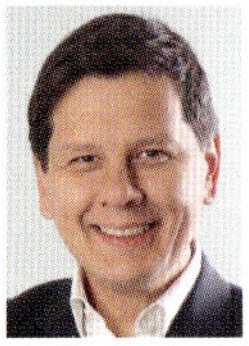

Andre Chen, DDS, MSc, PhD
Oral Surgery Specialist
Private Practice
International Advanced Dentistry
Academy Center for Continuing Dental Education
Av. da Liberdade 220, 1st Floor
1250-147 Lisboa
Portugal
Email: ac@iadlisbon.com

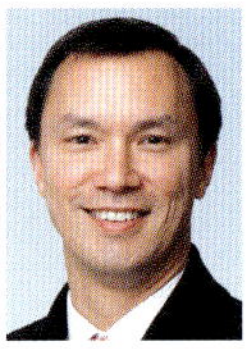

Stephen Chen, BDS, MDSc, FRACDS, PhD
Clinical Associate Professor
Melbourne Dental School
Faculty of Medicine, Dentistry and Health Sciences
The University of Melbourne
720 Swanston Street, Carlton, VIC 3053
Australia
Email: schen@periomelbourne.com.au

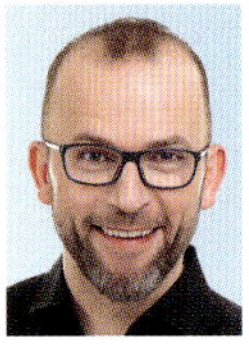

Krzysztof Chmielewski, DDS, MSc
SmileClinic Chmielewski & Karczewska
Advanced Implant Center
Karola Szymanskiego 2
80-280 Gdańsk
Poland
Email: krischmielewski@me.com

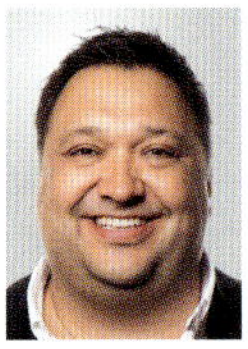

Karim Dada, Dr, DDS, MS
Private Practice
62 Bd de la Tour-Maubourg
75007 Paris
France
Email: dr.kd@me.com

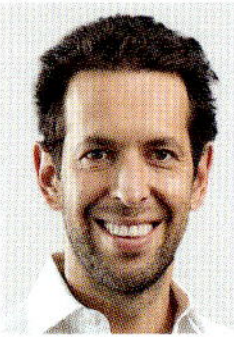

Gary Finelle, DMD
Private practice Dental7Paris
59 Av de la Bourdonnais
75007 Paris
France
Email: gary.finelle@dental7paris.com

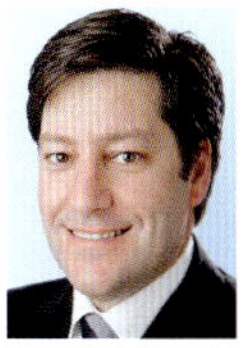

German O. Gallucci, DMD, PhD
Raymond J. and Elva Pomfret Nagle
Endowed
Associate Professor and Chair Department of
Restorative Dentistry and Biomaterials
Sciences
Harvard School of Dental Medicine
188 Longwood Avenue
Boston, MA 02115
United States of America
Email: german_gallucci@hsdm.harvard.edu

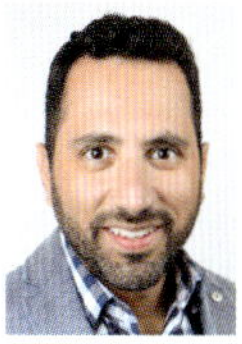

Luiz Gonzaga, DDS, MS
Clinical Associate Professor
Center for Implant Dentistry
Department of Oral and Maxillofacial Surgery
College of Dentistry
University of Florida
1395 Center Drive, Room D7-6
Gainesville, FL 32610-0434
United States of America
Email: lgonzaga@dental.ufl.edu

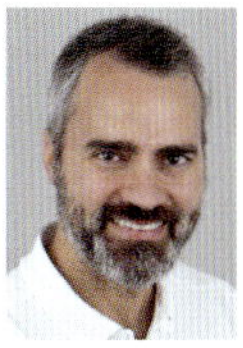

Oscar Gonzalez-Martin, DDS, PhD, MSc
Private practice, Atelier Dental Madrid
C/Blanca de Navarra 10
28010 Madrid
Spain
Email: oscar@atelierdentalmadrid.com

Visiting lecturer
Department of Restorative Dentistry and
Biomaterials Sciences
Harvard School of Dental Medicine
188 Longwood Ave
Boston, MA 02115
United States of America
Email: oscar_gonzalez-martin@
hsdm.harvard.edu

Visiting lecturer
University Complutense Madrid
Department of Periodontology
Plaza Ramon y Cajal
28040 Madrid
Spain

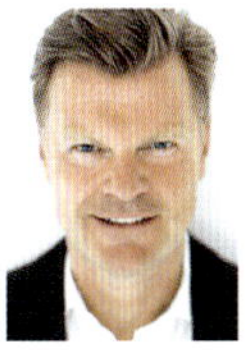

Arndt Happe, PD, Dr med dent
Private Practice Dr. Happe & Kollegen
Specialist in Implantology, Oral Surgeon
Schützenstr. 2
48 143 Münster
Germany
Email: a.happe@dr-happe.de

Clinic for Dental Prosthetics
Center for Dental, Oral and Maxillofacial
Medicine
University Hospital Ulm
Albert-Einstein-Allee 11
89081 Ulm
Germany

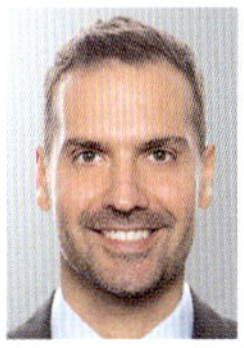

Alejandro Lanis, DDS, MS
Director Advanced Graduate Education in
Implant Dentistry
Assistant Professor in Restorative Dentistry
and Biomaterials Sciences
Harvard School of Dental Medicine
188 Longwood Avenue
Boston, MA 02115
United States of America
Email: alejandro_lanis@hsdm.harvard.edu

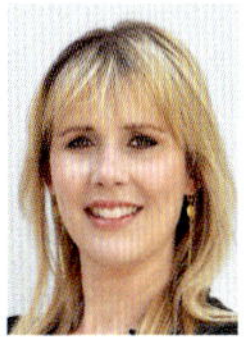

Amélie Mainjot, DDS, MSc, PhD
Professor and Head, Dental Biomaterials
Research Unit
University of Liège
Head of Clinic, Department of Fixed
Prosthodontics
University Hospital Center (CHU) of Liège
Department of Dentistry
Quai G. Kurth, 45
4000 Liège
Belgium
Email: amelie.mainjot@uliege.be

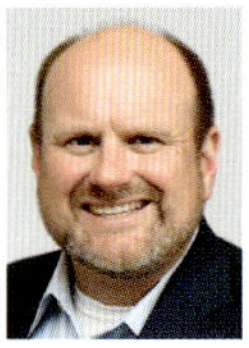

William Martin, DMD, MS, FACP
Clinical Professor and Director
Center for Implant Dentistry
Department of Oral and Maxillofacial Surgery
College of Dentistry
University of Florida
1395 Center Drive, Room D7-6
Gainesville, FL 32610
United States of America
Email: wmartin@dental.ufl.edu

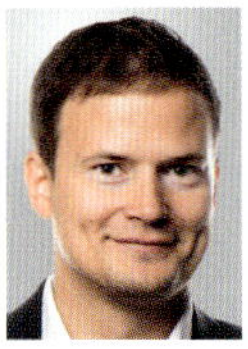

Léon Parienté, Dr, DDS
Private Practice
62 Bd de la Tour-Maubourg
75007 Paris
France
Email: drpariente@gmail.com

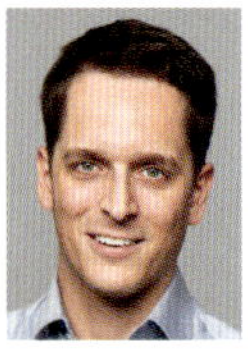

Stefan Röhling, DDS, PD, Dr med dent
Specialist in Oral Surgery
Senior Clinical Lecturer/Consultant Oral Surgeon
Private dental practice Gahlert & Röhling
Theatinerstraße 1
80333 Munich
Germany
Email: sr@oralchirurgie-t1.de

Senior Oral Surgeon and Associate Professor
Clinic of Oral- and Maxillofacial Surgery
Hightech Research Center
University Hospital Basel, Kantonsspital Aarau
Tellstrasse 25
5001 Aarau
Switzerland

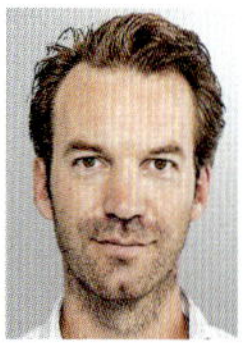

Björn Roland
Dental Design Björn Roland GmbH
Raiffeisenstraße 7
55270 Klein-Winternheim
Germany
Email: br@dental-design.de

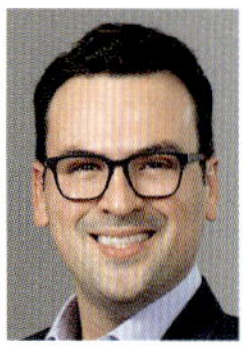

André Barbisan De Souza, DMD, MSc
Adjunct Professor
Nova Southeastern University College of Dental Medicine
3020 North Military Trail Ste 200
Boca Raton, FL 33431
United States of America
Email: andrebarbisan@gmail.com

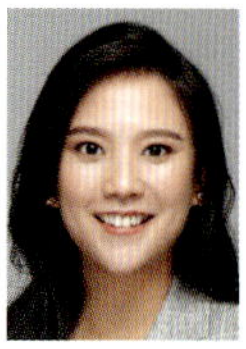

Teresa Chanting Sun, DDS, MS
Specialist in Periodontology
Department of Periodontology
Mackay Memorial Hospital
92 Zhongshan North Road Section 2
104 Taipei City
Taiwan

Clinical Assistant Professor
School of Dentistry
National Defense Medical Center
and Tri-Service General Hospital
161 Minquan E Road Section 6
114 Taipei City
Taiwan
Email: teresasun2015@gmail.com

Table of Contents

1 Introduction

A. Hamilton, F. Lambert

Once a tooth is indicated for extraction and immediate replacement with a dental implant, one of the first and most important clinical decisions to make is to select an appropriate protocol for implant placement and loading. The success of this protocol is determined by four main parameters: biological, prosthetic, and esthetic outcomes, as well as patient satisfaction (as per patient-reported outcome metrics). The selected protocol should combine the maximally predictable short- and long-term outcomes with the lowest surgical morbidity and highest efficiency (Buser and coworkers 2017a).

Our continuously better understanding of the biology of immediate placement has had a significant impact on the evolution of immediate placement and loading protocols and procedures. The advantages of immediate placement are well documented; they include shorter overall treatment times, limitation to a single surgical session, and maximum availability of potential bone volume (since the extraction socket will not yet have undergone the inevitable post-extraction resorption) (Hämmerle and coworkers 2004; Chen and Buser 2008). Immediate implant placement and loading is a desirable protocol—provided that the appropriate clinical indications are present.

However, several limitations have been reported for this approach. Immediate placement is made more complicated by the morphology of the socket and the surrounding alveolar bone. Achieving the ideal three-dimensional position of the implant while obtaining primary stability can be a challenge. Immediate placement does not limit the alveolar bone resorption associated with tooth extraction (Araújo and coworkers 2005). Unless addressed by proper patient selection and adjunctive regenerative procedures, this bone resorption may lead to midfacial recession and esthetic compromises (Chen and Buser 2014).

Considerable research into immediate placement and immediate loading in partially edentulous patients has been published over the last two decades. Overall, the literature reports this to be a predictable treatment approach, with implant survival rates comparable to delayed protocols using contemporary treatment approaches (Gallucci and coworkers 2018). However, the diversity of surgical and prosthetic techniques in terms of adjunctive procedures and factors can make clinical decisions difficult.

These adjunctive factors include:

- Type of surgery (flapless versus open-flap procedures)
- Alveolar ridge preservation (socket grafting versus no graft)
- Type of graft (*autologous, allograft, or xenograft*)
- Use of connective tissue graft (CT) for soft tissue augmentation
- Simultaneous connection of a provisional prosthesis (immediate loading)

There seems to be a trend for studies of immediate (type 1A) implant placement that use adjunctive regenerative procedures to minimize and compensate for resorption of the facial tissues (flapless, bone graft, and CT graft) to exhibit less variability in terms of esthetic outcomes (Chen and Buser 2008; Seyssens and coworkers 2021)

The focus of the present Volume 14 of the ITI Treatment series is on modern treatment protocols for immediate implant placement following the flapless extraction of a tooth. The reduced surgical trauma and morbidity associated with this approach offer distinct biological advantages and provide greater patient benefits than more invasive approaches.

This volume therefore aims to provide a comprehensive overview of immediate implant placement and loading protocols for the replacement of single teeth requiring extraction. The current literature on immediate implant placement and immediate loading is outlined to provide the biological understanding that underpins these concepts, together with a review of the success of immediate tooth-replacement protocols (Chapter 2).

The main objective of this volume is to highlight the importance of patient and site selection in conjunction with comprehensive treatment planning, and to provide the reader with a risk assessment tool that will aid in decision-making (Chapter 3).

Even if the sites for immediate implant placement and loading are carefully selected, these interventions are technically complex, with many variations in proposed treatment protocols. The second objective of this volume is therefore to describe the key aspects of both the surgical and loading procedures, in order to provide protocols that optimize the final outcome (Chapter 4).

This volume also provides step-by-step reports of clinical cases performed by experts in the field, exploring a range of indications and applications for immediate implant placement and loading protocols (Chapter 5).

The final chapter discusses typical complications associated with immediate implants and provides recommendations on how to prevent them (Chapter 6).

2 Evolution of Immediate Implant Placement and Loading

A. Hamilton, F. Lambert, M. Baćević, M. Araújo,
S. Chen, G. Gallucci

2.1 Evolution of Implant Placement Protocols

The original protocol for implant placement required a healed alveolar ridge and involved a two-stage surgical procedure (Schroeder and coworkers 1976; Brånemark and coworkers 1977). Even though the Tübingen immediate implant, which allowed implant placement into fresh extraction sockets, was introduced soon thereafter (Schulte and coworkers 1978), immediate implants presented a more challenging option to traditional (delayed) implants for decades to follow. Techniques based on the principles of guided bone regeneration (GBR) (Dahlin and coworkers 1988; Dahlin and coworkers 1989) were also investigated at that time and applied to peri-implant extraction defects of immediate implants in combination with open-flap procedures (Lazzara 1989; Becker and Becker 1990; Lang and coworkers 1994).

Early on, studies had shown that implants placed into fresh extraction sockets could successfully achieve osseointegration (Barzilay and coworkers 1988; Barzilay and coworkers 1991; Paolantonio and coworkers 2001), but higher implant failure rates were also reported (Schwartz-Arad and Chaushu 1997, Mayfield 1999). By the late 1990s, new studies had emerged to demonstrate that not only immediate implant placement was possible but also immediate loading (of the implants) (Wöhrle 1998). However, initial clinical results with immediate implants or immediate loading were not always satisfactory, particularly in regard to esthetic outcomes (Chen and coworkers 2004).

The introduction of implants with moderately rough surfaces provided a better understanding of the bone/implant interface and healing processes, as well as occlusion and proper prosthetic design. Along with the improvement of implant design, immediately placed and loaded implants slowly gained acceptance among the scientific community and among clinicians (Avila and coworkers 2007). Following the accumulation of an extensive body of evidence, both immediate implant placement and immediate loading have become accepted clinical procedures within the indicated conditions.

A widely adopted classification of 4 categories for the timing of implant placement after tooth extraction (type 1 to type 4) was first established at the 3rd ITI Consensus Conference (Hämmerle and coworkers 2004) and further modified in Vol. 3 of the ITI Treatment Guide series (Chen and Buser 2008), which classified immediate implant placement following tooth extraction as type 1 (Fig 1).

The main benefit of type 1 (immediate) implant placement lies in the reduced number of surgical procedures, shorter overall treatment times, reduced recovery times, and—in certain circumstances—the ability to immediately restore the implant, leading to high patient satisfaction as well as positive effects regarding the maintenance of the peri-implant softtissue architecture.

A biological understanding of immediate implant placement relies on the biology of socket healing. Post-extraction socket healing is a biological process where several processes develop continuously, despite being arbitrarily assigned to distinct phases, namely: hemostasis and coagulation, inflammatory, proliferative, and modeling and remodeling phases (de Sousa Gomes and coworkers 2019).

Immediately after tooth extraction, the socket is filled with blood; a blood clot is formed soon thereafter. The wound starts to attract inflammatory cells that infiltrate the clot and embark on phagocytosis—removing bacteria and clot structures—as well as on the production of different growth factors. At the same time, new blood vessels start to sprout, and loosely organized granulation tissue intensely infiltrated by inflammatory cells and fibroblasts replaces the initial blood clot, which undergoes coagulative necrosis (Cardaropoli and coworkers 2003).

The granulation tissue is progressively replaced by immature connective tissue (provisional matrix) rich in cells and collagen fibers organized in a woven pattern. Subsequently, undiffer-

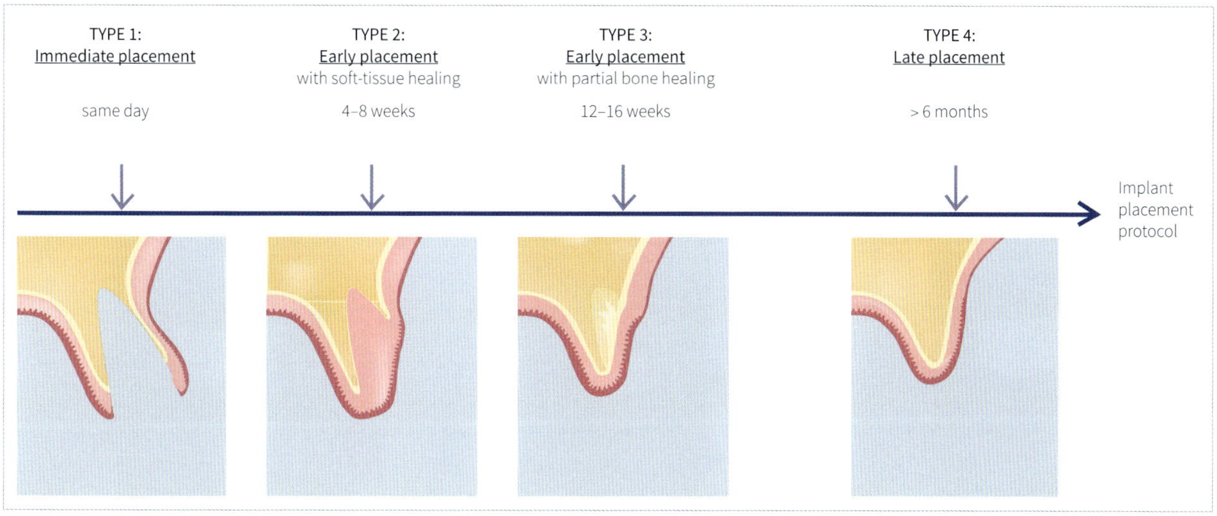

Fig 1 Timing of implant placement.

entiated mesenchymal cells penetrate the fibrous tissue and start differentiating into bone-forming cells, which promote the mineralization of the organic matrix to form the so-called woven bone. Woven bone progressively becomes replaced by mature lamellar bone tissue/bone marrow, and the alveolar ridge, at the socket wall, undergoes dimensional alterations (Figs 2a-b) (Araújo and Lindhe 2005).

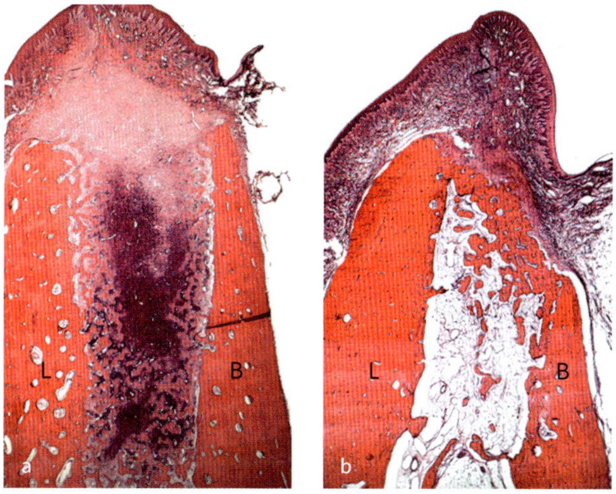

Figs 2a-b Macroscopic histological images demonstrating the bone modelling 1 week (a) and 8 weeks (b) following tooth extraction demonstrating resorption of the thin facial bone visible on the right side of the images.

Use this QR code to view a computer-animated 3D film on osseointegration.

Use this QR code to view a 3D animation about socket healing.

Most dimensional changes following tooth extraction occur in the first three months after tooth removal (Schropp and coworkers 2003) and continue as long as the modeling phase takes place, although with lesser intensity. Post-extraction dimensional alterations seem to be related to several factors, such as the individual healing properties of a patient, anatomical or pathological site characteristics, and the extent of surgical trauma and tissue destruction induced during the extraction procedure (Araújo and coworkers 2015).

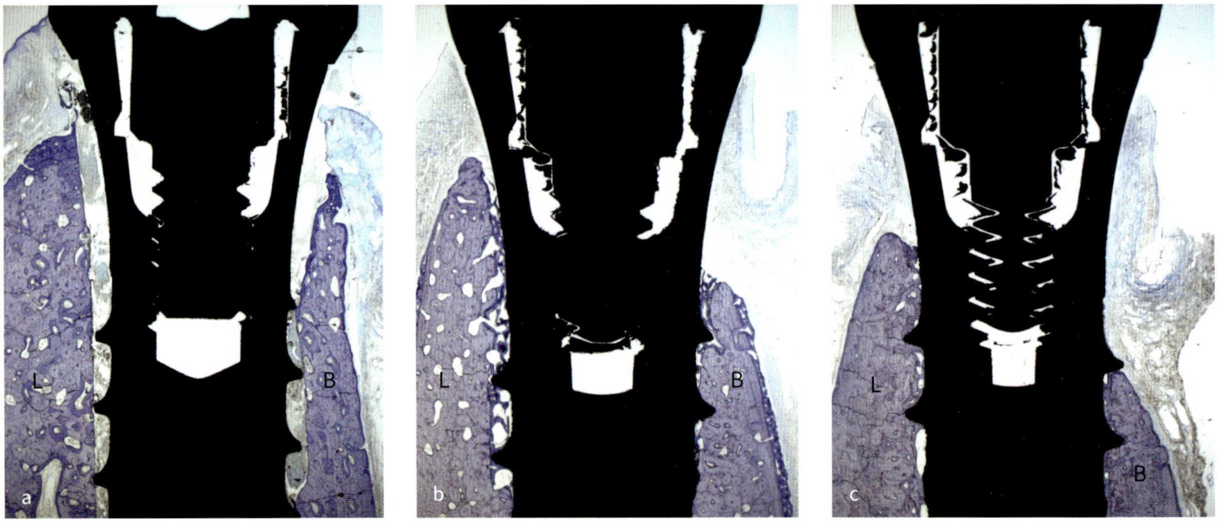

Figs 3a-c Resorptive changes after tooth extraction occur independently of the timing of implant placement and immediate implants fail to prevent them. Baseline (a), 4 weeks (b), and 12 weeks (c) after tooth extraction demonstrating resorption of the thin facial bone visible on the right side of the images adjacent to the immediately placed implants.

Although all these factors may vary, a mean hardtissue reduction of 3.8 mm (29–63%) in width and 1.24 mm (11–22%) in height during the first six months of healing was reported in a systematic review evaluating post-extraction hard and soft tissue dimensional changes (Tan and coworkers 2012).

The following resorption patterns have been observed:

- Greater resorption in width than height (Johnson 1969)
- The mandibular bone resorbs faster than the maxillary bone (Atwood 1971)
- The molar area endures more resorption than the frontal area (Pietrokovski and Massler 1967)
- Greater vertical changes occur in multiple adjacent extraction sites compared with single-tooth extraction sites (Lam 1960)
- The buccal plate is resorbed first (Cawood and Howell 1988)

Thin buccal walls, intrinsically present in the anterior maxilla, are especially prone to resorption. Araújo and coworkers (2005) hypothesized that the coronal part of buccal bone plate was often made only of bundle bone, which is a part of the periodontium and thus a tooth-dependent structure. Removing a tooth renders this bone useless, and its resorption is a natural consequence. Studies have shown that thin facial bone (< 1 mm) at the socket is likely to resorb three times more in the apicocoronal plane than thick facial bone (≥ 1 mm) when immediate implants are placed (Ferrus and coworkers 2010).

Additionally, damaged facial bone with fenestrations or any kind of dehiscence in the bone walls will make the bone weaker and more prone to resorption (Kan and coworkers 2007), while sites presenting thick buccal bone exhibit less dimensional changes of the alveolar ridge after tooth extraction (Chappuis and coworkers 2013; Chappuis and coworkers 2015). Other risk factors include a thin periodontal phenotype (Evans and Chen 2008; Cordaro and coworkers 2009) and inadvertent facial malposition of the implant within the socket at placement (Chen and coworkers 2007; Evans and Chen 2008).

Once it had been demonstrated that the osseointegration of implants placed in fresh extraction sockets was a predictable outcome (Chen and coworkers 2004) and took place irrespective of the gap between the implant surface and the bony socket walls, studies proceeded to investigate the physiological process of socket healing combined with immediate implant placement. Initially, proponents of immediate implants as a novel therapeutic concept argued that it may counteract post-extraction buccal-bone resorption, benefiting from the supporting role of the tooth and hence providing better esthetic outcomes (Lazzara 1989; Denissen and coworkers 1993). However, subsequent studies yielded contradictory results, namely that resorptive changes after tooth extraction occur independently of the timing of implant placement and that immediate implants fail to prevent them (Botticelli and coworkers 2004; Araújo and coworkers 2005; Chen and coworkers 2007) (Figs 3a-c) (Araújo and coworkers 2006).

These findings led researchers to combine immediate implants with alveolar ridge preservation procedures that involve grafting the peri-implant socket defect with bone substitutes to limit post-extraction remodeling and to achieve a better long-term functional and esthetic outcomes of implant restorations (Chen and coworkers 2004).

Most evidence on immediate implants involves maxillary anterior teeth (Zhou and coworkers 2021), where esthetic outcomes play a key role for success. One of the early limitations of immediate placement was the use of coronally advanced full-thickness mucoperiosteal flaps to achieve submerged healing with or without concomitant bone grafting. Implants were also often placed in compromised sockets with thin or absent buccal plates. Although such procedures produce successful outcomes in terms of osseointegration and implant survival, esthetic limitations and—most commonly—midfacial recession were frequently reported with 20–30% of immediate implants at risk of midfacial mucosal recession of 1 mm or more (Chen and Buser 2009; Chen and Buser 2014).

Various alveolar-ridge preservation techniques and protocols have been described, aimed at minimizing dimensional changes and esthetic challenges. These include particulate bone grafts or substitutes and socket-sealing techniques using connective tissue grafts, a barrier membrane, or plugs. Among other opinions, the 2019 European Workshop in Periodontology Consensus statements indicated that alveolar ridge preservation via socket grafting limits horizontal and vertical post-extraction bone resorption, compared to tooth extraction alone (Avila-Ortiz and coworkers 2019; Tonetti and coworkers 2019). The same workgroup also concluded that socket grafting in conjunction with immediate implant placement is an integral component of the procedure in most cases.

Current evidence seems to indicate a trend toward better outcomes when implants are placed immediately in a flapless approach combined with socket grafting, plus connective-tissue grafting in patients with a thin soft tissue phenotype (Seyssens and coworkers 2020; Seyssens and coworkers 2021).

2.2 Evolution of Implant Loading Protocols

The biological process of osseointegration of a dental implant follows a pattern similar to that of bone fracture healing.

One prerequisite for direct bone fracture healing is wound stabilization and rigid fixation, with excessive loads at the wound interface leading to delayed healing or non-union (Marsell and Einhorn 2011). With dental implants, this stabilization is achieved through the insertion of an endosseous implant with a diameter slightly larger than that of the osteotomy. This provides primary stability, which is a requirement for osseointegration and long-term implant success.

The original loading protocols for endosseous implants proposed by Per-Ingvar Brånemark and André Schroeder required an undisturbed healing time of three to four months prior to loading (Schroeder and coworkers 1976; Adell and coworkers 1981; Buser and coworkers 2000). The protocols were proposed based on their understanding of osseointegration at the time, which involved a necrotic border zone around the implant due to the surgical trauma of the osteotomy preparation. It was suggested that the necrosis and replacement of the bone adjacent to the implant was inevitable, and it was recommended to leave the implant undisturbed throughout this process until osseointegration had occurred, as minor movements would inhibit osteogenesis and jeopardize osseointegration (Albrektsson and coworkers 1981; Schroeder and coworkers 1981).

Over the next few decades, our understanding of the physiology of the osseointegration process evolved, and clinical studies soon emerged to challenge this paradigm by demonstrating that implants in fully edentulous sites could be immediately loaded when four implants were placed with cross-arch splinting (Ledermann 1979; Babbush and coworkers 1986).

The concept of immediate loading continued to evolve (Schnitman and coworkers 1990). By the late 1990s, interest had turned to a challenging clinical scenario in which an immediate provisional prosthesis was connected to an implant placed in a fresh extraction socket in the anterior maxilla (Wöhrle 1998). Implant technology had improved to the point where the healing period prior to loading could be reduced, with immediate loading considered predictable given a proper indication, with results comparable to conventional loading protocols (Cochran and coworkers 2004; Gallucci and coworkers 2014; Gallucci and coworkers 2018).

This was underpinned by advances in two areas:

- A research focus on the reduction of surgical trauma and subsequent necrosis to the surrounding bone during osteotomy preparation and insertion of a dental implant (Eriksson and Albrektsson 1983; Möhlhenrich and coworkers 2015; Bernabeu-Mira and coworkers 2021)
- Research on the regeneration of bone adjacent to the implant during the osseointegration process, where surface technology was identified as a key component (Salvi and coworkers 2015; Bosshardt and coworkers 2017).

Osseointegration is now recognized as a dynamic process in which the resorption of damaged bone and the apposition of new bone through regeneration occur simultaneously. This follows current mechanobiological models of bone fracture healing, which recognizes that the physiologically complex healing process involves both biological and mechanical aspects (Ghiasi and coworkers 2017).

It is generally established that mechanical stability throughout the osseointegration process is required for short- and long-term clinical success (Listgarten and coworkers 1991; Albrektsson and Zarb 1993). Mechanical stability is required to limit micromovements from direct or indirect forces being applied to the implant that would result in fibrous encapsulation and implant failure. As osseointegration occurs, the initial primary mechanical stability—by which the implant resists movement from loading in the initial healing phase—is substituted for secondary stability (Fig 4) where the newly regenerated bone has matured to the point where it can contribute to the stability of the implant under loading conditions (Bosshardt and coworkers 2017).

With this transition from primary to secondary implant stability, a dip in the overall mechanical stability of the implant occurs. This constitutes a risk factor for implant failure if excessive loads are applied at this point in the healing process (Raghavendra and coworkers 2005; Oates and coworkers 2007; Lang and coworkers 2011).

Immediate loading of dental implants may present some advantages, mainly in that it eliminates the need for removable transitional appliances, which are often inconvenient for the patient to wear and can be deleterious to the underlying surgical site if the transitional appliance is tissue-supported. An immediate implant-supported provisional restoration also provides an opportunity to provide prosthetically guided soft tissue healing, which can assist in maintaining the pre-extraction soft tissue architecture. While these objectives can also be achieved with alternatives (bonded bridges, custom healing abutments), immediate provisionalization of immediately placed dental implants provides the most efficient pathway.

Contemporary protocols for immediate implant placement recognize that the preservation of the soft tissue contours

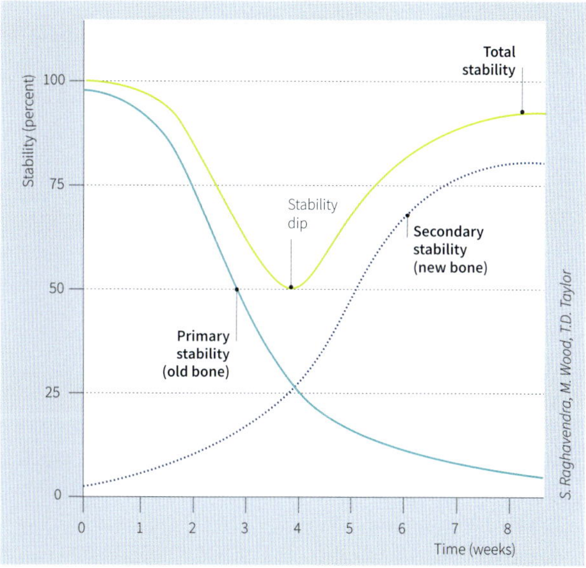

Fig 4 Illustration of the gradual rise in secondary stability as the primary stability Is reduced. The rate of increase in secondary stability can be influenced by the implant's surface characteristics, surgical trauma, and the biological capacity of the patient.

and architecture at the time of extraction can provide predictable results in the context of prosthetically guided soft tissue healing (Schubert and coworkers 2019). An immediately loaded provisional or custom healing abutment with an appropriately shaped emergence profile will support the marginal soft tissue while containing the grafting material and blood clot and minimizing contamination by saliva. With biocompatible materials, soft tissue adhesion can also promote soft tissue stability and help minimize post-extraction ridge alterations.

2.3 Current Concepts and Definitions of Implant Placement and Loading Protocols

The current classification of implant placement and loading protocols was defined in a 2018 systematic review by Gallucci and coworkers and adopted by the 2018 ITI Consensus Conference. In this new classification, the relationship between these two treatment concepts is combined into one classification system (Table 1) with the relative timelines illustrated in Figure 5. This approach recognizes that these two events occur for every implant that is placed and that they are not independent of each other, but rather co-dependent variables that influence success and outcomes. Twelve different combinations of implant placement and loading were described, as follows:

Type 1A: Immediate placement + immediate restoration/loading
Type 1B: Immediate placement + early loading
Type 1C: Immediate placement + conventional loading
Type 2A: Early placement with soft tissue healing + immediate restoration/loading
Type 2B: Early placement with soft tissue healing + early loading
Type 2C: Early placement with soft tissue healing + conventional loading
Type 3A: Early placement with partial bone healing + immediate restoration/loading
Type 3B: Early placement with partial bone healing + early loading
Type 3C: Early placement with partial bone healing + conventional loading
Type 4A: Late placement + immediate restoration/loading
Type 4B: Late placement + early loading
Type 4C: Late placement + conventional loading.

In this classification, previous definitions of the timing of implant placement and loading were adopted from previous ITI Consensus Conferences, as follows:

IMPLANT PLACEMENT PROTOCOLS

- ***Late implant placement:*** Dental implants are placed after completely bone healing, more than six months after tooth extraction
- ***Early implant placement:*** Dental implants are placed with soft tissue healing or with partial bone healing, four to eight weeks or twelve to sixteen weeks after tooth extraction
- ***Immediate implant placement:*** Dental implants are placed in the fresh socket on the same day of tooth extraction

(Chen and Buser 2009; Chen and coworkers 2004; Hämmerle and coworkers 2004).

Table 1 Classification combining implant placement and loading time

		Loading protocol		
		Immediate restoration/loading (type A)	Early loading (type B)	Conventional loading (type C)
Implant placement protocol	Immediate placement (type 1)	Type 1A	Type 1B	Type 1C
	Early placement (type 2-3)	Type 2-3A	Type 2-3B	Type 2-3C
	Late placement (type 4)	Type 4A	Type 4B	Type 4C

Gallucci, Hamilton, Zhou, Buser and Chen 2018. 6th ITI Consensus Report. Group 2. Article 2

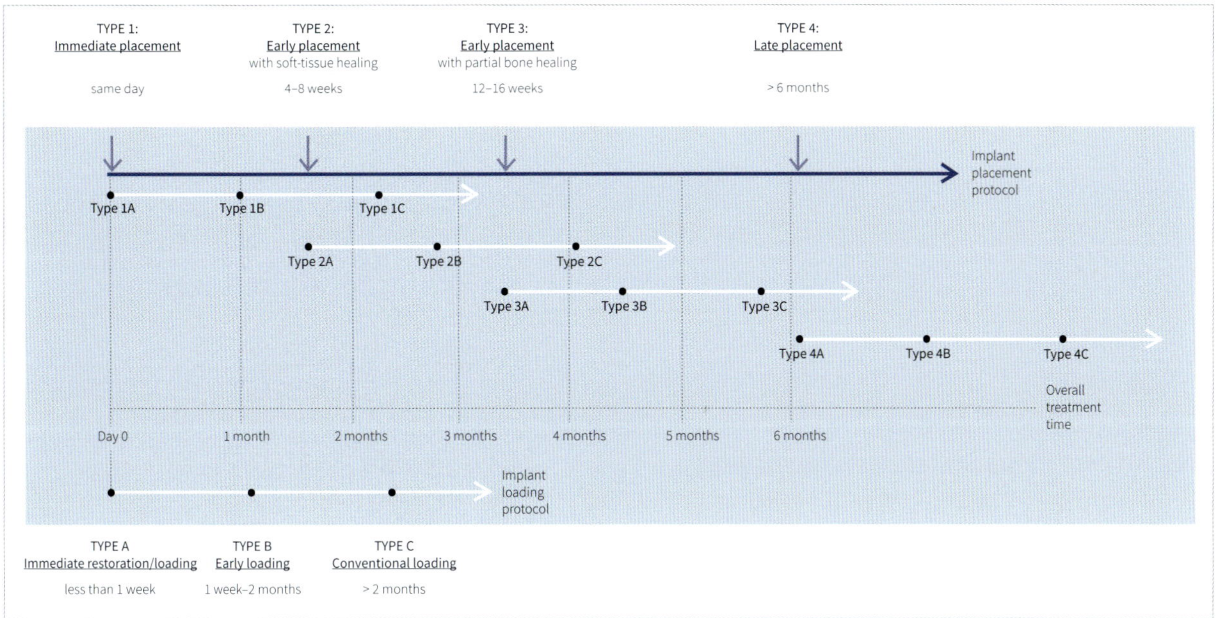

Fig 5 Timeline based on the definitions of implant placement protocols and implant loading protocols (after Zhou and coworkers 2021).

IMPLANT LOADING PROTOCOLS

- ***Conventional loading:*** Dental implants are allowed a healing period of more than two months after implant placement with no connection to the prosthesis.
- ***Early loading:*** Dental implants are connected to the prosthesis between one week and two months after implant placement.
- ***Immediate loading:*** Dental implants are connected to the prosthesis within one week after implant placement.

This is in line with the publications of the previous ITI Consensus Conferences (Benic and coworkers 2014; Chiapasco 2004; Cochran and coworkers 2004; Gallucci and coworkers 2014; Gallucci and coworkers 2009; Ganeles and Wismeijer 2004; Grutter and Belser 2009; Morton and coworkers 2004; Papaspyridakos and coworkers 2014; Roccuzzo and coworkers 2009; Schimmel and coworkers 2014; Schrott and coworkers 2014; Weber and coworkers 2009).

Thus, for immediate implant placement, three subcategories were listed:

- ***Type 1A:*** Immediate placement + immediate restoration/loading
- ***Type 1B:*** Immediate placement + early loading
- ***Type 1C:*** Immediate placement + conventional loading

The analysis of the survival rates of each of these treatment protocols based on this new classification follows in the next section.

2.4 Proceedings of the 6th ITI Consensus Conference

2.4.1 Consensus Statements Regarding Implant Placement and Loading Protocols

1. The newly proposed classification assessing both the timing of implant placement and loading combinations allows for comprehensive treatment selection.
2.
   a. Type 1A (immediate placement + immediate restoration) is a clinically documented protocol. The survival rate was 98% (median: 100%; range: 87–100%).
   b. Type 1B (immediate placement + early loading) is a clinically documented protocol. The survival rate was 98% (median: 100%; range; 93–100%).
   c. Type 1C (immediate placement + conventional loading) is a scientifically and clinically valid protocol. The survival rate was 96% (median: 99%; range: 91–100%).
3.
   a. Type 2-3A (early placement + immediate restoration/loading) presents clinically insufficient documentation.
   b. Type 2-3B (early placement + early loading) presents clinically insufficient documentation.
   c. Type 2-3C (early placement + conventional loading) is a scientifically and clinically valid protocol. The survival rate was 96% (median: 96%; range: 91–100%).
4.
   a. Type 4A (late placement + immediate restoration/loading) is a clinically documented protocol. The survival rate was 98% (median: 99%; range 83–100%).
   b. Type 4B (late placement + early loading) is a scientifically and clinically valid protocol. The survival rate was 98% (median: 99%; range: 97–100%).
   c. Type 4C (late placement + conventional loading) is a scientifically and clinically valid protocol. The survival rate was 98% (median: 100%; range: 95–100%).
5. When considering placement/loading protocols, there are factors that can prevent achievement of the intended treatment. These factors include:
   a. Patient-related factors
   b. Lack of primary stability
   c. The need for bone augmentation

2.4.2 Clinical Recommendations Regarding Implant Placement and Loading Protocols

Immediate implant placement and immediate restoration/loading is considered a complex surgical and prosthodontic procedure. Clinicians performing this procedure need to have sufficient training, experience, and clinical skill to be able to undertake the necessary diagnostic procedures and to perform the treatment.

The ITI recommends that the type 1A protocol should only be considered if there are demonstrable patient-centered advantages, such as esthetic requirements or a clinical indication to reduce surgical morbidity (Morton and coworkers 2018). For example, there seems to be little advantage in connecting an immediate provisional restoration to an immediately placed implant in a first-molar site. Although it has been clinically documented (Atieh and coworkers 2010), there is little patient-centered advantage to this approach over conventional placement and loading protocols.

The following clinical conditions are recommended for the type 1A protocol (Morton and coworkers 2014; Morton and coworkers 2018):

- ***Intact socket bone walls.*** In particular, the status of the facial bone wall is critical to esthetic outcomes. Diagnostic CBCT scans are often able to evaluate the condition of the facial socket wall; however, it can often be obscured by metal artifacts from a post within a root canal. The facial bone wall can also be damaged as a result of the extraction procedure. Therefore, the facial bone should be definitively evaluated following tooth extraction.

- ***Facial bone at least 1 mm thick.*** Clinical studies have demonstrated that thin facial bone (< 1 mm) is prone to significant vertical crestal resorption (Chen and coworkers 2007; Ferrus and coworkers 2010; Sanz and coworkers 2017). If this resorption is extensive, bone grafts placed into the facial peri-implant defect may not be fully contained within the bone walls and are therefore prone to resorption. This may result in incomplete bone fill within the peri-implant defect (van Steenberghe and coworkers 2000; Chen and coworkers 2007; Juodzbalys and Wang 2007), exposure of the rough surface of the implant crestally, and recession of the midfacial peri-implant mucosa.
- ***Thick soft tissue phenotype.*** Sites with a thin soft tissue phenotype run a greater risk of recession of the midfacial mucosa, which may have adverse implications for final esthetic outcomes (Evans and Chen 2008; Cordaro and coworkers 2009). Cases with a thin soft tissue phenotype should be avoided unless additional interventions promote thickening of the facial gingiva. Such additional interventions may include intentional decoronation and submergence of the root to promote gingival overgrowth, soft tissue thickening (Langer 1994) incorporating connective tissue grafts into the soft tissue marginal area on the facial aspect of the socket (Kan and coworkers 2005; Chen and coworkers 2009; Kan and coworkers 2009), or grafting of the supracrestal region with small-particle bone substitutes that promote soft tissue thickening (Chu and coworkers 2012; Chu and coworkers 2015).
- ***No acute infection at the site.*** Sites with acute infection should not be considered for the type 1A protocol as there is likely to be damage to one or more socket walls, and the inflammation of the soft tissues may lead to significant recession.
- ***Sufficient bone volume apical and lingual to the socket.*** This is to allow the implant to be placed with primary stability. This is an essential requirement to ensure that the implant can then be connected to a provisional restoration. CBCT scans provide essential information establishing this requirement.
- ***Resistance to rotational torque.*** The implant should resist the torque that is likely to be applied to the abutment screw of the provisional restoration. This largely depends upon the recommendations of the implant manufacturer, which with current implant systems should be in the range of 25-40 Ncm or ISQ value > 70.
- ***Occlusal scheme that protects the provisional restoration*** during function. Cases should therefore be selected where direct occlusal contact between the provisional restoration and opposing dentition can be avoided.
- ***Patient compliance.*** The patient should be prepared to follow postoperative instructions. The critical factor is to avoid direct masticatory function on the provisional prosthesis.

2.5 Proceedings of the 7th ITI Consensus Conference

In the 7th ITI Consensus Conference in 2023, the literature specifically on type 1A immediate implant placement and immediate loading in the anterior maxilla (teeth 15 to 25) was assessed and new consensus statements as well as clinical recommendations were made as an update to those from the 6th ITI Consensus Conference, in which all implant placement and loading protocols were assessed.

2.5.1 Consensus Statements Regarding Type 1A Immediate Implant Placement and Immediate Loading

The following consensus statements were developed from the two systematic reviews that assessed selection criteria and implant survival (Hamilton and coworkers 2023) and clinical performance (Wittneben and coworkers 2023) of immediately placed and immediately loaded dental implants (type 1A) for single-tooth replacement in the anterior maxilla (teeth 15 to 25) (region of esthetic significance). All implants included in the two reviews exhibited a minimum of 12 months of follow-up.

SYSTEMATIC REVIEW PAPER 1

***Hamilton** A, Gonzaga L, Amorim K, Wittneben JG, Martig L, Morton D, et al. Selection criteria for immediate implant placement and immediate loading for single tooth replacement in the maxillary esthetic zone: a systematic review and meta-analysis. Clin Oral Implants Res. 2023; 34 [forthcoming].*

Preamble

The following consensus statements are based on a systematic review that assessed implant survival with type 1A (immediate implant placement and immediate restoration/loading) protocol for implant replacement of single teeth in the anterior maxilla (teeth 15 to 25), with a minimum of 12 months of follow-up. The review also assessed the reported patient and site-specific selection criteria that may influence survival outcomes. The review is based on data from 43 prospective (11 randomized controlled trials, RCTs, and 6 clinical controlled trials, CCTs) and 25 retrospective studies with a total of 2,531 implants with a mean follow-up of 2.6 years.

Consensus statements

1. The type 1A protocol for replacement of a single tooth in the anterior maxilla (teeth 15 to 25) is predictable with high implant survival rates. This is based on studies with highly selective populations, with favorable patient and site-specific characteristics. When failures occur, the majority are within the first 6 months of implant placement. This statement is supported by 43 prospective (including data from 11 RCTs, 6 CCTs) and 25 retrospective studies.
2. Multiple patient and site-specific factors are relevant in the selection and completion of a type 1A protocol for the replacement of a single tooth in the anterior maxilla (teeth 15 to 25 FDI). These include:
   a. General factors
      - Medical status (63 studies)
      - Periodontal disease (54 studies)
      - Occlusal scheme (57 studies)
      - Parafunction (26 studies)
   b. Site-specific factors
      - Facial bone wall (60 studies)
      - Endodontic infection (42 studies)
      - Bone for anchorage (37 studies)
      - Soft tissue quality (25 studies)
      - Gingival margin position (22 studies)
   c. Treatment factors
      - Mucoperiosteal flap (63 studies)
      - Damage during tooth extraction (59 studies)
      - Gap between the facial bone and implant (56 studies)
      - Primary implant stability (42 studies)

3. The type 1A protocol may not be able to be completed in all selected sites due to intraoperative procedural events mostly related to the extraction of the tooth or lack of primary implant stability. This statement is supported by 23 prospective studies (including data from 11 RCTs and 2 CCTs).
4. A chronic periapical infection associated with the tooth to be extracted is not a contraindication for the type 1A protocol provided there is sufficient bone to achieve primary implant stability. This statement is supported by 29 prospective (including data from 9 RCTs and 3 CCTs) and 13 retrospective studies.
5. With regards to implant position, the presence of at least a 2 mm gap between the implant and the facial bone increases implant survival when the type 1A protocol is utilized. This statement is supported by 13 prospective (including data from 5 RCTs and 2 CCTs) and 7 retrospective studies.

SYSTEMATIC REVIEW PAPER 2

***Wittneben** JG, Molinero-Mourelle P, Hamilton A, Alnasser M, Obermaier B, Morton D, et al. Clinical performance of immediately loaded single implants in the esthetic zone. A systematic review and meta-analysis. Clin Oral Implants Res. 2023; 34 [forthcoming].*

Preamble

The following consensus statements are based on a systematic review that assessed the clinical performance of dental implants used according to the type 1A (immediate implant placement and immediate restoration/loading) protocol for replacement of single teeth in the esthetic zone (anterior maxilla, teeth 15 to 25).

The statements are based on up to 38 prospective (including 10 RCTs) and 25 retrospective studies with a follow-up of being 12 and 96 months.

Consensus statements

1. The type 1A protocol, when utilized in the esthetic zone, is a clinically viable treatment option. However surgical, technical, and biological complications can occur. This statement is supported by 63 studies (10 randomized controlled trials, 28 prospective and 25 retrospective studies) with a follow-up ranging from 12 to 96 months. Surgical (mean per year, 5.86%; 38 clinical studies) technical (mean, 3.27%; 25 clinical studies) and biological (mean, 2.18%; 29 clinical studies) complications may occur.
2. For the type 1A protocol, survival is not influenced by the type of implant (bone level versus parallel walled versus tapered design). This statement is supported by 63 studies (10 randomized controlled trials, 28 prospective and 25 retrospective studies) with a follow-up ranging from 12 to 96 months.
3. For the type 1A protocol there was an increase in PES (pink esthetic score) when the space between the implant and the facial bone of the residual socket was grafted with autologous bone or bone substitute. This statement is supported by 35 studies (7 randomized controlled trials, 12 prospective and 16 retrospective studies) with a follow-up ranging from 12 to 96 months.
4. For the type 1A protocol, the flapless approach provides good esthetic outcomes (papilla height, PES, and WES). This statement is supported by 11 clinical studies for papilla height, 31 clinical studies for PES and 16 clinical studies for WES.
5. For the type 1A protocol, differences in survival are not influenced by type of retention (screw- or cement-retained) when focusing on the final restoration. This statement is supported by 29 clinical studies.

2.5.2 Clinical Recommendations Regarding Type 1A Immediate Implant Placement and Immediate Loading

The replacement of a single tooth in the anterior maxilla (teeth 15 to 25 FDI) with the type 1A protocol is a complex procedure with high patient-centered benefits. It should be considered as the treatment of choice when ideal conditions are present. Ideal site conditions include:

- Healthy adjacent teeth
- Intact facial bone
- No acute infection
- Ability to place the implant in the correct three-dimensional position for restoration
- Anticipated stability of the implant to allow immediate restoration

Multiple patient- and site-related factors need to be considered for this treatment in order to achieve predictable long-term functional and esthetic outcomes. If the criteria for the type 1A protocol are not met, alternative treatment options must be considered.

Patients undergoing implant therapy should have no medical or psychological contraindications to complex oral surgical and restorative procedures. Patients should have realistic expectations about the final outcomes, be fully informed, and have consented to undergo the type 1A protocol.

1. **What clinical experience is recommended for the type 1A protocol?**
   The type 1A protocol is classified as a complex procedure in the ITI SAC Classification (Dawson and coworkers 2021) and should be performed by clinicians experienced in surgical and restorative implant procedures. These clinicians should have skills specific to tooth extraction and immediate implant placement, hard and soft tissue augmentation procedures, and immediate loading/restoration of implants. A team approach is often needed.

> The SAC Classification in Implant Dentistry 2nd Edition
> Anthony Dawson, William Martin and Waldemar Daudt Polido
> *To view this material, you need to be an ITI Member.*

2. **How should a patient be clinically assessed for the type 1A protocol?**
   A thorough clinical examination should be performed for the proper assessment of the patient and site. The patient should be assessed with the ERA (Esthetic Risk Assessment: ITI TG 10; SAC, 2nd edition) and Risk assessment for immediate implant placement in single-tooth sites (Chapter 5.2; Hamilton and coworkers 2023) to determine the patient and site-specific risk factors for immediate implant placement.
3. **What radiographs are recommended to properly assess a site for the type 1A protocol?**
   Radiographic assessment of the site and relevant surrounding tissues with a good quality periapical radiograph and a cone-beam computed tomography (CBCT) scan is strongly recommended. The following radiographic criteria should be fulfilled:
   - An intact or minimally damaged facial bone plate
   - Sufficient bone available to provide primary stability in an ideal 3D position
   - Health of the adjacent teeth
4. **Is software planning recommended for the type 1A protocol?**
   When a CBCT (digital volume) has been captured, the use of implant planning software is strongly recommended in order to evaluate the site and simulate the ideal 3-dimensional implant position. This allows the following to be analyzed:
   - The tooth-alveolus axis relationship to allow planning for optimal 3D restoration-driven implant placement
   - The gap between the implant and the facial bone wall at the level of the planned implant shoulder position
   - Abutment options
5. **What restorative preparation should there be prior to commencing treatment?**
   The prior fabrication and use of a traditional or computer guided surgical template is highly recommended to achieve an optimal restoratively driven three-dimensional implant position. A provisional crown, shell crown or matrix should be prepared prior to tooth extraction according to the desired method for fabrication of the planned immediate implant restoration. An alternative provisional prosthetic replacement of the tooth should be prepared and available in the event the treatment cannot be completed due to intraoperative events.
6. **How should the tooth be extracted when utilizing the type 1A protocol?**
   A minimally traumatic tooth extraction with a flapless approach is recommended and all efforts should be made to preserve bone and soft tissue integrity. Special instrumentation may be required to achieve this goal. Debridement of the socket should be performed. The integrity of the socket walls should be confirmed following extraction.
7. **What should be done if the facial bone is compromised when the tooth is extracted?**
   If the facial bone is compromised during and following tooth extraction, the extent of the defect must be assessed. If a minor defect in the facial bone is present, the type 1A protocol may still be considered. However, the risk of esthetic complications is increased and additional adjunctive hard and soft tissue regenerative procedures may be required. In larger defects, alternative treatment protocols to type 1A must be considered.
8. **Can the type 1A protocol be done in the presence of chronic periapical infection?**
   The type 1A protocol can be selected for teeth presenting with chronic periapical infections. However, it is recommended that this is only considered when the following conditions exist:
   - Absence of a fistula
   - Infection can be completely debrided
   - There is sufficient bone remaining to provide primary implant stability
9. **How big should the facial gap be?**
   The facial gap should ideally be > 2 mm in width at the level of the implant shoulder. However, this may not always be possible, and ultimately needs to be considered in relation to the likely functional loading, implant diameter, and the dimensions of the socket.
10. **What should be done when the facial bone or soft tissues are thin?**
    The following treatment can be considered:
    - In thin tissue phenotype situations, or when facial bone is thin (less than 1 mm), the type 1A protocol can still be considered. However, in addition to grafting

of the gap, adjunctive soft tissue grafting may be required to compensate for anticipated post-extraction dimension changes. This will increase the complexity of the procedure and risk of adverse outcomes.
- Alternative implant placement and loading protocols may also be considered to reduce the risk.

11. **What steps should be done for connection of the provisional crown to the implant?**
Immediate placement of a provisional restoration is well documented. This can be performed according to previous published consensus statements. The following factors should be considered:
    - Screw retention is recommended.
    - Emergence profile should be appropriate (not over- or undercontoured).
    - Time frame should be from implant placement to 1 week after placement.
    - Highly polished surface of the provisional is required.
    - The occlusion scheme should be without any eccentric contacts.
    - Light proximal contacts should be present.
    - The provisional restoration should be inserted and the retaining screw (abutment or prosthetic) torqued according to guidelines published by each manufacturer.

12. **What should be done if the type 1A protocol cannot be completed at the time of surgery?**
If the type 1A protocol cannot be completed, the implant can be placed with simultaneous grafting and allowed to heal without loading the implant. If the implant cannot be placed, an early placement protocol can be considered. Alternatively, the socket may be grafted and followed by late implant placement.

2.6 Evidence for Type 1A Protocols: Immediate Implant Placement + Immediate Loading

For the type 1A protocol, Hamilton and coworkers (2023) identified 43 prospective (including data from 11 randomized controlled trials and 6 controlled clinical trials) and 25 retrospective cohort studies that fulfilled the inclusion criteria. These studies comprised 2,531 implants that were observed for a mean follow-up period of 2.6 years (SD: 2.3 years; range: 1–18 years). The weighted mean survival rate was 97,7% (95%-CI: 96.6%–98.4%).

In 23 studies, there was sufficient documentation to undertake an intention-to-treat (ITT) analysis. ITT is a statistical concept that calculates the proportion of the study population who complete the study without any major protocol violations (Gupta 2011). In the context of the type 1A protocol, not every implant intended for immediate placement and loading could be treated according to the protocol. The ITT analyses indicated a range of 85–100% of sites successfully treated according to the stated protocol. The main reasons for not proceeding with this protocol included: insufficient intact facial bone walls following extraction and lack of sufficient insertion torque following implant placement (Gallucci and coworkers 2018; Hamilton and coworkers 2023).

The clinical implications are significant. For a type 1A protocol, careful case selection is required, and clinicians should be aware (and patients advised) that there is a chance that the condition of the socket following extraction will not lend itself to immediate implant placement or that the criteria for the delivery of a provisional restoration immediately after implant placement may not be met. Therefore, contingency plans need to be made to amend the treatment plan, should it be impossible to proceed with immediate placement or immediate restoration/loading (Morton and coworkers 2018; Morton and coworkers 2023).

The majority of studies on the type 1A protocol have been limited to the maxillary incisors, canines, and premolars (Zhou and coworkers 2021). Very few studies reported a type 1A protocol for molar teeth, which is due to the limited patient-centered benefit and increased loading risks in this area. Only 2 studies were reported on the anterior mandible, with a low number of implants. This is likely related to the anatomical constraints in this region and limited mesiodistal space for single-tooth replacements.

High survival rates for immediate implants have been widely documented. However, risk factors for implant failure and esthetic complications have also been identified. In a systematic review comparing different implant placement and loading protocols, the reported mean implant survival rate for the type 1A protocol in partially edentulous patients assessed in 24 studies with a combined total of 1067 implants was 98.4% (range: 87.5–100%) with a median of 100% and a mean follow-up period of 28.9 months (Gallucci and coworkers 2018). For the type 1C protocol, 16 studies were evaluated with a total of 963 implants and a mean survival rate of 96% (range: 91.3–100%) after a mean follow-up period of 38.4 months (Gallucci and coworkers 2018).

The loading protocol was a driving factor for the increased variation in outcomes observed with the type 1A compared to the type 1C protocol. The potentially increased risk associated with immediate loading is specific to patients, locations, and sites and should be weighed together with the patient-centered benefits. When analyzed by location, the type 1A protocol has mostly been investigated in the maxillary anterior region. Immediate loading of immediately placed implants in the posterior molar regions has not been sufficiently documented to be recommended as a routine procedure. Where immediate implant placement is desired in posterior sites, the type 1C protocol with a customized healing abutment should be considered.

The esthetic outcomes of immediately placed implants have also been reported to be favorable (Chen and Buser 2014: Wittneben and coworkers 2023). However, an increased variability of esthetic outcomes was found compared to type 2 and type 3 placement protocols. It was suggested that variations in adjunctive procedures performed simultaneously with implant placement, as well as variation in the site-specific inclusion criteria, contributed to the variation in esthetic outcomes.

Midfacial recession of > 1 mm was the most frequently reported esthetic complication with immediate implant placement. Site-specific risk factors for midfacial recession following immediate implant placement have been reported, including defects of the facial bone plate, thin facial bone, and thin soft tissue phenotype.

Treatment variables contributing to esthetic risk have also been identified, including malposition of the implant, Implant size, grafting the buccal gap, a flapless surgical approach, connection of an immediate provisional, and connective tissue grafting. When the type 1A protocol is being utilized, the variability of esthetic outcomes was found to be reduced when combined with a flapless procedure, grafted buccal gaps, and connective tissue grafting.

2.7 Evidence for Type 1B Protocols: Immediate Implant Placement + Early Loading

Gallucci and coworkers (2018) identified relatively few studies on immediate placement and early loading in partially edentulous patients. Only one controlled clinical trial and two non-comparative studies were identified, comprising 43 implants. The weighted mean survival rate was 98.2% (median: 100%; range: 93.75–100%) with a mean follow-up period of 28 months (SD: 27.7 months; range: 12–60 months). There was insufficient data for an ITT analysis.

Due to the paucity of evidence, the authors concluded that while the type 1B protocol is clinically documented, it lacks sufficient evidence to be clinically and scientifically validated. Clinicians should therefore be cautious in recommending this protocol for implant placement and loading (Morton and coworkers 2018). When the literature is restricted to single-tooth replacements by intraoral location, no studies reported on the outcomes of type 1B protocols (Zhou and coworkers 2021).

2.8 Evidence for Type 1C Protocols: Immediate Implant Placement + Conventional Loading

A total of 6 comparative studies (5 randomized controlled trials, 1 controlled clinical trial) and 10 non-comparative studies were identified in the systematic review of Gallucci and coworkers (2018). Of 963 implants placed with a type 1C protocol, 24 implants failed, yielding a weighted survival rate of 96% (median: 99.2%; range: 91.3–100%). The mean follow-up period was 38.7 months (SD: 34.3 months; range: 12–120 months). The authors concluded that this protocol was scientifically and clinically validated and could be recommended, provided that strict inclusion and exclusion criteria were adopted (Morton and coworkers 2018).

In all, 5 studies provided sufficient data for an ITT analysis. Between 84.2% and 100% of sites could be treated as intended, according to the study protocols (median: 85.2%). Reasons for not proceeding with the intended treatment included sites with alveolar bone defects and loss of the facial bone wall encountered following tooth extraction, inadequate bone volume apical to the socket for primary stability, and gaps of < 1 mm between the implant and the facial bone wall.

Although clinically and scientifically validated, clinicians should be aware that between 15% and 20% of implants may be impossible to place according to the type 1C protocol. Strict inclusion and exclusion criteria should be observed to achieve predictable outcomes. If a type 1C protocol cannot be carried out, the clinician can abort the procedure or graft the socket with a suitable bone substitute for ridge preservation (Darby and coworkers 2009).

When identifying local site-related risk factors, type 1C protocols were scientifically and clinically validated in the anterior and posterior maxilla, clinically documented in the posterior mandible, and clinically insufficiently documented for anterior mandible (Zhou and coworkers 2021). This protocol is largely indicated for posterior tooth replacements where immediate loading presents greater risks with fewer benefits, provided the local site-specific factors are favorable for immediate implant placement.

3 Preoperative Analysis and Treatment Planning

F. Lambert, A. Hamilton, A. De Souza, W. Martin

Preoperative patient- and site-specific analysis is one of the key aspects of predictable success with immediate implant treatment. As discussed in Chapter 2, our understanding of the principles of wound healing and of changes in the surrounding alveolar bone following tooth extraction has shaped our current thinking regarding implant placement protocols. They are partly determined by the genetic sequence of events in the wound-healing cascade, but also largely influenced by the surrounding hard and soft tissues.

The anatomy of the socket also influences the predictability of obtaining primary stability and the intraoperative conditions required for predictable immediate loading of a dental implant in a fresh extraction socket (immediately placed dental implant). This chapter reviews the current concepts in patient and site assessment/selection designed to minimize risk and provide predictable outcomes with immediate tooth replacement.

3.1 Patient Characteristics

3.1.1 Medical Status

The overall health of a patient should always be carefully assessed when selecting a dental implant procedure, given the inherent surgical risks. Regarding immediate placement and loading, patients with certain systemic conditions may have increased risks of an adverse event, implant failure, postoperative complications, and delayed or compromised wound healing (Bornstein and coworkers 2009).

Where local anatomical parameters permit flapless immediate placement, it can be associated with low surgical morbidity and with a reduced risk of postoperative bleeding, swelling, and pain. This can eventually be beneficial for patients who present with systemic conditions or who are taking medications that increase the surgical risk of bleeding, or who are otherwise poor candidates for invasive surgery.

However, systemic conditions that compromise wound healing and osseointegration may represent an additional risk in immediate placement or immediate loading. In osteoporosis patients taking antiresorptive medications, slower bone remodeling and soft tissue healing may delay the process of osseointegration; more conventional delayed implant placement and loading procedures may therefore be preferred.

The same applies to heavy smokers, or patients with certain immunodeficiency conditions, or poorly controlled diabetes, where healing delays may compromise the success of an immediate procedure. In patients with compromised healing, the risk-to-benefit balance should be assessed when establishing the treatment strategy, and a staged approach is recommended.

3.2 Esthetic Analyses and Esthetic Challenges

An Esthetic Risk Assessment (ERA) for the treatment of partially edentulous patients with dental implants was first introduced in Volume 1 of the ITI Treatment Guide (2004). It was developed to assist clinicians in the diagnosis and planning of partially edentulous patients for treatment in the esthetic zone, and to identify clinical factors or situations that could contribute to esthetic compromise. Understanding that implant therapy in the esthetic zone can be a challenging process, as patient demands on esthetics coupled with preexisting deficiencies in the anatomy could present obstacles to obtain ideal results, the ERA table has become a valuable tool to identify risk prior to initiating care.

In 2017, the ERA table was updated to reflect current practice trends and technology as discussed in detail by Martin and coworkers (2017) in Volume 10 of the ITI Treatment Guide. The ERA table can also be found in the second edition of the SAC Classification in Implant Dentistry (Dawson and coworkers 2021) (Table 1).

The ERA table identifies 13 clinical factors that can add risk to the ability to achieve ideal esthetic outcomes. In a specific clinical situation, there may be many more of these factors.

With the introduction of immediacy in the esthetic zone, several pre- and intraoperative factors require attention to minimize esthetic compromise and enhance overall success. Clinicians performing this type of rehabilitation must have a thorough understanding of hard and soft tissue biology and all available treatment modalities for a given clinical situation. For the purposes of this volume, the ERA table will be considered as a factor in the overall treatment of patients with dental implants.

When planning an immediate implant and restoration in the esthetic zone, it is also recommended to perform a conventional or digital smile analysis to set the final objective, to evaluate the clinical challenge, and to establish the optimal treatment strategy (Fig 1).

ITI Treatment Guide Vol. 1
Implant Therapy in the Esthetic Zone – Single-Tooth Replacements
Urs Belser and coworkers
To view this material, you need to be an ITI Member.

ITI Treatment Guide Vol. 10
Implant Therapy in the Esthetic Zone – Current Treatment Modalities and Materials for Single-Tooth Replacements
Vivianne Chappuis and William Martin
To view this material, you need to be an ITI Member.

The SAC Classification in Implant Dentistry 2nd Edition
Anthony Dawson, William Martin and Waldemar Daudt Polido
To view this material, you need to be an ITI Member.

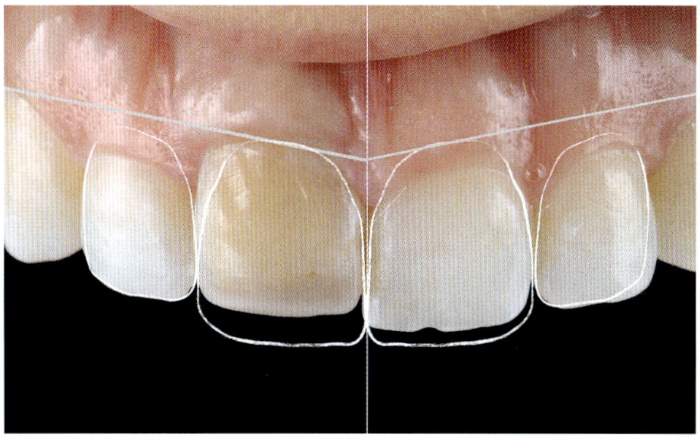

Fig 1 Clinical scenario: An ankylosed tooth 11 needs to be replaced. The gingival margin position may be considered as unfavorable when compared to the neighboring tooth margins. and a type II or III implant placement may be preferred. However, based on the digital esthetic analyses (line overlay), the cervical level of tooth 11 is correct; the neighboring tooth margins should be lengthened for a more harmonious smile. Eventually, immediate placement may be considered. (Esthetic analyses/Image courtesy of Prof Amélie Mainjot.)

Table 1 Esthetic Risk Assessment (ERA) table outlining the factors that can be assessed to determine the level of esthetic risk associated with implant tooth replacements irrespective of the protocol for implant placement or loading. (From Chappuis and Martin 2017; Dawson and coworkers 2021.)

Esthetic risk factor	Level of risk		
	Low	**Medium**	**High**
Medical status	Healthy, uneventful healing		Compromised healing
Smoking habit	Non-smoker	Light smoker (≤ 10 cigs/day)	Heavy smoker (> 10 cigs/day)
Gingival display at full smile	Low	Medium	High
Width of edentulous span	1 tooth (≥ 7 mm)[1] 1 tooth (≥ 6 mm)[2]	1 tooth (< 7 mm)[1] 1 tooth (< 6 mm)[2]	2 teeth or more
Shape of tooth crowns	Rectangular		Triangular
Restorative status of neighboring teeth	Virgin		Restored
Gingival phenotype	Low-scalloped, thick	Medium-scalloped, medium-thick	High-scalloped, thin
Infection at implant site	None	Chronic	Acute
Soft tissue anatomy	Soft tissue intact		Soft tissue defects
Bone level at adjacent teeth	≤ 5 mm to contact point	5.5 to 6.5 mm to contact point	≥ 7 mm to contact point
Facial bone-wall phenotype*	Thick-wall phenotype ≥ 1 mm thickness		Thin-wall phenotype < 1 mm thickness
Bone anatomy of alveolar crest	No bone deficiency	Horizontal bone deficiency	Vertical bone deficiency
Patient's esthetic expectations	Realistic expectations		Unrealistic expectations

* If three-dimensional imaging is available with the tooth in place
[1] Standard-diameter implant, regular connection
[2] Narrow-diameter Implant, narrow connection

3.3 Prosthodontic Planning

Contemporary implant planning recognizes the important relationship between the prosthodontic and biological outcomes to achieve long-term functional and esthetic success. The term "restoration-driven implant planning" is often used to highlight that this relationship begins with an understanding of the desired prosthodontic reconstruction. The design of the restorations is determined through a digital diagnostic tooth set-up, or alternatively, a conventional diagnostic wax-up, which can be scanned and digitized for implant planning (Figs 2a-b). This predetermined prosthodontic design is then used to assist in determining the most biomechanically suitable implant specification and position.

To visualize this relationship, it is recommended for the prosthodontic design to be registered and incorporated into a virtual implant-planning environment where it can be assessed in relation to the anatomical data acquired from a cone-beam computerized tomography (CBCT) scan (Figs 3a-c). During the virtual implant planning process, if anatomical challenges and limitations are present clinical decisions can be made regarding regenerative approaches with bone and soft tissue augmentation, or possible modification to the prosthetic planning.

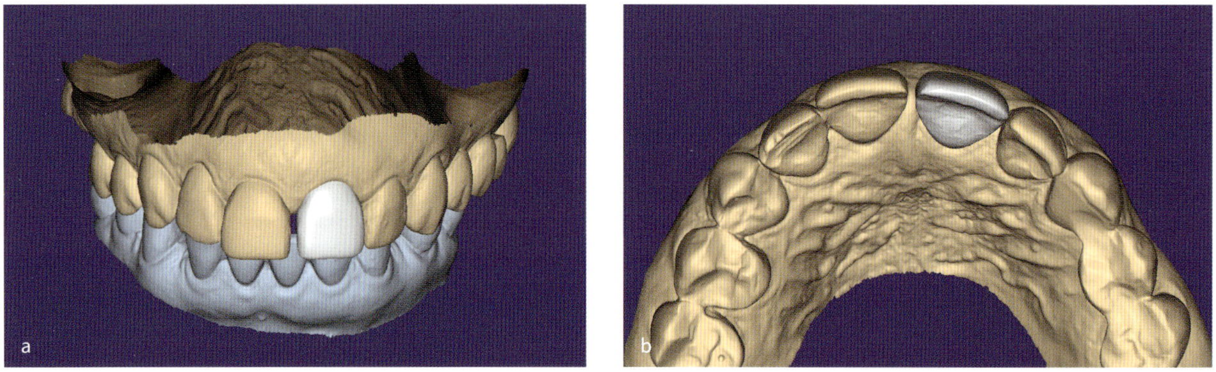

Figs 2a-b Digital diagnostic set-up for a fractured tooth 21.

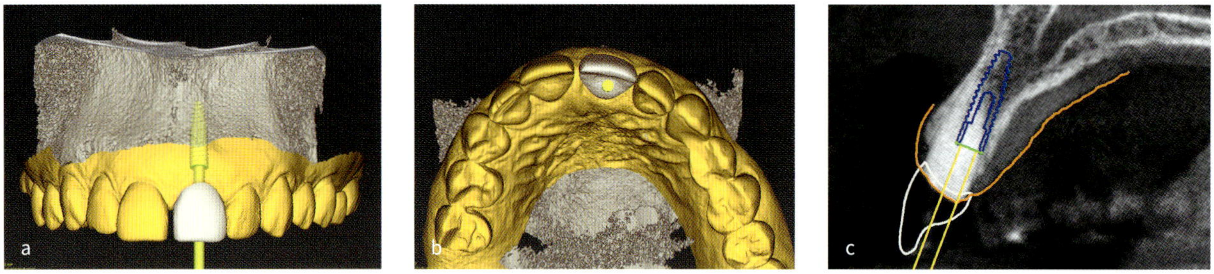

Figs 3a-c Comprehensive virtual implant planning for an immediate replacement of tooth 21. Registration of CBCT DICOM data with intraoral surface scans and a digital diagnostic set-up.

3.3.1 Diagnostic Wax-Up/Digital Diagnostic Set-Up

Determining the prosthodontic design is the first step in the planning process. In situations where immediate placement and restoration are planned, the existing tooth may supply this information, provided its clinical crown meets all of the objectives of the final restoration. If not, it is recommended to perform a diagnostic wax-up or digital diagnostic set-up to precisely determine and analyze the key determinants of implant planning:

- Incisal edge position
- Prosthetic volume
- Proposed mucosal margin position
- Interarch prosthetic space
- Deficiencies of the alveolar ridge and soft tissue

The diagnostic process should yield the external shape of the immediate provisional restoration. It may include a putty index of the diagnostic wax-up or a 3D-printed digital diagnostic set-up. Alternatively, the diagnostic tooth can be used in the design and fabrication of a shell temporary for direct pick-up, or it may be copied digitally for indirect fabrication of the provisional from an impression or intraoral scan made at the surgical appointment.

3.3.2 Occlusal Assessment

As part of the prosthodontic evaluation, it is imperative for the occlusion to be carefully assessed to determine the anticipated biomechanical loads on the planned rehabilitation. This will be equally important for planning the definitive restoration and for assessing the suitability of the site for immediate loading.

Although firm scientific evidence is lacking regarding the optimum occlusion for implant restorations, for single-tooth restorations it is generally accepted that an implant protected occlusion is ideal (Rilo and coworkers 2008; Koyano and Esaki 2015). This entails an absence of occlusal contacts in maximum intercuspation at light biting forces and only light contact at heavy biting forces, as well as the absence of excursive contacts, which should be distributed across the remaining natural dentition. This recommendation needs to be seen in the context of the patient's overall dentition, occlusal scheme, tooth being replaced, status of the adjacent teeth, and esthetic requirements. As such, the elimination of excursive occlusal contacts on the proposed restoration is not always desirable or even possible. However, this aspect should be taken into consideration when selecting an appropriate implant design, material, and diameter, as well as the prosthetic design and restorative materials.

All implants restored within the first week after implant placement are considered to be immediately loaded. The term "immediate loading" should still be applied for immediate provisional restorations that are completely free of occlusal contact, as it is recognized that during mastication and movements of the oral tissues, the restoration will still be loaded. However, we should distinguish whether the restoration is immediately loaded with occlusal contact, or immediately loaded without direct occlusal contact.

The majority of clinical studies on immediate loading of immediately placed implants in partially edentulous patients have reported no occlusal contacts on the provisional implant restoration in either maximum intercuspation or excursive movements (Zhou and coworkers 2021). This is to limit micromovement of the implant that may be caused by occlusal contacts, particularly in the presence of parafunction, leading to failed osseointegration. Literature on immediately loaded single implants with full occlusal contact is limited (Zhou and coworkers 2021).

Non-axial loading of immediately placed implants is likely to have the most detrimental effects and is more likely to be encountered in anterior teeth due to the angle of the alveolus relative to the clinical crowns, as well as the angle of occlusion formed by the vertical and horizontal overlap. Teeth that are the sole determinants of anterior guidance during excursive mandibular movements are the most subject to non-axial loading. When these teeth are planned for replacement, immediate loading would be contraindicated unless the guidance can be temporarily transferred to another tooth by flattening and shortening the cusps or incisal edge of the immediate provisional restoration, which may result in esthetic compromises (Fig 4). The full range of mandibular movements should be carefully assessed for contacts in excursion, including all paths into and returning from mandibular crossover positions.

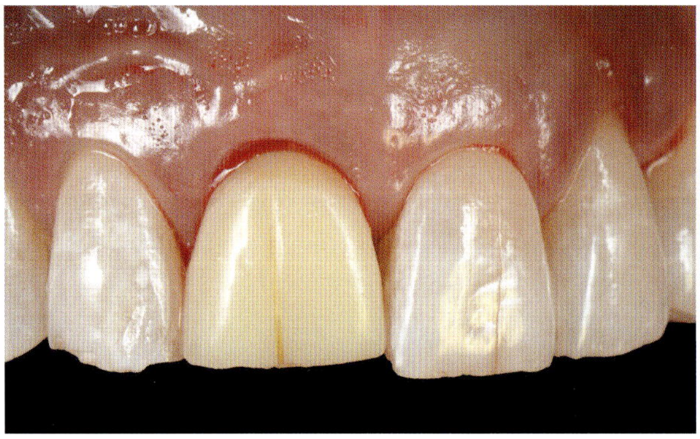

Fig 4 Shortening of an immediate provisional restoration on an immediately placed implant 11 to relieve any protrusive contacts.

The presence of occlusal parafunction, as determined by signs of attrition or a history of tooth fractures, also present as a risk factor for implant failure with immediate loading. Fremitus and mobility of adjacent teeth should also be considered risk factors in the occlusal assessment and may preclude an implant-protected occlusal scheme.

3.3.3 Alternative Provisional Restorations (Plan B)

As a part of planning for the immediate implant and loading protocol (type 1A), it should be recognized that if preoperative risk factors are identified or intraoperative criteria are not met, immediate loading of immediately placed implants may not be possible or recommended. It is advisable to discuss this with the patient before initiating treatment and to keep a pathway for an alternative interim tooth replacement readily available.

The alternative solutions for interim tooth replacement during early or conventional implant loading protocols are highlighted in more detail in Chapter 10 of Volume 10 of the ITI Treatment Guide (Martin and coworkers 2017). They may involve one of the following:

- Indirect resin-bonded provisional fixed bridge
- Direct resin-bonded provisional fixed bridge
- Conventional fixed provisional bridge (where adjacent teeth are planned for restoration with crowns)
- Removable suspension bridge (ESSIX-style retainer)
- Removable partial denture
- Orthodontic retention

Although the literature on type 1A protocols demonstrates comparable survival rates, this does not exclude additional risks when immediately loading an immediately placed implant. Where suitable alternative fixed provisional restorations are readily available during the healing phase, such as when adjacent teeth are already planned for crowns and a provisional fixed bridge can be provided, type 1C protocols may be more justifiable. In this case, prosthetically guided soft tissue healing, socket management, and grafting should be delivered using an appropriately designed and shaped pontic. This pontic should support the mucosal tissues and contain any graft biomaterials in the socket in the same manner as an immediately loaded provisional restoration (Figs 5a-j).

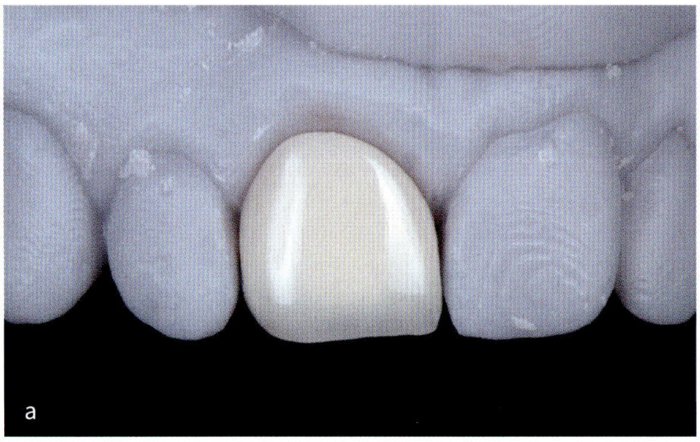

a

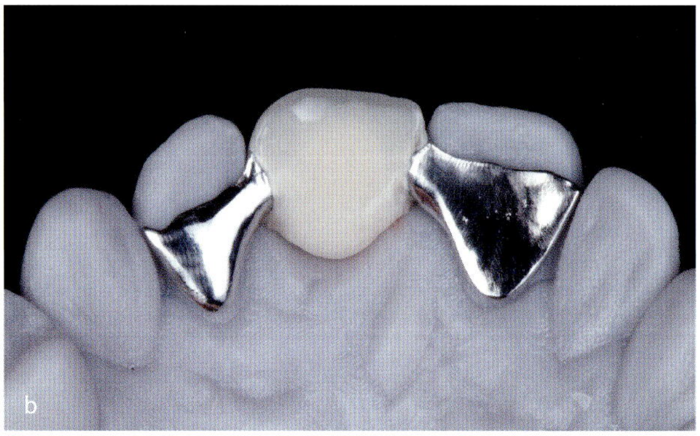

b

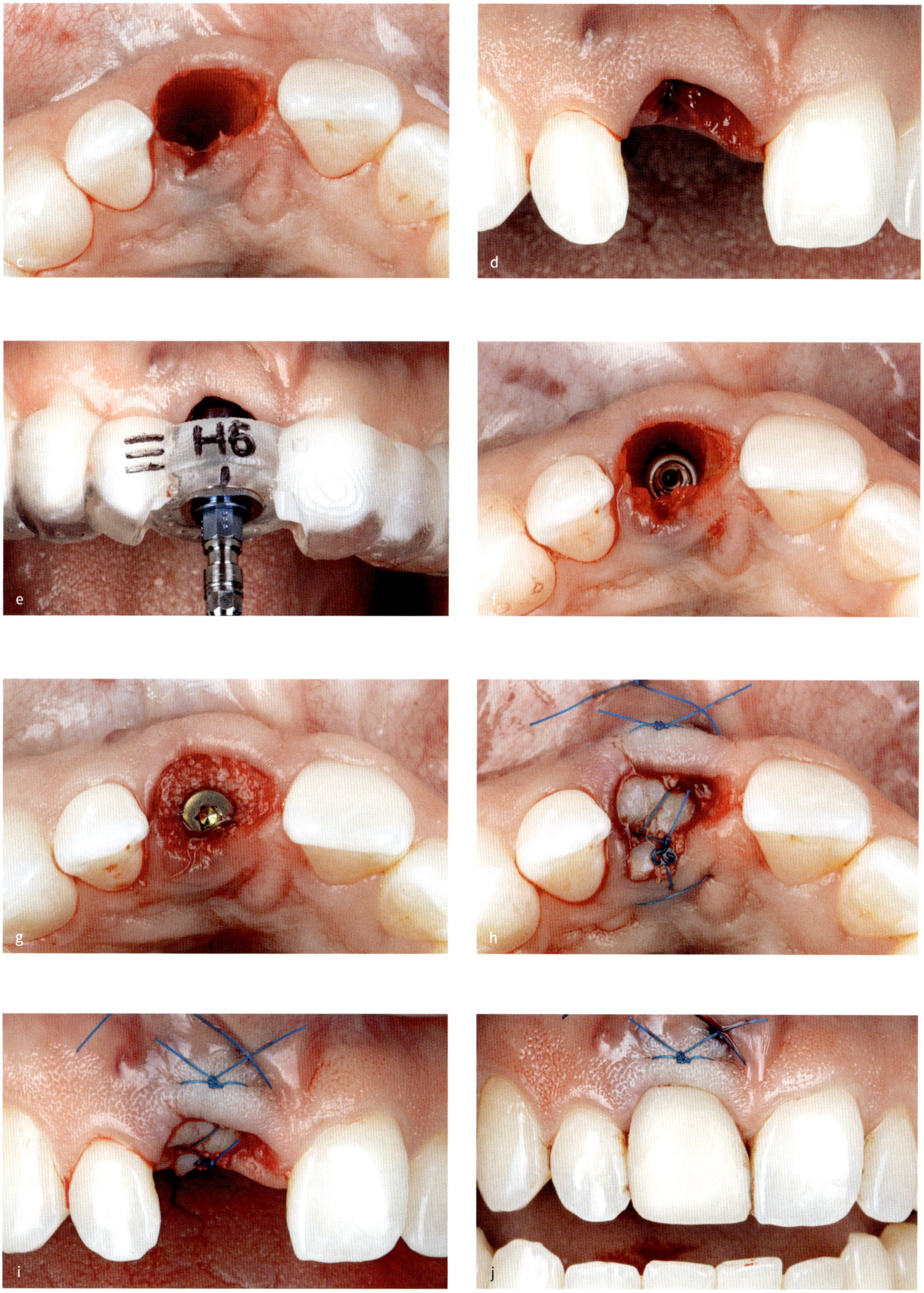

Figs 5a-j Resin-bonded bridge pontic used to provide prosthetically guided soft tissue healing over an extraction socket and immediately placed implant.

3.4 Surgical Planning

Surgical planning according to the predetermined prosthodontic design of the implant restoration is based on esthetic and functional analyses, an assessment of local bone anatomy and volume using 3D imaging (CBCT), and a clinical evaluation of the soft tissue conditions. As part of the planning process, the suitability for immediate placement and immediate loading will be determined, together with specific procedural details including the length, diameter, design, and position of the implant and the need for adjunctive surgical procedures.

3.4.1 Bone Conditions

Planning for immediate placement involves careful evaluation of the site-specific bony anatomy. A comprehensive preoperative 3D radiographic examination (e.g., by CBCT) should be performed to evaluate whether the alveolar bone is adequate to satisfy the criteria for immediate placement. Although 2D plain-film radiographs are commonly used in implant dentistry, when considering flapless immediate placement, it is highly recommended to consider 3D imaging as a routine primary imaging modality (Bornstein and coworkers 2017).

Bone anatomy and type of socket. To obtain primary stability in immediate placement, both in the anterior and in the posterior regions, several anatomical considerations should be preoperatively evaluated. Important site-specific landmarks such as the nasal floor, maxillary sinus floor, mandibular canal, accessory canals, lingual concavity, etc., should be identified when planning for immediate placement. Moreover, the socket anatomy and its relationship with the alveolar and basal bone are also determinants in evaluating the possibility to immediately place and load an implant. These characteristics are different in the anterior and in the posterior regions.

Anterior region. In the anterior maxilla, the anatomy, shape, and availability of basal and palatal bone are the most crucial bone structures for the anchorage of an immediate implant. In a clinical study, Botelho and coworkers (2020) found that the basal bone has a trapezoidal shape with a larger dimension in the lateral incisor site and smaller dimensions in the canine sites. Along with larger root dimensions, this makes it more difficult to obtain primary stability in the canine area compared to central or lateral incisors. In these areas, the maxillary nasal floor will be the apical boundary and, together with root length, will determine the height of the basal bone (Figs 6a-c)

Other factors such as root shape, length, and position related to the alveolar process are also important. A CBCT study by Kan and coworkers (2011a) demonstrated the relationship between sagittal root position and the alveolar bone housing.

Root positions are classified as class I to class IV:

- Class I: Root positioned against the facial cortical bone
- Class II: Root positioned in the middle of the alveolar housing without engaging either the facial or the palatal cortical plates at the apical third of the root
- Class III: Root is positioned against the palatal cortical plate
- Class IV: At least two thirds of the root engages both the labial and the palatal cortical plates.

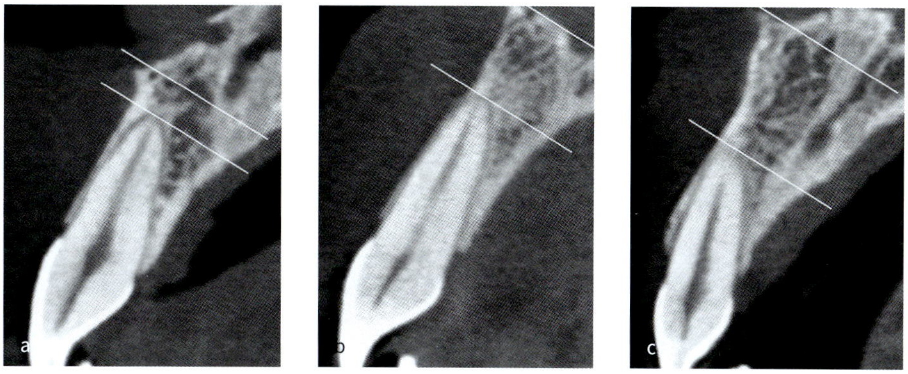

Figs 6a-c CBCTs of central incisors demonstrating variability in available apical bone for primary stability of immediately placed implants which is related to the root length and proximity of the nasal floor.

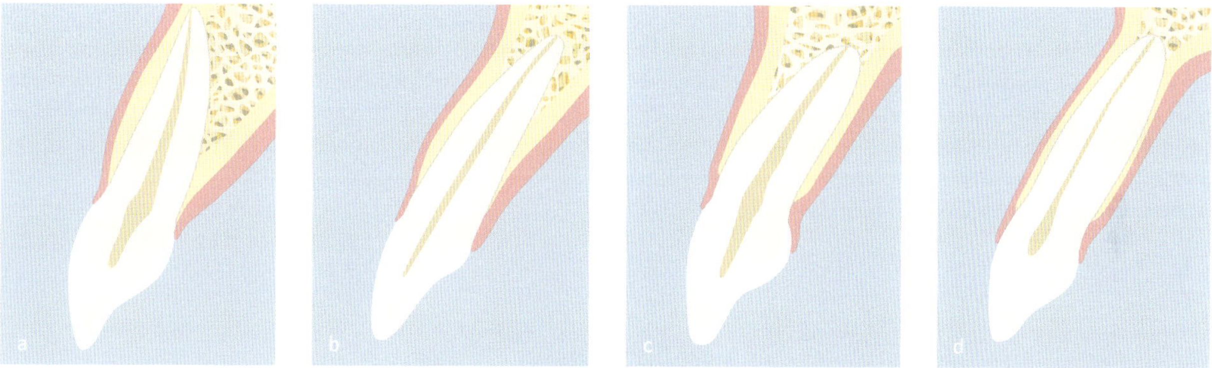

Figs 7a-d Classes of sagittal root positions related to the alveolar bone housing. Left: Class I sagittal root position. Middle left: Class II sagittal root position. Middle right: Class III sagittal root position. Right: Class IV sagittal root position.

Based on the results of this study, in the maxillary anterior region, class I was the most predominant root position, accounting for 86.5% in central incisors, 76% in lateral incisors, and 81% in canines (Figs 7a-d) (Kan and coworkers 2011a).

These findings demonstrate the significance of the palatal bone for primary stability in the anterior maxilla in most clinical scenarios. However, it also highlights the thin facial wall. Caution should be exercised in class IV root position, which is unsuitable for immediate placement due to the lack of labial or palatal bone (Fig 8).

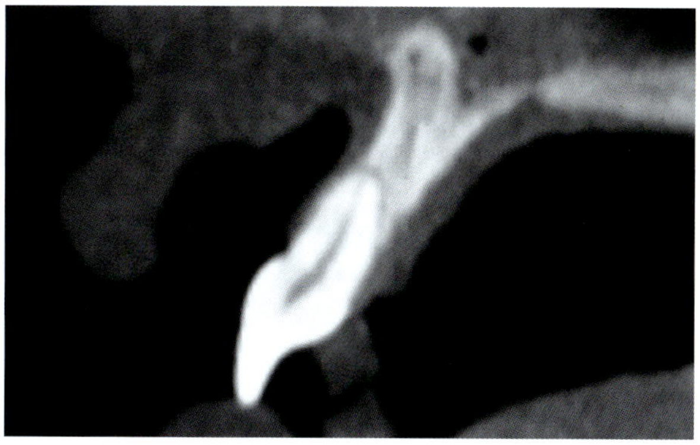

Fig 8 A class IV root position. It is not a result of pathological bone loss but due to a genetic variation of the local anatomy and alveolar bone contours in the presence of healthy periodontal tissues.

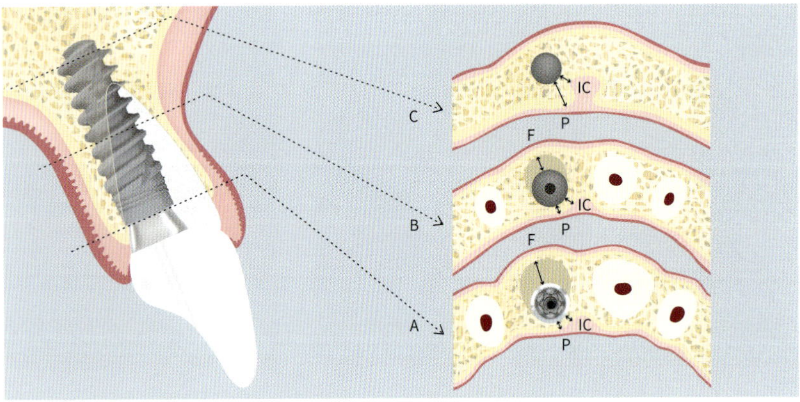

Fig 9 The proximity of the incisal canal to an immediately placed central incisor implant should be carefully evaluated along the entire length of the implant. It is best visualized in axial CBCT cross-sections.

When replacing missing maxillary incisors with dental implants, the nasopalatine canal and its incisive foramen are critical anatomical structures to be considered during implant planning and surgery. Fenestrations or dehiscences into the nasopalatine canal and incisive foramen should be avoided, as these can increase the risk of implant failure, bleeding, and neurosensory disturbances. Hamilton and coworkers (Hamilton and coworkers 2022) found that the nasopalatine canal is often closer than 0.5 mm to the regular implant virtually planned at the most coronal aspect in the maxillary central incisor position (Fig 9).

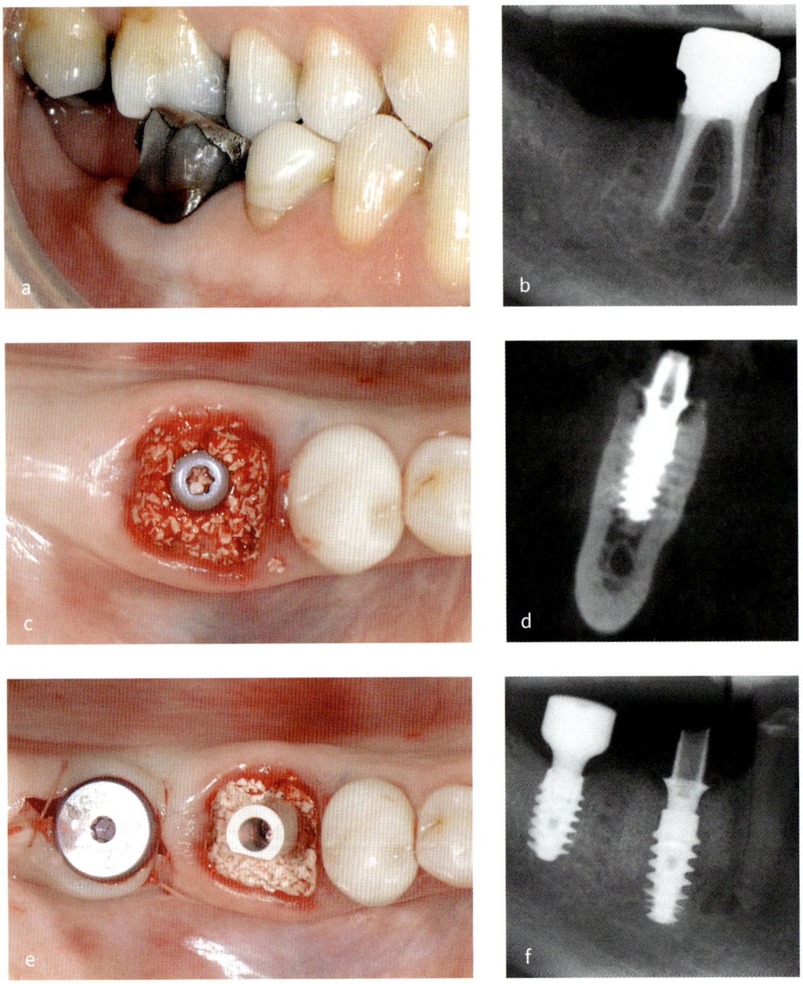

Figs 10a-f Immediate placement in the region of the mandibular first molar. The interproximal septum and the available bone in the apical region allowed immediate placement.

Posterior region. In posterior sites, the anatomy of the alveolar process is distinctly different from anterior sites. This may impact the survival and success of immediate implants but also the technical difficulty of immediate placement (Zhou and coworkers 2021). In premolar areas, the roots are wider buccolingually and narrower mesiodistally. Here primary stability can be achieved even with long roots by engaging the interproximal bone walls. In multirooted molar sites, the width and height of the interradicular septum bone plays an important role for immediate placement (Figs 10a-f, 11a-f). Therefore, root trunk height and root divergency should be evaluated to decide whether the site is suitable for immediate placement (Figs 12a-c).

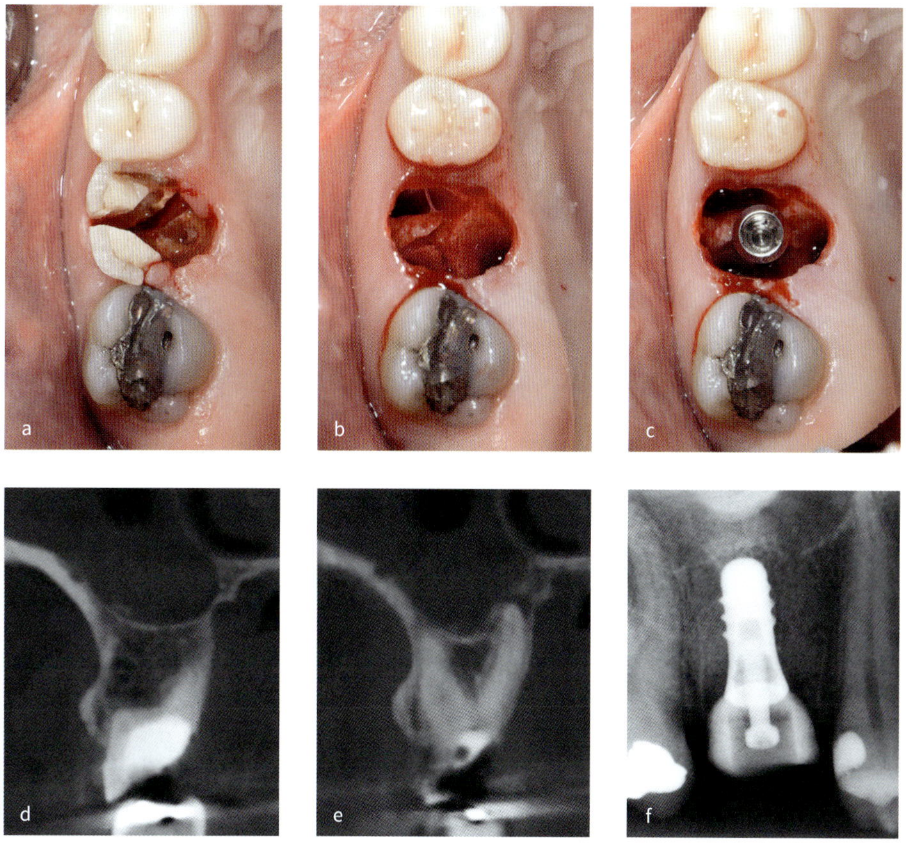

Figs 11a-f Immediate placement in the region of the maxillary first molar. The interproximal septa and the available bone in the apical region allowed immediate placement.

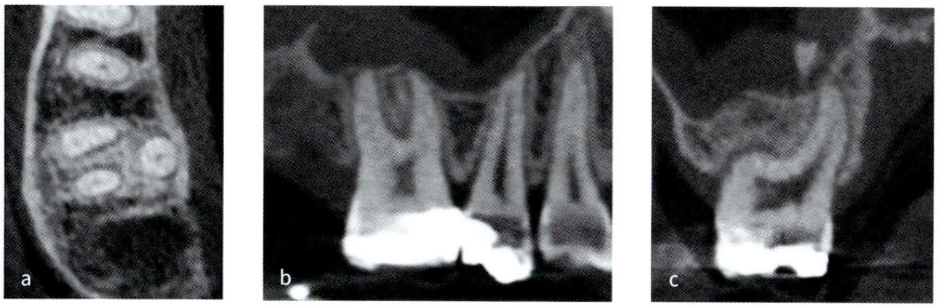

Fig 12a-c CBCT of tooth 16: axial (a), tangential (b), and cross-sectional (c) views. The tooth has a high root trunk, narrow interseptal bone, and sinus proximity. These local bone conditions do not allow immediate placement.

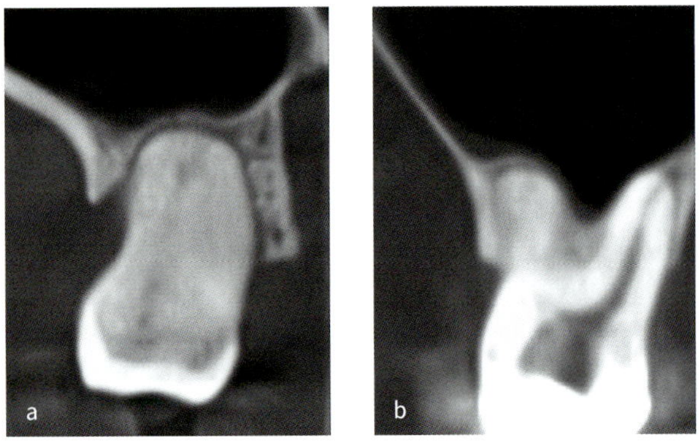

Fig 13a-b CBCT of a maxillary molar showing close contact with the maxillary sinus. Immediate placement would be contraindicated here.

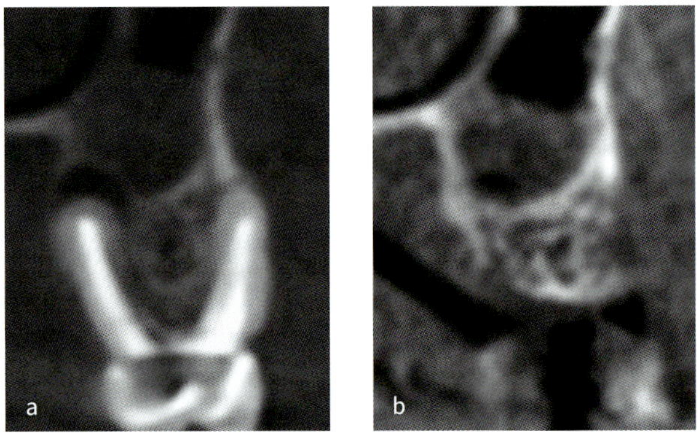

Figs 14a-b CBCT of a maxillary first molar. Cross-sectional view before (a) and six months after (b) tooth extraction.

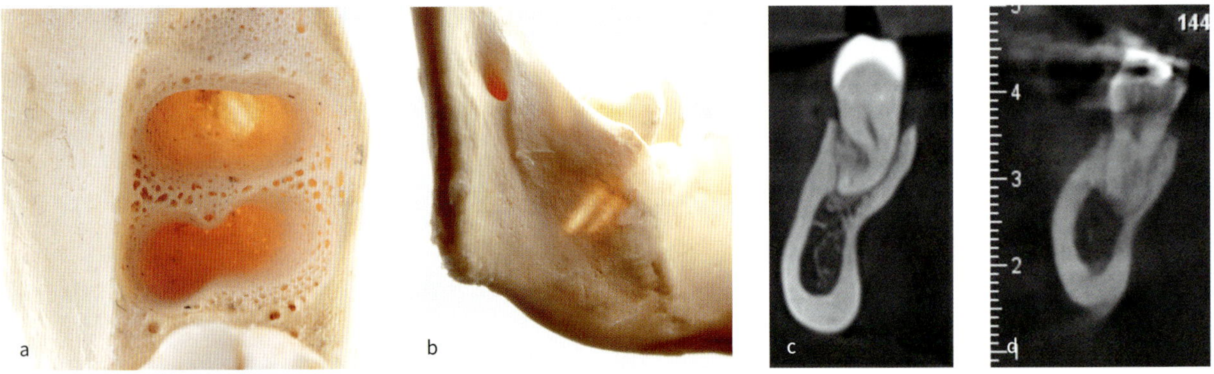

Figs 15a-d Dry skull and CBCT images showing the proximity of the root apices of a lower molar to the submandibular fossa, where apical engagement of bone for immediate placement beyond the root apices is contraindicated.

In the posterior maxilla, the main anatomical structure limiting bone height is the maxillary sinus cavity. The roots of maxillary molars are frequently in close contact with the floor of the maxillary sinus, and preoperative 3D imaging is required for adequate assessment (Figs 13a-b). Previous studies have demonstrated that the proportion of molar roots protruding into the sinus varies from 26% to 50% depending upon patient population and age (Ok and coworkers 2014; Tian and coworkers 2016; Zhang and coworkers 2019).

Chen and coworkers (2020) demonstrated that after extracting of a molar, the change in vertical bone height was about 35% if no regenerative procedure was performed (Chen and coworkers 2021). This was predominantly attributed to losses on the coronal aspect of the alveolar ridge, with slight sinus pneumatization in the middle portion of the ridge (Figs 14a-b).

In the posterior mandibular area, the relationship between the tooth and these anatomical structures should be identified prior to tooth extraction and immediate placement: submandibular and sublingual fossa (risk of lingual cortical perforation and arterial damage during surgery) (Figs 15a-d); mandibular canal, mental foramen, and anterior loop extension of the mandibular canal anterior to mental foramen (risk of nerve damage) (Figs 16a-d).

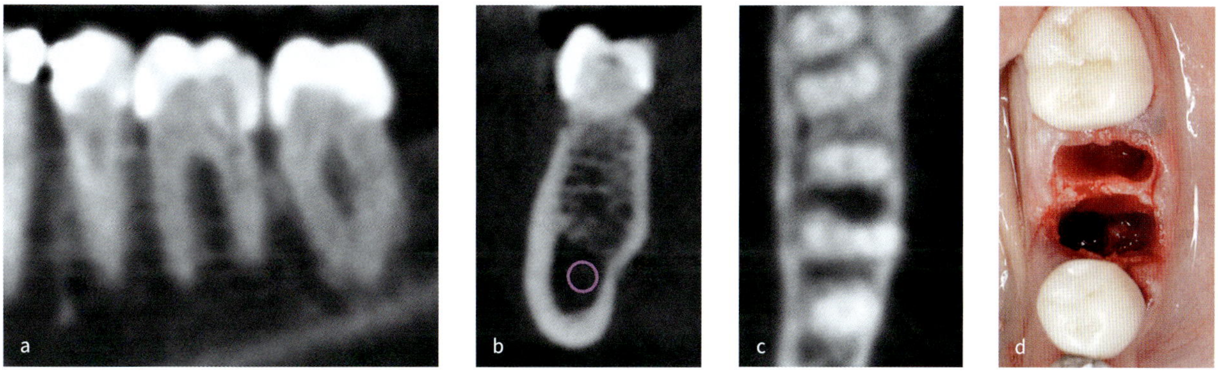

Figs 16a-d CBCT of a mandibular first molar with panoramic (a), cross-sectional (b), and axial (c) views before extraction, and an occlusal clinical view (d) of the socket anatomy following tooth extraction.

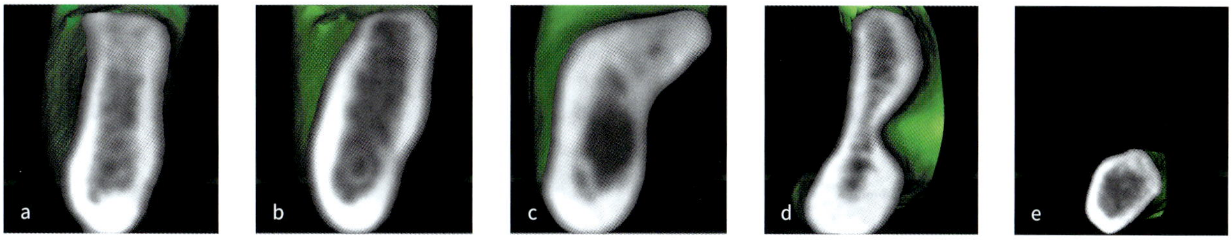

Figs 17a-e Various cross-sectional shapes of the mandible in relation to the tooth socket. S-shape (c) and hourglass (d) shapes may present anatomical challenges for immediate placement.

Gallucci and coworkers (2017) classified the morphology of the mandibular posterior alveolar bone into five categories: straight, oblique, S-shape, hourglass, and basal bone. Their study demonstrated that the straight ridge morphology was most prevalent (53.6%), which facilitates immediate placement. S-shape or hourglass alveolar ridge morphologies were less prevalent and carried a higher risk of damage on adjacent anatomical structures. In healed sites, this classification also applies to immediate implant procedures, as the implant often needs to be anchored in the basal bone (Figs 17a-e).

3D imaging is also recommended for posterior mandibular sites and helps identify structures such as the mandibular canal (containing the inferior alveolar nerve), sublingual and submandibular fossae (lingual concavities). The latter is in close proximity to the lingual artery, where damage can lead to critical hemorrhage (Braut and coworkers 2012).

The mental foramen (containing the mental nerve) and its anterior loop, which can extend from 5 to 9 mm from the foramen itself, should be identified radiographically. For immediate placement in the posterior mandible, the relationship of the socket and its surrounding alveolar bone with the previously mentioned anatomical landmarks should be part of a careful preoperative evaluation.

Whether an anterior or a posterior immediate implant is considered, it is important to determine bone availability for primary stability by preoperative 3D imaging. Bone anchorage can be found in the apical, palatal/lingual, or lateral bony aspects of the socket.

Bone phenotype (thickness of the facial bone plate) and integrity. It has been demonstrated that after a tooth extraction, the alveolar socket undergoes a series of events resulting in significant alveolar ridge resorption (Araújo and Lindhe 2005). Resorption is most prominent in the crestal region, on the facial aspect of the alveolar socket. The dimensional change resulting from this physiological wound healing alters the facial contour of the alveolar process. Immediate placement in fresh extraction sockets will cause the same resorptive processes and does not prevent the previously mentioned bone alterations (Araújo and coworkers 2005; Araújo and coworkers 2019).

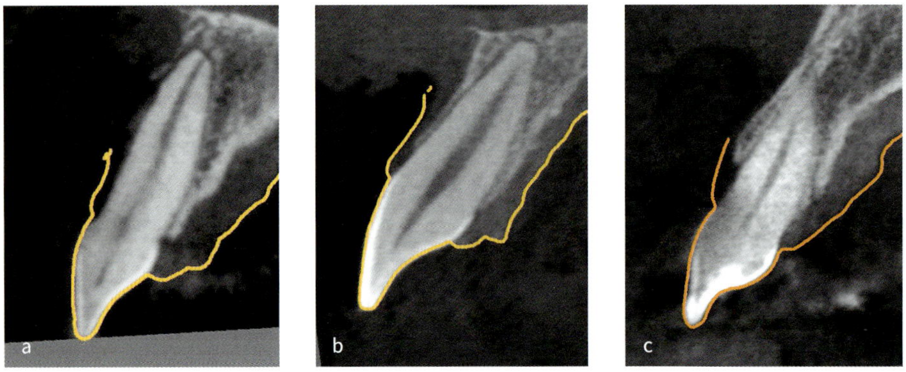

Figs 18a-c CBCT tangential slices through a maxillary central incisor with the outline of the intra-oral scan demonstrating (a) absent labial bone, (b) 0.5 mm thickness of midfacial labial bone, and (c) 1.7 mm thickness of midfacial labial bone.

The thickness and integrity of the facial bone is one of the most crucial factors in determining the extent of alveolar bone remodeling (Chappuis and coworkers 2013). Patients with a thin phenotype (less than 1 mm of facial bone thickness) run a higher long-term risk of biological complications, with significant impact on soft tissue support and esthetic outcomes. Thus, adjunctive procedures such as socket management or soft tissue grafting need to be considered to mitigate the consequences of alveolar bone resorption when an implant is placed in a fresh extraction socket (Levine and coworkers 2017: Araújo and coworkers 2019).

Facial bone plate thickness. Midfacial recession can occur when immediate implants are placed in the presence of a thin (1 mm or less) or missing facial bone plate (Levine and coworkers 2014; Tonetti and coworkers 2017). Clinical studies using CBCT scans to examine the facial bone on immediate implants have shown a significant relationship between recessions of the midfacial mucosa and a lack of a visible facial bone walls on the CBCT images (Januário and coworkers 2011; Miyamoto and Obama 2011: Vera and coworkers 2012).

Preoperative planning for immediate implants should include a CBCT showing the presence and thickness of the facial bone. Moreover, in a CBCT study, Chappuis and coworkers (2013) found that patients with less than 1 mm of bone thickness (thin bone phenotype) exhibited greater vertical bone loss than patients with more than 1 mm of facial bone (thick bone phenotype). In the anterior maxilla, most patients (80% to 95%) present with thin facial bone thickness of less than 1 mm (Braut and coworkers 2011; Januário and coworkers 2011) (Figs 18a-c).

Systematic reviews have demonstrated that socket management using biomaterials (socket grafting) and connective tissue grafting were the most effective in mitigating the risk of facial recession, especially in sites with a thin bone phenotype (Seyssens and coworkers 2021).

Therefore, immediate placement in sites with a facial bone thickness of less than 1 mm should be considered at risk for midfacial recession and simultaneous adjunctive procedures (socket management/soft tissue grafting) should be considered in order to decrease the risk.

Facial bone plate integrity. Immediate placement in sites with damaged facial socket bone also carries a risk of midfacial recession. Kan and coworkers (2007) demonstrated that 8.3% of immediate implants placed in sites with minor facial dehiscence (isolated at the facial aspect of the facial bone) developed midfacial mucosal recession greater than 1.5 mm one year later. They also showed that 42.8% of sites with a moderately large dehiscence (defect extended to the mesial or distal aspect) demonstrated recession of greater than 1.5 mm. All (100%) sites with a large dehiscence (defect extended to the mesial or distal mesial and distal aspect of the adjacent teeth) developed recession of greater than 1.5 mm up to one year later. Thus, damage to the facial bone represents a significant risk factor for soft tissue recession, the risk increasing with the size of the dehiscence defect of the facial socket bone.

Following tooth extraction, the shape and size of the facial bone defect also seems to influence the predictability of immediate placement (Kan and coworkers 2007). The facial bone defect was categorized a V-, U-, or Ultra-U (UU)-shaped using a bone-sounding technique on the midfacial, mesial and distal aspects, based on the following description (Figs 19a-c).

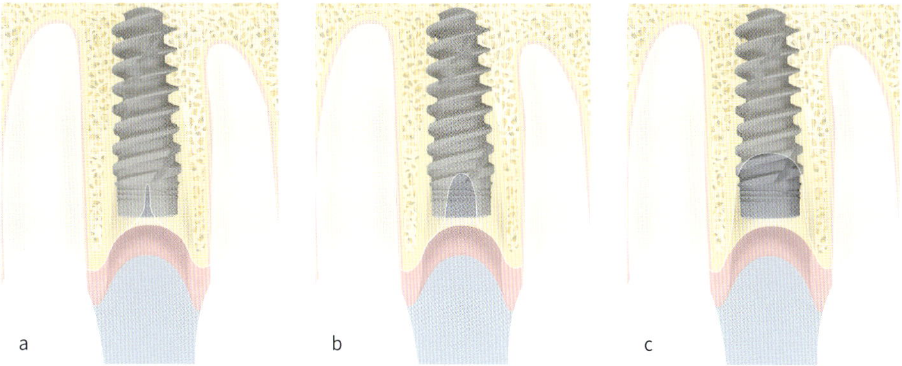

Figs 19a-c V-shaped defect, isolated at the facial aspect of the facial bone (a). U-shaped defect, extended to the mesial or distal aspect of the failing tooth (b). UU-shaped defect, extended to the mesial or distal mesial and distal aspect of the adjacent teeth (c).

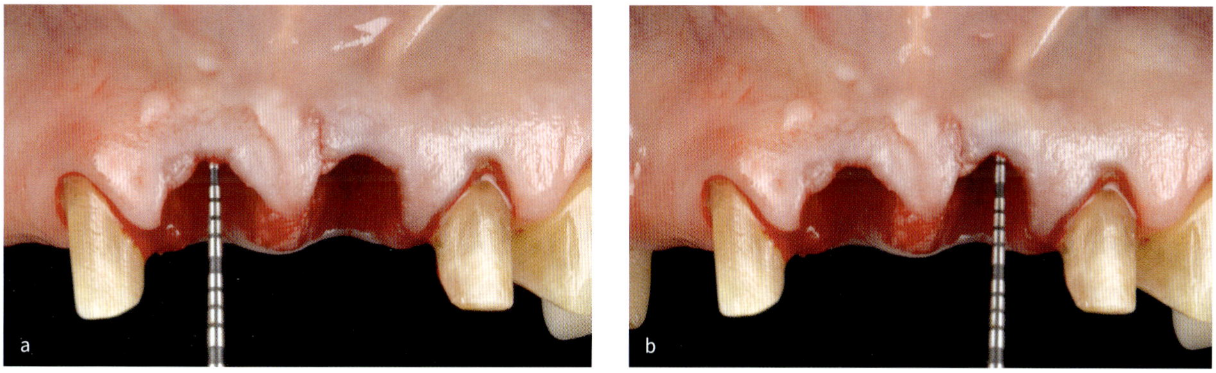

Figs 20a-b Extraction sockets. Facial bone inspection with a periodontal probe.

Small V-shaped defects present a lower risk of midfacial recession on immediate placement when combined with guided bone regeneration. However, facial soft tissue dehiscence was frequently reported after 1 year of function on sites with U-shaped or UU-shaped defects. The extent of the facial defects will increase with post-extraction remodeling, as extensively discussed in Chapter 2.

To evaluate the extent and shape of the facial bone defect in cases of flapless extraction, bone integrity (vertical and mesiodistal extension) should be inspected with a periodontal probe (Figs 20a-b).

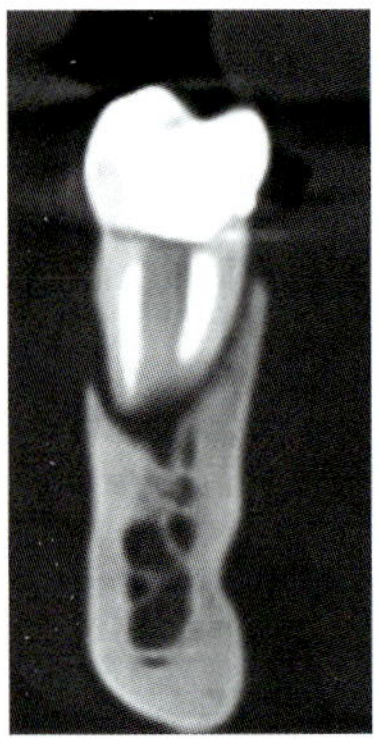

Fig 21 Buccal alveolar-ridge deficiency in the molar region.

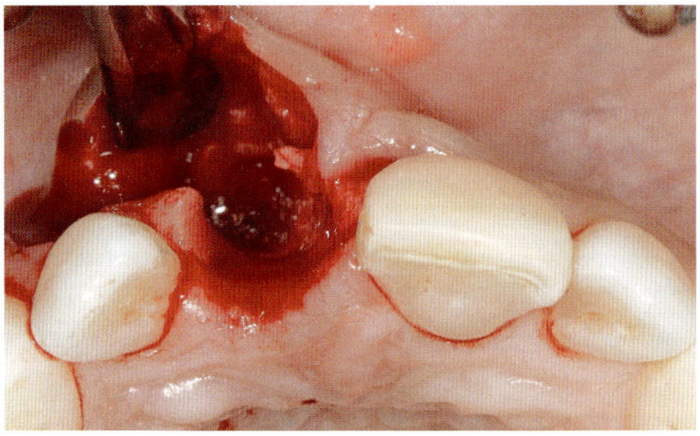

Fig 22 Labial alveolar-ridge deficiency in the anterior region.

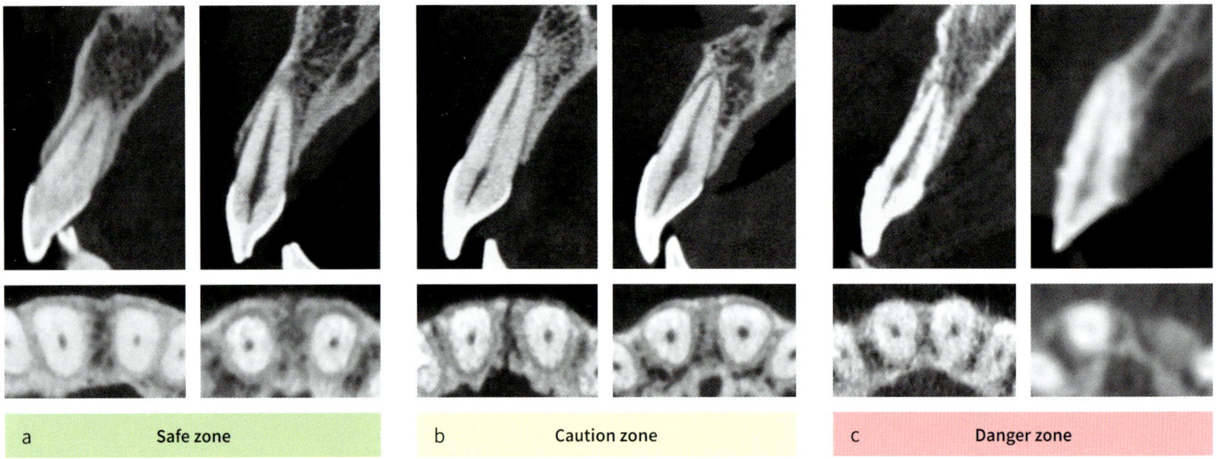

Figs 23a-c Assessment of root position and dimensions of the alveolar bone in cross-sectional CBCT images. Root positioned entirely within the alveolar housing with adequate labial, palatal, and apical bone for immediate placement (a). Root positioned entirely within the alveolar housing with slightly reduced labial, palatal, or apical bone; increased risk associated with immediate placement (b). Root projecting outside of the alveolar housing or significant compromise in the labial, palatal, or apical bone; high risk associated with immediate placement (c).

Therefore, a failing tooth with a large U-shaped or UU-shaped defect is contraindicated for immediate placement (Figs 21 and 22). Minor V-shape facial bone dehiscences are a risk factor for midfacial recession, and alternative implant placement protocols such as early placement should be considered. Where immediate placement is still the preferred treatment option in these situations, and esthetic risk is determined to be low, adjunctive procedures including socket management should be performed to mitigate the anticipated dimensional changes and recession.

Socket position within the bone envelope. Assessing the position of the socket and proposed implant within the alveolar housing is important when selecting an appropriate timing for implant placement (Buser and coworkers 2017). This can be observed on the axial sections of the 3D images at the various levels of the alveolar process.

The roots of maxillary anterior teeth are typically located in the facial half of the alveolar process, following the facial inclination of the facial bone (Kan and coworkers 2011). When the roots are located entirely within the alveolar housing, the facial and palatal bony contours are relatively parallel arcs, with the interproximal bone extending to the facial contour of the alveolar housing (Figs 23a-c).

This arrangement means a relatively narrow mesiodistal dimension of the thin facial bundle bone. If the alveolar process has a reduced buccolingual dimension or the roots are located facial to the alveolar process, the labial bone will exhibit labial scalloping and an increased mesiodistal dimension of the thin facial bone.

The alveolar bone proper (bundle bone) is an avascular structure that depends on the periodontal ligament for nutrition.

If, after extraction, the socket is located further outside the bony envelope, more extensive alveolar bone resorption can be expected.

Even under conditions of minimally traumatic extraction and maintenance of the alveolar bone proper, the integration of any grafting material in the gap between an immediately placed implant and facial wall depends upon the blood supply and nutrition of the interproximal bone and periosteum. Therefore, the further the root is positioned outside of the alveolar bony envelope, the greater will be the reduction in the regenerative potential of the facial bone (Figs 24a-b).

CBCT axial sections allow an analysis of prospective socket remodeling by assessing the presence and thickness of the facial bone, as well as the relationship of the root prominence to the alveolar housing. If the root and facial bone wall protrude from the bony envelope, particularly when combined with a reduced facial-lingual dimension of the interproximal bone and alveolar housing, the regenerative potential of the socket is low, and immediate implants should be avoided.

Facial defect. Although it was demonstrated that an empty marginal defect wider than 1 mm may heal with new bone, use of a graft does not promote healing but plays the role of a defect "filler" material (Botticelli and coworkers 2004). However, implants being positioned in the socket and the gap between the facial bone and an immediately placed implant play a critical role in the regeneration of the bone of the remaining socket (Caneva and coworkers 2010; Tomasi and coworkers 2010). Implants should be planned with a palatal/lingual implant position allowing for a gap of at least 2 mm between the implant and facial bone plate. This will optimize the osteogenic potential of the buccal defect and allow for socket grafting, which helps limit post-extraction bone remodeling and is well documented in alveolar ridge preservation procedures (Avila-Ortiz and coworkers 2019; Levine and coworkers 2022).

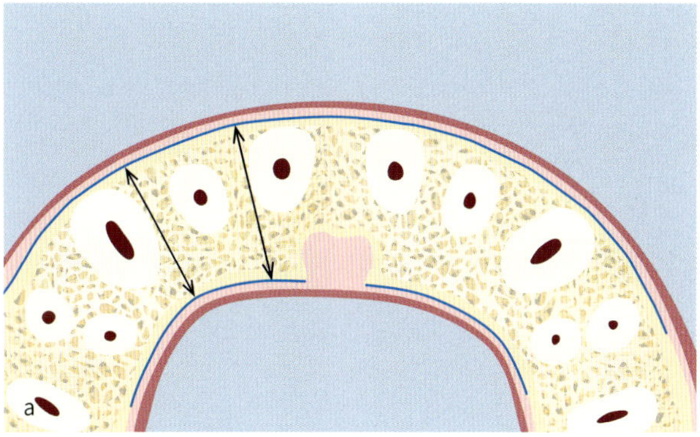

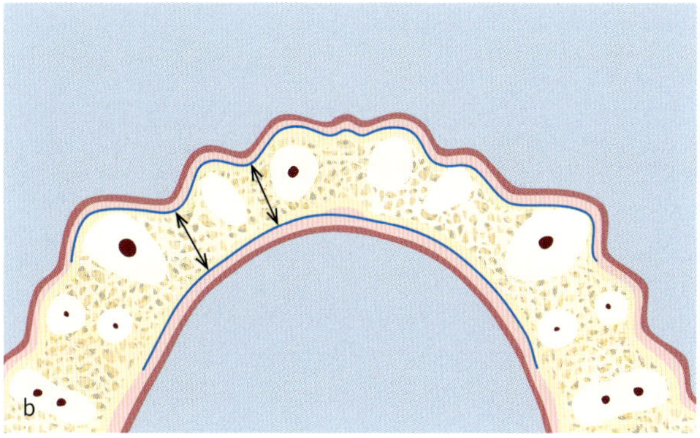

Figs 24a-b Root position and labial prominence in relation to the alveolar housing. Where the interproximal bone peaks extend to the most labial aspect of the root surface (a), there is a greater regenerative potential than in (b), where greater dimensional changes in the alveolar ridge following tooth extraction may be expected.

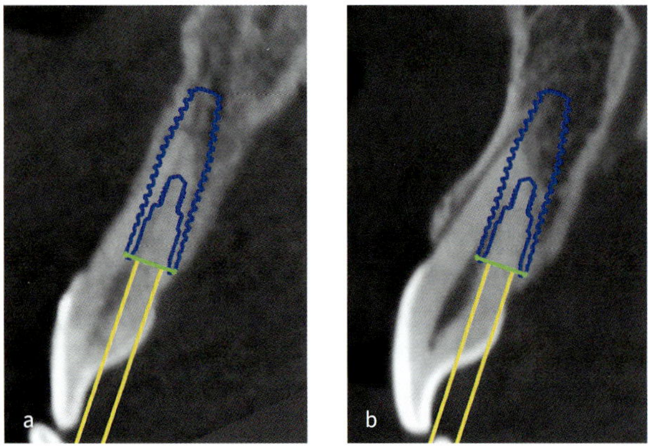

Figs 25a-b Digital planning of an immediate implant. Limited horizontal gap compromising socket management and the horizontal gap (a). Adequate horizontal gap distance for socket grafting (b).

The latest evidence suggests that socket grafting may contribute to horizontal bone preservation and soft tissue stability at the midfacial aspect of immediate implants and should therefore be routinely considered as an adjunct to immediate placement in clinical practice (Seyssens and coworkers 2021).

A reduced horizontal gap of less than 2 mm can result from facial implant positioning, whether due to the anatomy of the alveolar process or to an increased implant diameter. If the implant is placed too close to the facial bone, the potential for socket grafting is reduced, and significantly less facial bone can be expected after healing (Caneva and coworkers 2010), with a compromised esthetic result (Figs 25a-b).

A facial gap of less than 2 mm is considered high risk, as it is not possible to effectively graft the gap and provide a site that will predictably regenerate bone in light of the anticipated facial bone resorption (Figs 26a-b).

Alveolar crest status. Several local conditions can lead to periodontal bone loss, such as periodontal disease, root fracture, periapical lesions, or external root resorption. They should be identified by a 3D radiograph (CBCT) prior to tooth extraction and immediate placement. Orofacial or mesiodistal bone deficiencies may make immediate placement impossible or unsuitable from a biological and esthetic perspective. Deficiencies in the alveolar bone crest on the facial, lingual/palatal, or interproximal aspects of the extracted tooth will require flap elevation and simultaneous guided bone regeneration. In such a clinical scenario, other treatment approaches such as socket grafting or type II/type III implant placement are advised.

The level of the papillae around a single implant depends on the bone levels on the mesial and distal aspects of the adjacent teeth, as well as on its relationship to the contours of the restoration and the contact point (Kan and coworkers 2003). Therefore, interproximal bone loss around the tooth due to previous infections or traumatic extraction could result in undesirable black triangles after healing (Figs 27a-b).

To our knowledge, the regeneration of crestal bone in areas with interproximal bone loss is not predictable and is unlikely to occur.

3.4.2 Soft Tissue Status

The soft tissue status should be considered when deciding on the treatment strategy for immediate implants, both in the anterior and posterior regions, to minimize the impact of mucogingival defects on the longevity and esthetics of the tooth replacement. When planning implant treatment, gingival esthetic parameters should be carefully evaluated preoperatively to determine and predict the desired position of the facial mucosal margin of the tooth being replaced. Where achieving harmony in the gingival and mucosal architectures is a challenge, adjacent periodontal plastic surgical procedures or prosthetic soft tissue replacements can be considered.

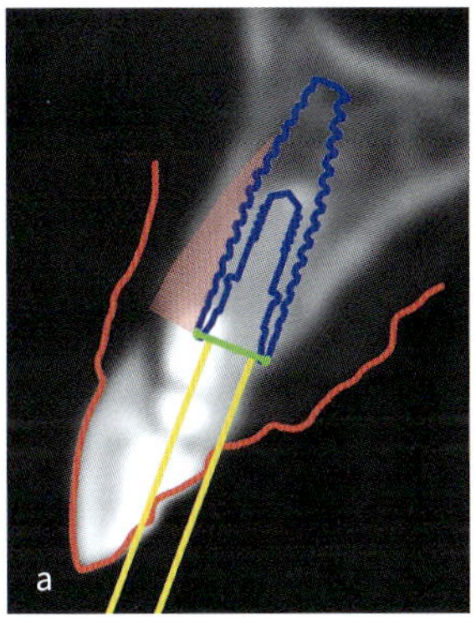

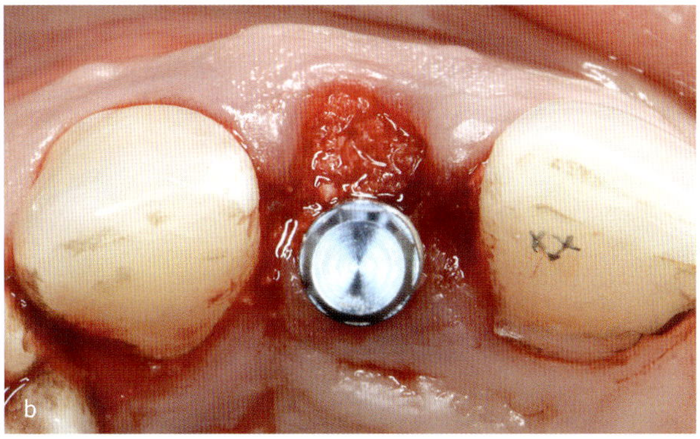

Figs 26a-b Digital implant planning displaying a horizontal gap of more than 2 mm (a) and allowing socket grafting simultaneously with implant placement using demineralized bovine bone mineral (DBBM) (b).

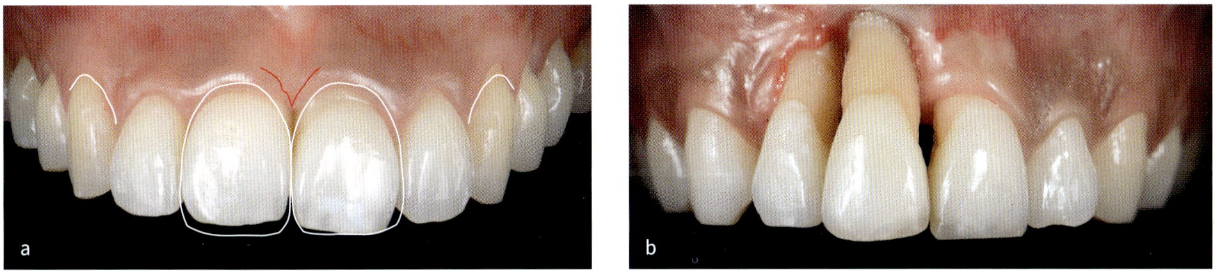

Fig 27a-b Alveolar crest conditions. Limited loss of the interproximal papilla (a). Severe loss of crestal tissues (b).

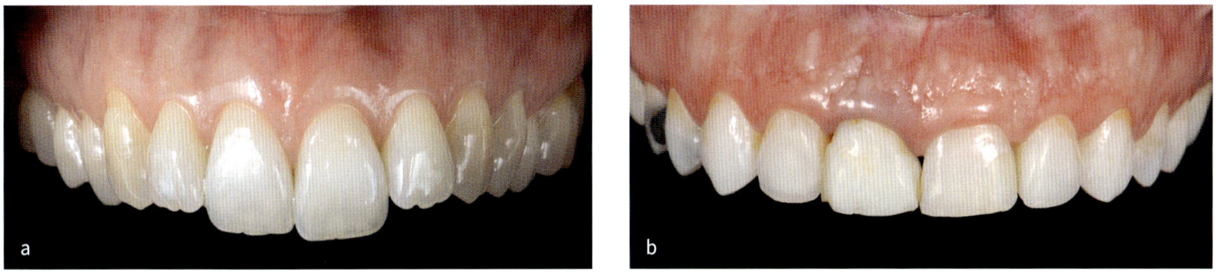

Figs 28a-b Gingival morphology or phenotype. Thin/scalloped soft tissue phenotype (a). Thick/flat soft tissue phenotype (b).

Gingival phenotype. The gingival phenotype is currently defined as the three-dimensional gingival thickness and width of the keratinized tissue, and is classified as thin/scalloped, thick/flat, or medium (De Rouck and coworkers 2009) (Figs 28a-b). A thin phenotype increases the risk for gingival recession and compromised soft tissue response following surgical or restorative therapy (Romandini and coworkers 2021).

Immediate implants placed in sites with a thin gingival phenotype are also associated with significantly more recession of the midfacial mucosa than sites with a thick gingival phenotype (Kan and coworkers 2003; Kan and coworkers 2011a). The gingival phenotype can be reproducibly assessed by using a periodontal probe to measure the gingival thickness, observing the periodontal probe shining through the gingival tissue after being inserted into the sulcus. If the probe is visible, the gingival thickness is below 1 mm, and the phenotype is considered thin. It is considered thick when the probe is not visible (Jepsen and coworkers 2018) (Figs 29a-b).

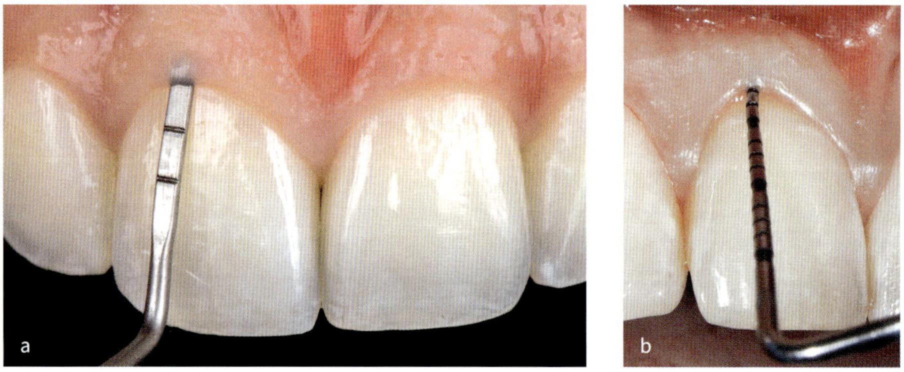

Figs 29a-b Periodontal probe visible through the gingival margin, indicating a thin gingival phenotype (a). Periodontal probe not visible through the gingival margin, indicating a thick gingival phenotype (b).

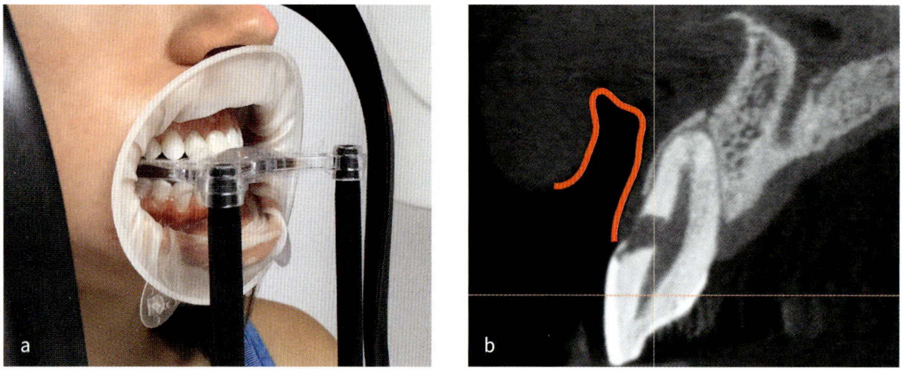

Figs 30a-b Lip retractors used during CBCT exposure will help visualize the labial soft tissue thickness and its relationship to the facial bone crest.

Metal-free lip retractors used during CBCT acquisition for implant planning can also help to visualize the labial soft tissue thickness relative to the facial bone and determine the phenotype (Januário and coworkers 2008) (Figs 30a-b).

A thin/scalloped marginal gingiva should be regarded as a risk for recession, particularly in areas of esthetic importance. A recent systematic review concluded that the placement of a connective tissue graft contributes to midfacial soft tissue stability following immediate placement and should be considered when an elevated risk for midfacial recession (thin soft tissue phenotype, less than 0.5 mm facial bone thickness) is expected in the esthetic zone (Seyssens and coworkers 2021) (Figs 31a-c).

Therefore, despite the limited evidence, immediate placement in patients with a thin soft tissue phenotype should be considered at risk for midfacial recession and, in esthetic cases, simultaneous soft tissue grafting should be considered to decrease the risk.

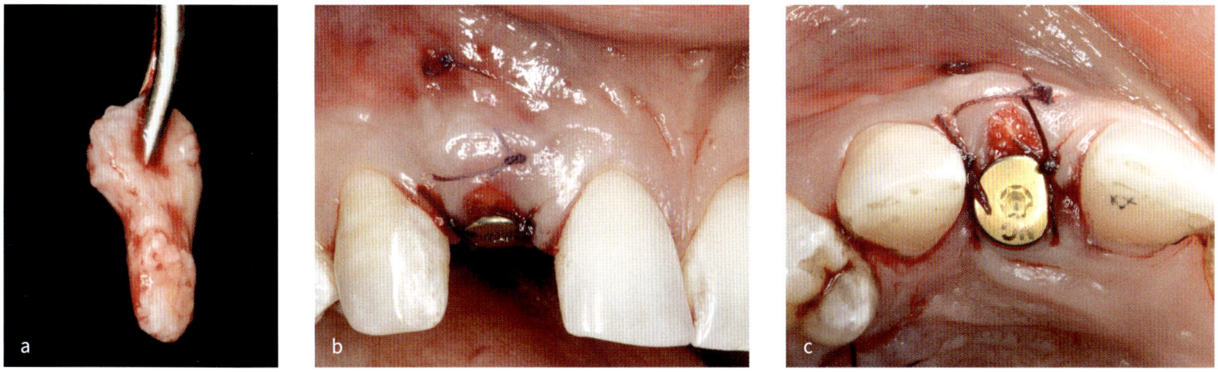

Figs 31a-c Subepithelial connective tissue graft and simultaneous immediate placement on a patient with a thin soft tissue phenotype.

Soft tissue deficiencies. Midfacial recession is a common complication following immediate placement of a single implant (Kan and coworkers 2003; Kan and coworkers 2011a; Chen and Buser 2014; Yuenyongorarn and coworkers 2020). According to Cosyn and coworkers (2012), several factors contribute to such complications; the risk can be mitigated with proper case selection (intact facial bone wall, thick gingival phenotype). The authors also emphasize the potential benefit of flapless surgery and immediate restoration.

Consequently, in cases of an existing recession/soft tissue deficiency on the failing tooth, immediate placement should not be recommended, and early implant placement or alveolar ridge preservation should be preferred to improve the soft tissue condition (Figs 32a-c).

In the presence of a minor recession (less than 1 mm) or a limited amount of keratinized tissue, immediate placement might be considered in combination with soft tissue grafting (Figs 33a-d).

It is commonly accepted that the amount of keratinized tissue around dental implants contributes to peri-implant health (Souza and coworkers 2016), and strategies for keratinized tissue augmentation are often suggested (Thoma and coworkers 2018; Tavelli and coworkers 2021). In the absence of keratinized gingiva around a failing tooth to be replaced by an implant, efforts should be made to improve the future peri-implant soft tissue contour; immediate placement should be avoided, and early or late implant placement is preferred.

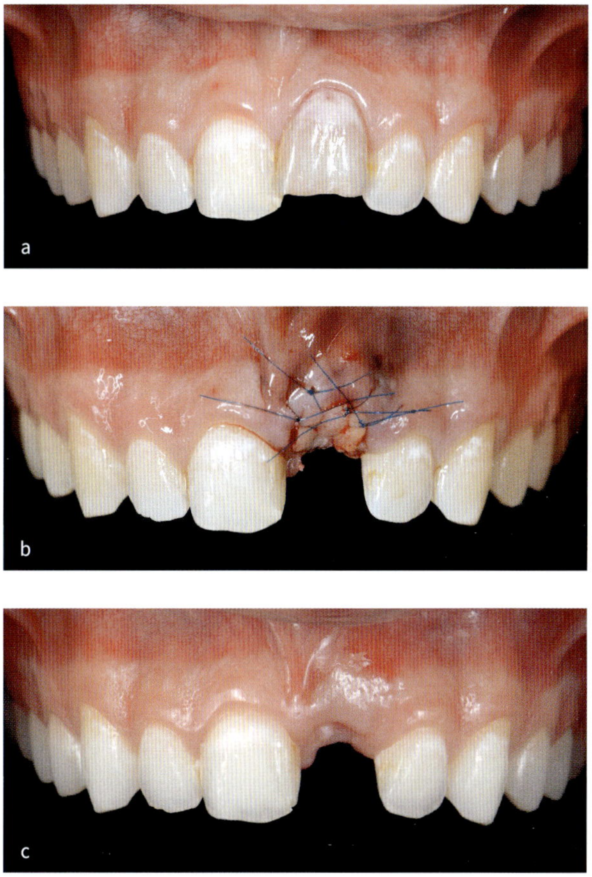

Figs 32a-c Severe gingival recession and soft tissue deficiency, which would contraindicate immediate placement. In this case, implant placement was delayed. An alveolar ridge preservation procedure combined with a connective tissue graft was considered to improve the soft tissue situation.

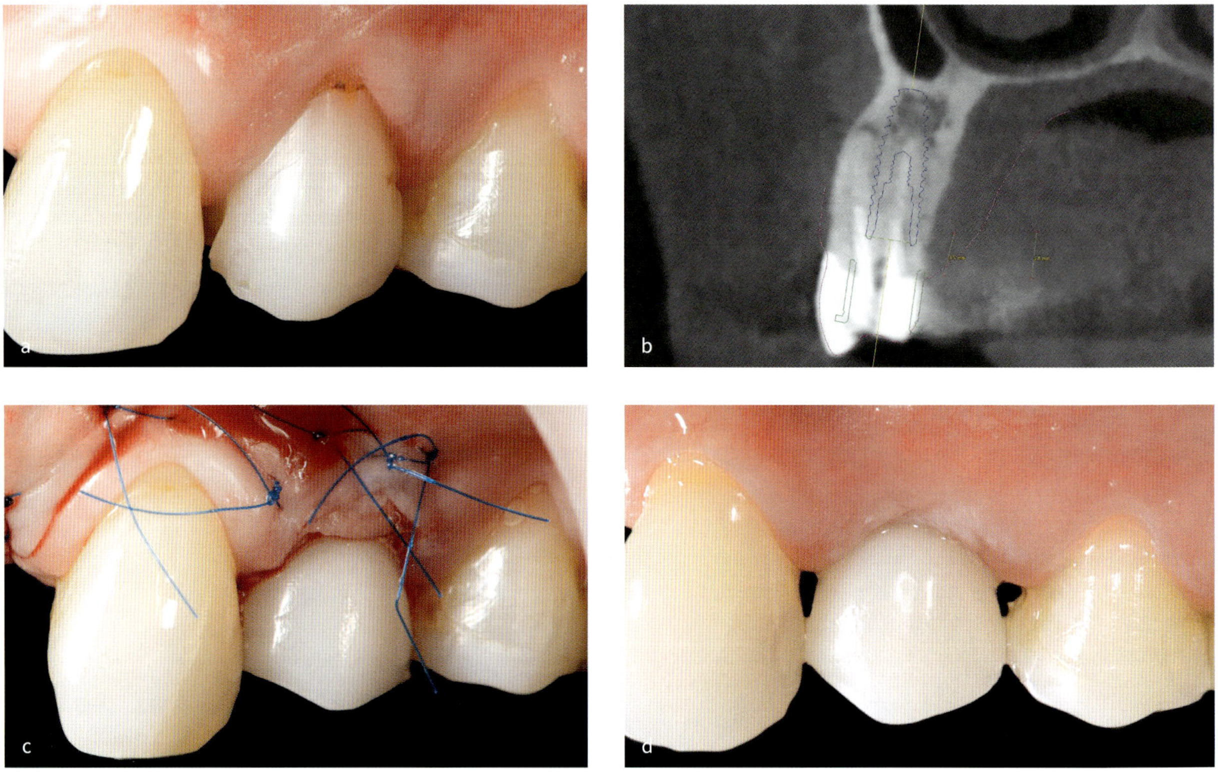

Figs 33a-d The alveolar ridge and socket allowed for an immediate implant; however, because of the minor recession combined with a limited amount of keratinized tissue, a soft tissue graft was considered.

3.4.3 Preoperative Infections

The presence or a history of infection should be clinically and radiographically identified in the preoperative examination. Local infections from endodontic lesions, root fractures, periodontal diseases, root resorption, etc., affect the hard and soft tissue at the implant site or adjacent structures, potentially causing undesirable outcomes. The type of local infection should be properly diagnosed as chronic or acute, or both.

Endodontic infection. Acute endodontic infection leads to significant tissue swelling and suppuration, which, combined with a high bacterial load, present a risk for implant failure and esthetic complications with immediate placement. Endodontic infections may also lead to alveolar bone crest deficiencies at the facial, lingual/palatal, or interproximal areas of the extracted tooth and may result in future peri-implant complications (Figs 34a-b and 35a-b). An unfavorable orofacial or mesiodistal bone situation as a result of infection may create anatomical conditions in which immediate placement is no longer possible or unsuitable from a surgical, biological, or esthetic perspective. Here, other approaches such as socket grafting or type II or III implant placement are advised.

However, chronic infections of a root apex contained within the bony envelope with no significant alveolar bone deficiency do not increase the risk of implant failure or esthetic complications, provided that sufficient remaining apical bone can provide primary implant stability. Indeed, evidence suggests that implants can be placed in sites with chronic periapical lesions (Crespi and coworkers 2010; Truninger and coworkers 2011; Jung and coworkers 2013; Chrcanovic and coworkers 2015). However, the site must be carefully debrided to remove all granulation tissue prior to implant placement.

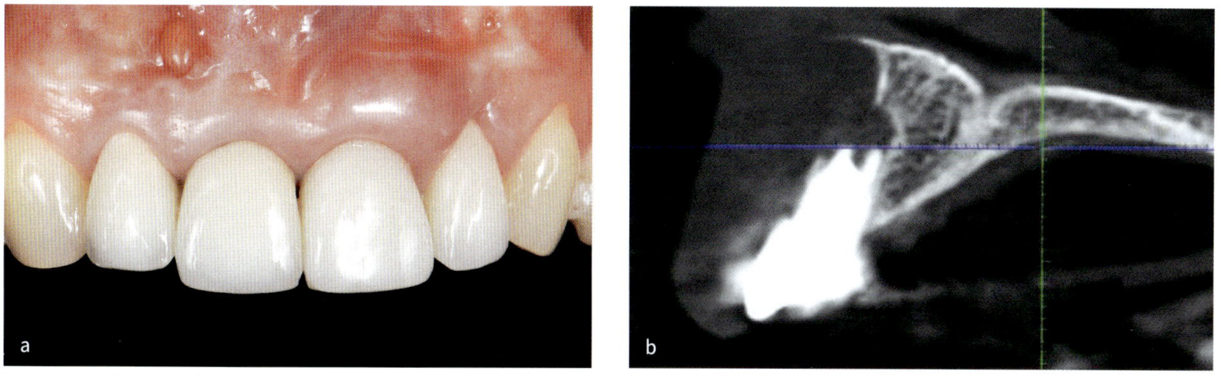

Figs 34a-b Endodontic infection: Chronic suppurating fistula (a) associated with a large buccal fenestration (b).

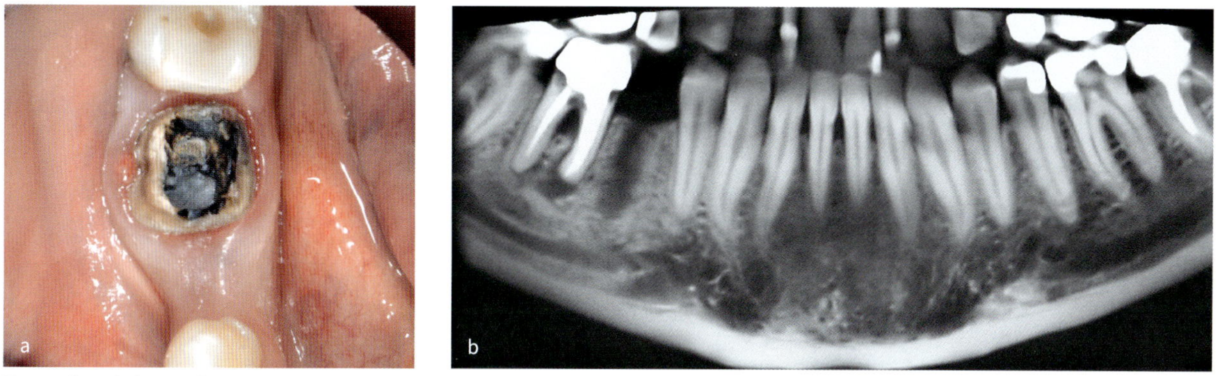

Figs 35a-b Endodontic infection combined with interradicular lesions and soft tissue inflammation.

Periodontal disease. For patients with periodontal disease, the infection should be resolved prior to implant placement (Romanos and coworkers 2019) throughout the mouth. Strict plaque control and adequate oral hygiene should be in place for the long-term success of an implant treatment. If the tooth to be replaced is periodontally compromised (e.g., by fissures, terminal periodontitis) but provides adequate bone for immediate placement, the periodontal inflammation should be controlled. Localized subgingival instrumentation is advisable a few days ahead of the surgery to obtain healthier soft tissue. As this may lead to soft tissue recession, the implant and restoration should be planned accordingly.

Patients with a history of periodontal disease may also present with already compromised gingival esthetics due to recession and the loss of papillae. The risk of further esthetic complications following tooth extraction is increased due to marginal bone loss, with a more coronal position of the papillae or facial mucosa of the tooth to be extracted. Here, tooth extraction and early or late implant placement with socket management would be recommended for a more predictable visualization of the final esthetic outcome.

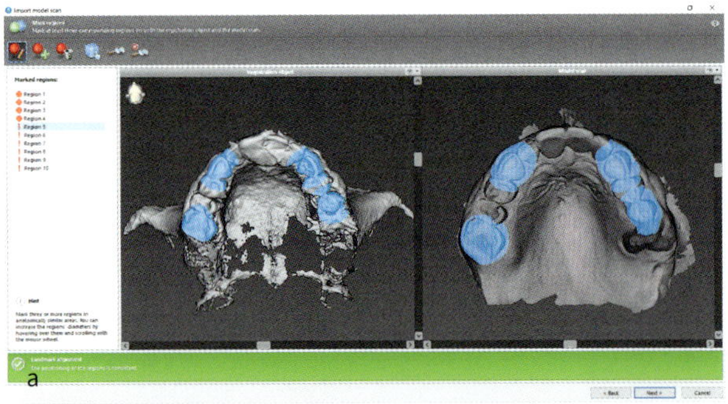

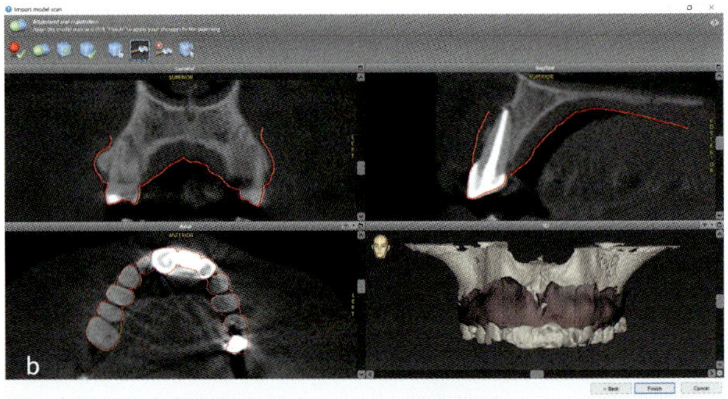

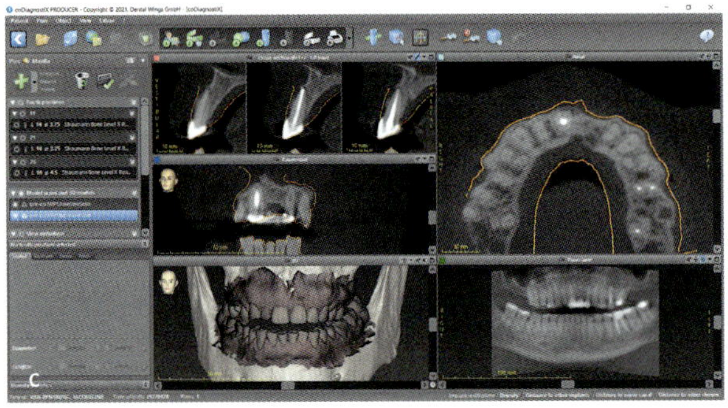

Figs 36a-c Registration of CBCT DICOM data together with intraoral STL data using common reference points (a). Verification of registration accuracy (b). Virtual patient with combined data sets providing the information required for comprehensive prosthetically driven virtual implant planning (c).

3.4.4 Virtual Implant Planning and 3D Positioning

Virtual implant planning with CBCT (DICOM file) and a digital tooth set-up (STL file) superimposed helps visualize a prosthetically driven implant position related to the adjacent anatomical structures. This tool combines all anatomical aspects (soft tissue, alveolar bone, and tooth location) and assists the implant surgeon in determining the optimal implant position (Figs 36a-c).

In addition, virtual planning can assess the likelihood of primary stability for immediate provisionalization or loading and opens the possibility for fully guided implant placement. During virtual implant planning, the implant position should be prosthetically driven, and the amount of palatal/lingual, basal, and interproximal bone engagement should be carefully evaluated.

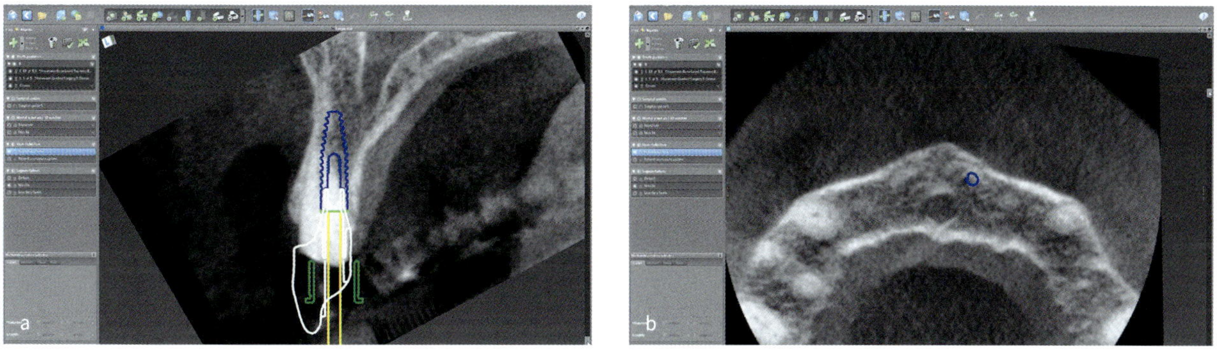

Figs 37a-b Two dimensional axial and cross-sectional images of virtual implant planning. Three-dimensional assessment of the anatomical structures and their relationship to the virtually planned implant is better visualized through rotation around the axis of a virtually planned implant and scrolling through axial cross-sectional images as visible in the QR code videos below.

Use this QR code to view a highlight video showing the rotation around the axis of a virtually planned implant to facilitate the three-dimensional assessment of the anatomical structures in relation to the implant position.

Use this QR code to view a highlight video scrolling through axial cross-sectional images of a virtually planned implant to facilitate the three-dimensional assessment of the anatomical structures in relation to the implant position.

The virtual planning should be visualized in all views, as individual 2D cross-sections often misrepresent the relationship of the implant and the adjacent anatomical structures. Alignment of the cross-sectional view with the implant axis and rotation through the other views (Figs 37a-b) are recommended to assess whether the site is adequate for immediate placement. The amount of engagement of the planned implant with the surrounding bone should be sufficient to predictably achieve primary stability. Implant diameter, length, and position can be manipulated to increase the chances of primary stability and open the path toward immediate loading.

One of the most difficult steps during immediate placement is to assure optimal 3D implant positioning. The alveolar socket and surrounding anatomical structures are always a challenge when it comes to achieving predictable outcomes.

When performing virtual implant planning for a type 1A implant protocol, the positioning guidelines for ideal implant placement described in Volumes 1 and 10 of the ITI Treatment Guide should be followed. These guidelines delineate the comfort and danger zones established at the 3rd ITI Consensus Conference (Buser and coworkers 2004) for the orofacial, mediodistal, and apicocoronal implant positions and for implant angulation.

Compromising the ideal implant position to obtain primary stability and the insertion torque required for immediate loading, or to meet the biological requirement of placing the implant below the facial crest with immediate placement, should be avoided. Here, an alternative placement protocol, different implant macrodesign, or different loading protocols should be prioritized, as any compromises may result in a malpositioned implant, which is one of the primary causes of esthetic implant complications (Chackartchi and coworkers 2019).

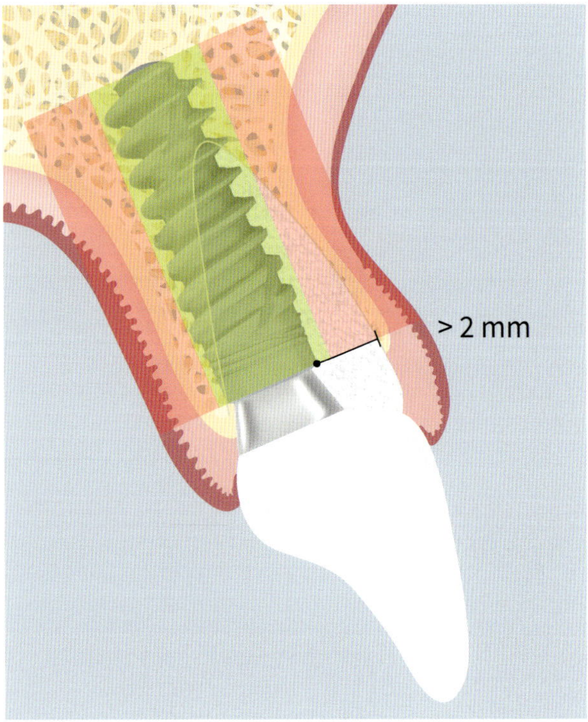

Fig 38 The ideal orofacial implant position is at least 2 mm palatal/lingual to the facial bone to allow for at least a 2 mm horizontal gap for augmentation.

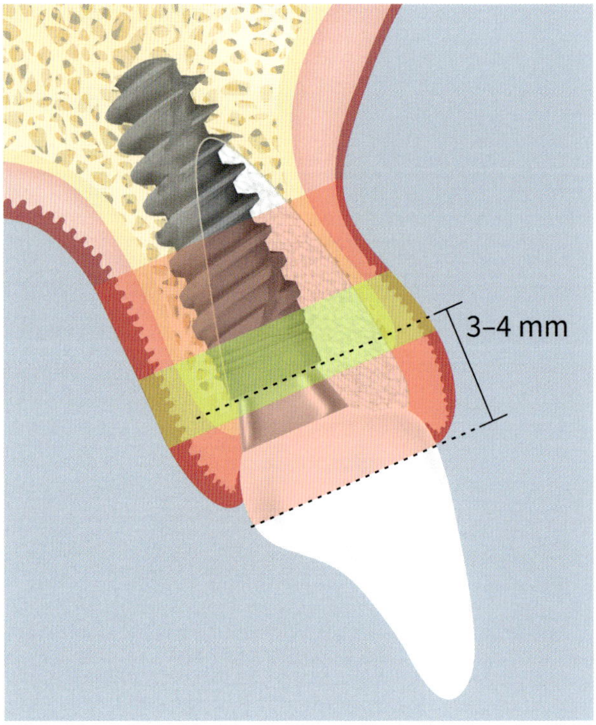

Fig 39 The apicocoronal position of an immediately placed implant should be no further than 3-4 mm apically to the mucosal margin while still below the apical and palatal bone crest.

The orofacial position of the implant is critical in immediate placement. There is a tendency to give immediate implants a more facial inclination and position to obtain better apical/palatal bone anchorage. However, facially positioned implants pose a high risk of peri-implant soft tissue recession and biological complications (Testori and coworkers 2018) (Fig 38).

The apicocoronal implant position should also be within the comfort zone, with a depth of 3 to 4 mm from the future restoration mucosal margin/zenith for bone-level implants (Fig 39).

This should correspond to a bone-level implant positioned at or below the level of the facial and palatal bone crest. If the facial or palatal bone crest is positioned further apically than the implant when planned in the ideal apicocoronal position relative to the proposed mucosal margin of the planned restoration, immediate placement would be contraindicated and early implant placement protocols would be recommended.

The implant should keep an adequate distance mesiodistally between the implant shoulder and adjacent teeth (at least 1.5 mm), and also between adjacent implants (at least 3 mm). Implants placed too close to adjacent teeth increase the risk of vertical bone loss and reductions in papilla height (Fig 40).

Ideally, the implant long axis should be positioned through the cingulum (or central fossa) or incisal edge position of the proposed final restoration (Fig 41).

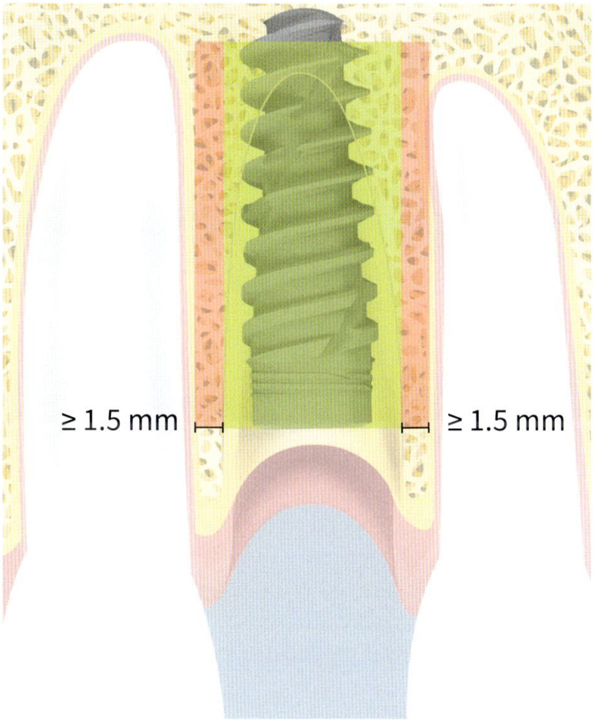

Fig 40 The mesiodistal position of an immediate implant should respect the bone support to the adjacent teeth with at least 1.5 mm of distance.

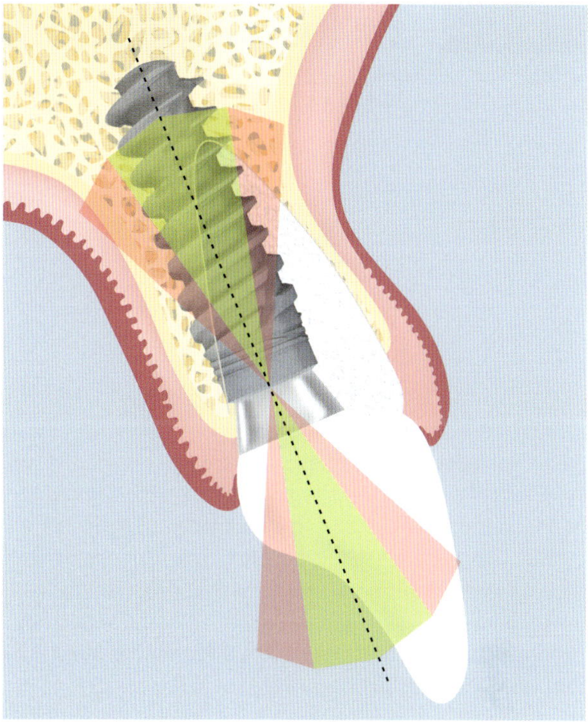

Fig 41 The implant inclination should be such that the implant engages with the apical and palatal basal bone, yet the access hole exits through the cingulum or incisal edge.

3.4.5 Implant Selection

For single-tooth immediate implants in the esthetic zone, a bone-level implant design with an internal conical connection is generally recommended. These implants have been shown to minimize bone resorption at the implant neck (Heitz-Mayfield and coworkers 2013), and they allow a customized transmucosal design—a particular advantage in the esthetic zone.

The implants should have surfaces conducive to new bone formation and osseointegration of the exposed part of the implant (Schwarz and coworkers 2007). Furthermore, an appropriate implant body and thread design can assist in achieving the primary stability required for immediate loading. Tapered implant designs—often with a more aggressive thread—are now often suggested by manufacturers for immediate implant protocols; however, the literature shows that adequate primary stability can also be achieved with parallel-wall designs (Jung and coworkers 2018).

3.5 Risk Assessment Table with Indications and Contraindications

When considering immediate implant treatment, an assessment of patient- and site-specific risk factors should be performed to examine the overall treatment risk against the clinical and patient related benefits. Two risk assessment tools for immediate implant placement and immediate loading of the partially edentulous patient (Tables 2 and 3) have been developed to function as a checklist of the most relevant clinical risk factors.

Not every risk factor is weighted equally when determining overall risk. When all of the clinical factors indicate a low risk (green column), this would indicate a condition where a type 1A protocol is the most desirable of treatment protocols and can be considered routine. Individual risk factors or combinations that indicate a medium risk should be carefully assessed, in light of the clinical and patient-related benefits, as to whether this treatment should be considered, and only provided where the clinician has appropriate experience.

Where any one individual factor indicates a high risk in the red column, a type 1A protocol would not be recommended, and alternative treatment protocols should be considered, as indicated by the decision tree for immediate placement and loading by Gallucci and coworkers (2022) (Fig 42). This decision tree offers a workflow based upon clinical factors seen during treatment and is divided into four sections:

- Preoperative assessment
- Intraoperative assessment
- Placement protocol
- Loading protocol

This table can be used as one component (scientific evidence) of an evidence-based approach to dental treatment.

Table 2 Risk assessment for **immediate implant placement** in single-tooth sites

	Low risk	Medium risk	High risk
Preoperative assessment			
Patient-related			
Medical status	Healthy, uneventful healing		Compromised healing
Esthetic risk	Low/medium esthetic risk	High esthetic risk	Significant esthetic compromise expected
Site-related			
Gingival-margin position	No recession	Minor gingival recession	Gingival recession ≥ 2 mm
Soft tissue quality	Thick gingival phenotype	Thin gingival phenotype or limited keratinized gingiva	No keratinized gingiva
Bone anchorage	Sufficient bone anchorage to achieve primary stability		Lack of bone anchorage to achieve primary stability
Facial bone wall	≥ 1 mm facial bone thickness	Facial bone plate < 1 mm thickness, or small fenestration or dehiscence defect	Significant fenestration or dehiscence of facial bone
Need for a mucoperiosteal flap	Sufficient alveolar bone for a flapless approach		Need for flapped bone augmentation
Socket position within alveolar envelope	Socket within the alveolar bone envelope		Socket and facial bone wall protruding out of the bone envelope
Presence of endodontic infection	No infection	Chronic periapical infection	Acute infection
Presence of periodontal disease	Periodontally healthy	Controlled periodontal disease	Active periodontal disease
Planning implant position	Ideal three-dimensional position with axis exiting through the cingulum or incisal edge		Facially positioned or over-angulated implant or excessive implant depth
Gap between facial bone and planned implant position	≥ 2 mm	1–2 mm	< 1 mm
Intraoperative assessment			
Extraction	Minimally invasive tooth extraction	Damage to surrounding soft tissue, including severed/detached papillae	Significant damage to soft tissue and surrounding bone
Primary implant stability	Primary stability achieved		Lack of primary stability
Final implant position	Ideal three-dimensional position achieved		Facially positioned or over-angulated implant or excessive implant depth

Table 3 Risk assessment for **immediate loading** of an immediately placed single implant

	Low risk	**Medium risk**	**High risk**
Preoperative assessment			
Patient-related			
Occlusal scheme	No direct occlusal contacts	Minimal occlusal contact and/or shared guidance	Main determinant of anterior guidance
Occlusal parafunction	Absent		Present
Site-related			
Bone anchorage	Sufficient bone anchorage to resist loading forces		Insufficient bone anchorage to resist loading forces
Tooth position	Incisor, premolars	Canine	Molars
Intraoperative assessment			
Primary implant stability	30–45 Ncm insertion torque	20–30 Ncm insertion torque	< 20 Ncm insertion torque

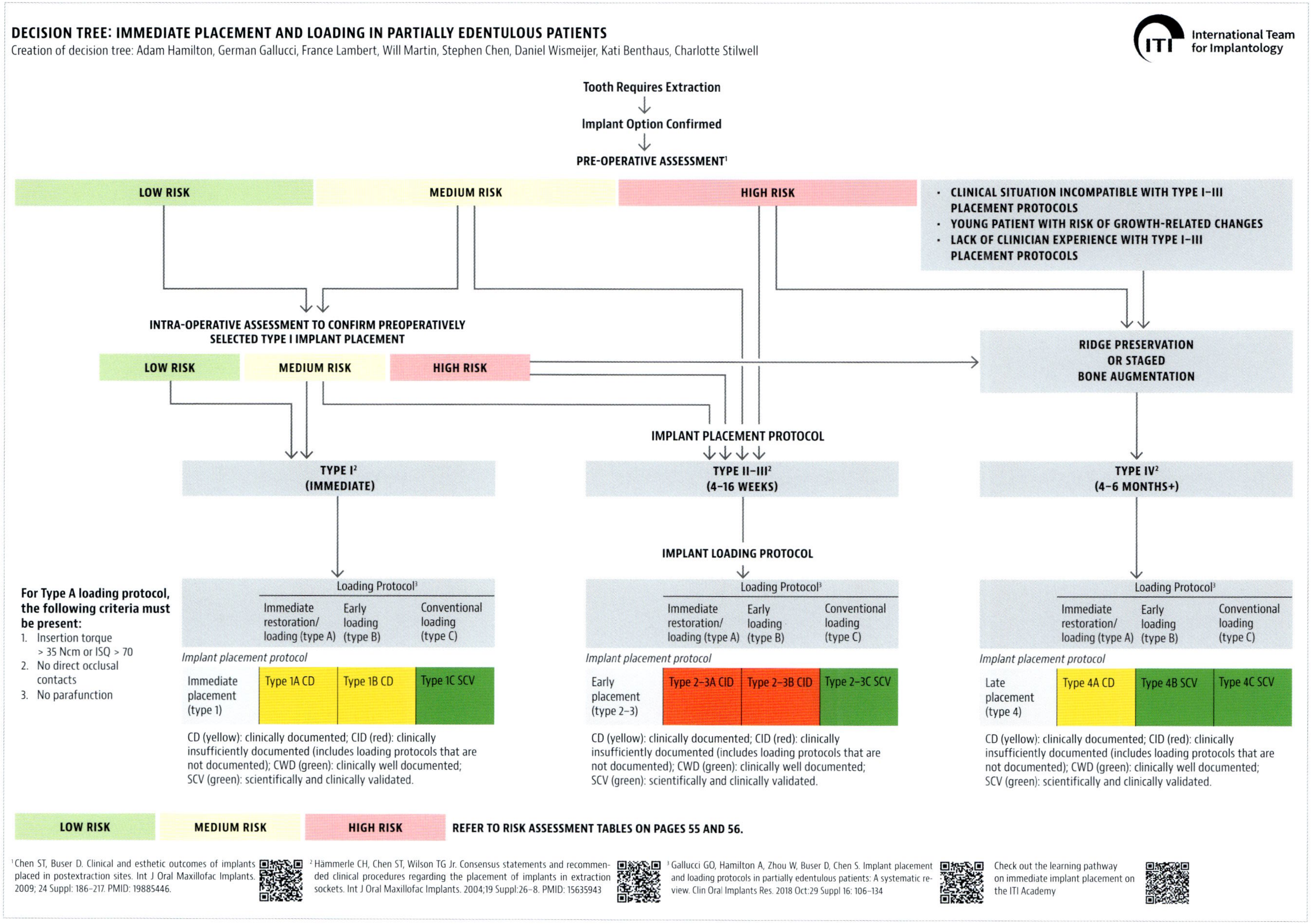

Fig 42 Decision tree for immediate implant placement and loading in single anterior sites.

4 Clinical Procedures

F. Lambert, A. Happe, A. Hamilton, O. González-Martín

Successful outcomes with immediate implant placement and immediate loading are not only determined by the patient and site characteristics, which are evaluated preoperatively, but also by the clinical decision making and execution of the surgical and prosthodontic procedures. Following careful evaluation of the suitability of a patient and site for immediate implant placement and immediate loading, the clinician will need to plan the specific surgical strategies and prosthodontic workflow. This chapter section aims to discuss the step-by-step surgical strategies for type 1A treatment protocols from extraction to immediate implant placement and immediate loading. The various treatment protocols will be outlined with supporting literature and illustrated with clinical examples.

4.1 Immediate Implant Placement

The surgical strategy in immediate implant placement is highly dependent on the preoperative clinical and radiological analyses. Surgical planning always involves a radiographic assessment of the site, preferably by 3D imaging with cone beam computed-tomography (CBCT) scans (Tahmaseb and coworkers 2014). This technology allows the clinician to consider potential difficulties during the extraction, to assess bone availability, and to evaluate the integrity, thickness, and nature of the facial bone plate, important for the prognosis of immediate implants (Elian and coworkers 2007).

Digital surgical planning based on the prosthodontic set-up is recommended prior to immediate implant placement to visualize the ideal implant position, to aid in the selection of the appropriate implant, and to anticipate potential technical difficulties. A meticulous assessment of the soft tissue conditions is also essential to appreciate the soft tissue phenotype, the gingival/mucosal cervical position, the presence of papillae, and the potential need for soft tissue management. In the esthetic zone, an esthetic analysis is also important to determine the expected outcomes and appreciate the surgical challenges. All these aspects will affect the surgical strategy for immediate implants.

4.1.1 Minimally Invasive Extraction

Extracting the tooth and preserving the bone structures of the alveolar socket—especially the facial bone plate and the septa—and the surrounding soft tissue is a key factor for success in immediate implant placement. Minimally invasive extraction is therefore recommended when considering immediate implants, in the anterior as well as in the posterior region.

A minimally invasive extraction does not usually involve the removal of the alveolar bone or the elevation of a flap. The extraction technique mainly depends on the root anatomy. With straight single-rooted teeth presenting enough remaining coronal structure, the luxation and the extraction can be performed directly by forceps (Figs 1a-l); however, the intensity and the extent of the tooth movement will need to be very controlled to avoid any fractures of the alveolar bone or of the roots. Specific instruments such as periotomes, delicate luxators, or the Benex (Zepf Dental, Seitingen-Oberflacht, Germany) might also decrease the trauma to the surrounding tissue damage (Fig 1c).

If the root anatomy is more complex or in the absence of an adequate coronal point of application, the hopeless tooth would have to be sectioned.

In the anterior region, the root can be sectioned in the mesiodistal or buccolingual direction to extract the root a piece at a time, minimizing the risk of damage to the alveolar bone (Fig 1d). The roots are then elevated with a thin luxator or periotome (Figs 1 e-j).

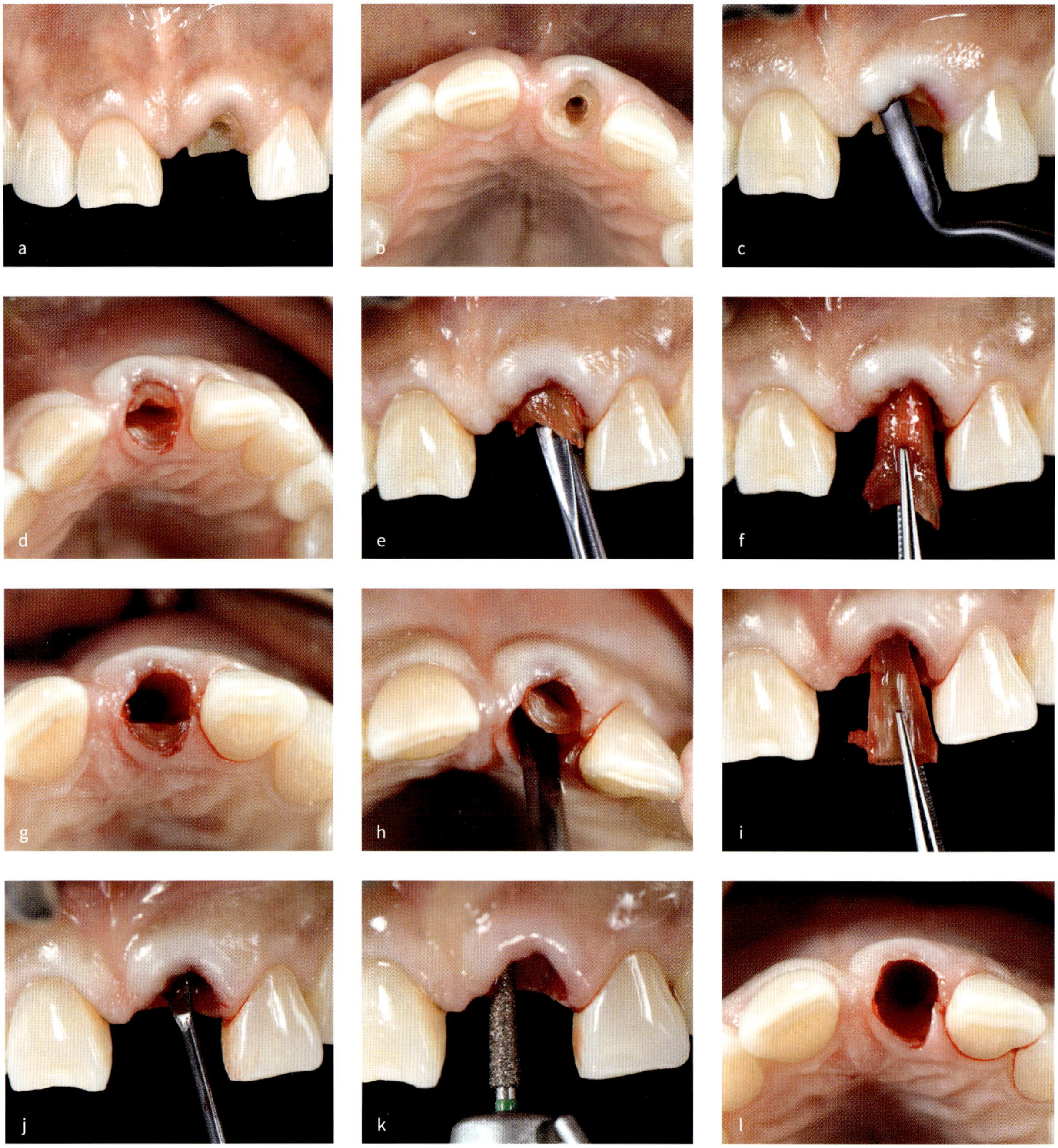

Figs 1a-l Step-by-step sequence of a minimally invasive extraction of a single-rooted tooth in the anterior maxilla. Facial and occlusal view of the baseline situation (a-b). Syndesmotomy using a periotome (c). Mesiodistal section of the root (d). Elevation and extraction of the facial root fragment (f). Occlusal view of the socket after extracting the facial root fragment (g). Elevation and extraction of the palatal root fragment (h-i). Removal of the granulation tissue with a Lucas curette (j). Removal of the intrasulcular and junctional epithelium with a diamond bur (k). Occlusal view of the debrided socket after extraction (l).

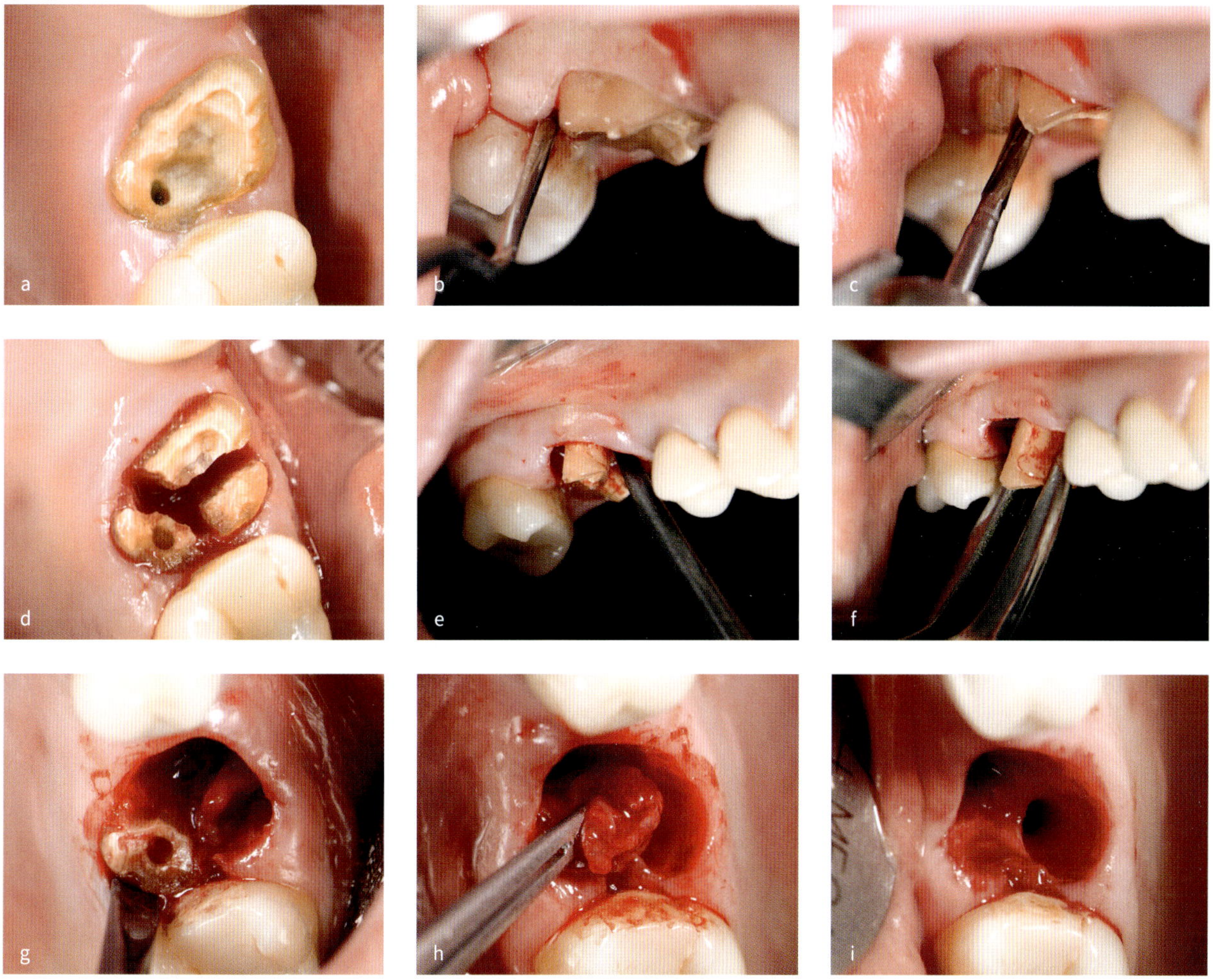

Figs 2a-i Minimally invasive extraction of an upper molar using root separation. Occlusal view of the baseline situation (a). Syndesmotomy using a periotome (b). Root sectioning using a Zekria bur (c). Occlusal view of the root sections (d). Elevation and extraction of the root fragments (e-g). Removal of the granulation tissue (h). Occlusal view of the socket after extraction. The hard and soft tissues have been preserved (i), (Surgery: Dr Bertrand Debaty.)

In the posterior region, multi-rooted teeth are usually subjected to root separation using a tapered conical bur (Zekrya; Dentsply-Maillefer, Ballaigues, Switzerland) (Figs 2a-i). After careful luxation, each root is extracted in the proper direction according to the root curvature, using a root forceps.

In case of the fracture of a root apex, a thin bur (Ariane-Z; Dentsply-Maillefer) can be used to produce a narrow furrow; the apex is then removed with a thin instrument, such as a luxator.

Some authors have suggested Piezosurgery for minimally invasive tooth extraction prior to immediate implant placement. Although they did not demonstrate the superiority of Piezosurgery for dental extraction, the risk of instruments slipping during the procedure is lower than when burs are used (Blus and Szmukler-Moncler 2010). Care must be taken to ensure copious irrigation and to avoid prolonged static use, as the instruments may overheat the bone and even cause necrosis (Cardoni and coworkers 2006; Schütz and coworkers 2012; Rashad and coworkers 2015; Lajolo and coworkers 2018).

4.1.2 Socket Assessment and Debridement

Once the tooth has been extracted, it is important to check the integrity of the facial bone wall and to debride the socket. An intact facial bone wall at least 1 mm in thickness after tooth removal is commonly cited as a prerequisite for immediate implant placement (Chen and Buser 2009; Esposito and coworkers 2010; Buser and coworkers 2017). However, 90% of anterior teeth in the maxilla exhibit a facial plate less that 1 mm in thickness (Braut and coworkers 2011). Although not an absolute contraindication for an immediate implant, thin facial bone must be considered in the surgical strategy; connective tissue grafting may be an option.

The granulation tissue must be carefully removed with a curette. Animal studies (Novaes and coworkers 1998) and clinical studies (Crespi and coworkers 2010; Bell and coworkers 2011; Truninger and coworkers 2011) have shown that placing implants in sockets affected by chronic periapical pathology can still be a safe and viable treatment option. However, it is important to thoroughly debride the socket and remove all granulation tissue with a surgical curette or rotary instrument.

In the cervical area, a large diamond bur can also be used remove not only the granulation tissue but also the intrasulcular and junctional epithelium. Leaving these inner epithelial tissues may induce soft tissue scarring, especially if a connective tissue graft is performed.

4.1.3 Flapless vs. Flapped

For many decades, traditional implant surgery involved a trapezoid full-flap design to gain access to the alveolar ridge and to provide an overview of the site. However, raising a traditional mucoperiosteal flap with releasing incisions and detachment of the periosteum from the bone has several drawbacks. Omitting the releasing incisions improves the blood supply, which is essential for uneventful healing (Kleinheinz and coworkers 2005). Moreover, bone denudation due to detachment of the periosteum may induce bone resorption. Animal studies have shown that the elevation of both full- and partial-thickness flaps results in bone loss and elevated osteoclastic activity (Fickl and coworkers 2011). This phenomenon has also been observed in clinical studies (Merheb and coworkers 2017). Avoiding releasing incisions also limits the risk for scarring and soft tissue recession.

Because of these biological effects, flapless surgery is most often considered for immediate implant placement, leading to esthetic outcomes that are superior to the traditional approach with a raised flap (Boardman and coworkers 2016). Therefore, current concepts consider a nearly or completely flapless approach. Some authors favor a fully flapless approach, not touching the peri-implant soft tissues at all and sealing the socket with a temporary restoration or anatomical healing abutments combined with a transmucosal connective tissue graft (Tarnow and coworkers 2014; Cosyn and coworkers 2016). Others use a minimally invasive surgical approach by creating a facial full- or split-thickness pouch in order to thicken the bone tissue with guided bone regeneration (GBR) or the soft tissue with autologous connective tissue grafts (Mankoo 2007; Grunder 2011; Tsuda and coworkers 2011) or biomaterials as substitutes (Happe 2021).

4.1.4 Osteotomy Preparation

IMPLANT POSITION

Assessing the anatomy of the available bone around the socket is important when planning the placement of an implant in its correct 3D position, to anticipate the expected primary stability (Kan and coworkers 2011a; Tahmaseb and coworkers 2014). The implant positioning must be very carefully planned. In the esthetic zone, following the socket anatomy, the implant will be anchored in the palatal or apical bone. In the posterior region, the interradicular septa will help ensure the primary stability of immediate implants. However, the need for sufficient bone anchorage and primary stability should not compromise the 3D position of the implant within the socket, which is a key factor for success (Chen and coworkers 2007; Tomasi and coworkers 2010).

In the buccolingual direction, the ideal position is in the palatal compartment of the socket, with the implant leaning on the palatal wall and leaving a gap of 2 to 4 mm from the facial wall. The remaining socket will be filled with a bone substitute. Vertically, the implant needs to be positioned deep enough—about 3 to 4 mm apically of the soft tissue margin—to allow the establishment of the biologic width and a proper emergence profile, from the palatally positioned implant neck to the more facial cervical line. Furthermore, the buccolingual inclination of the implant should be such that the access hole exits through the cingulum or incisal edge in anterior teeth and on the occlusal surface of posterior teeth. Optimal implant 3D positioning is described in detail in Chapter 3.

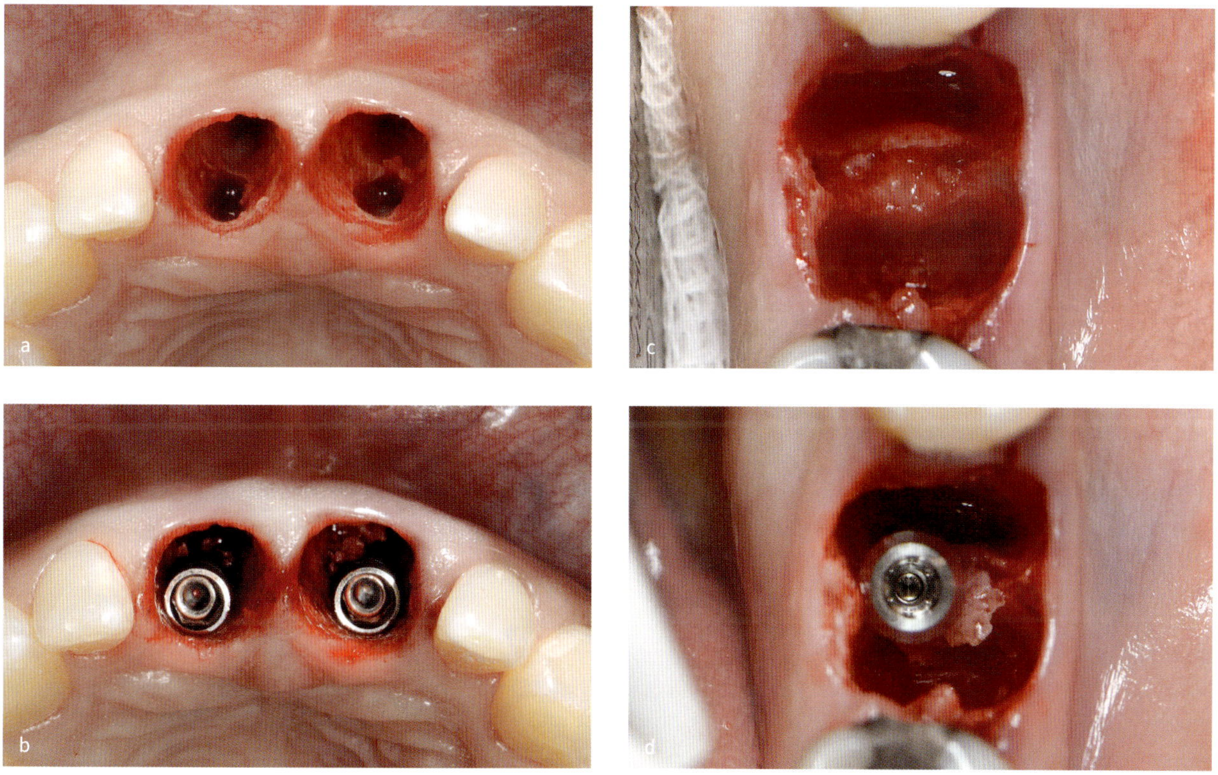

Figs 3a-d Osteotomies in the palatal wall of the sockets of teeth 11 and 21 (a-b). Implant insertion in the interradicular septa of tooth 46 (c-d).

DRILLING SEQUENCE AND IMPLANT SELECTION

To ensure the primary implant stability (above 25 Ncm of insertion torque) recommended to consider an immediate restoration, the drilling protocol can be adjusted. The implant bed can be underprepared at the discretion of the surgeon to match the bone quality.

Although implant selection is usually determined based on presurgical planning, the final decision is taken at the time of the surgery; implant length, diameter, or design can always be adapted to the prevailing surgical conditions. Tapered implants—some with an enhanced thread design—are often suggested for immediate implant placement, as in-vitro and clinical studies have emphasized the relevance of a tapered implant design for primary stability (Romanos and coworkers 2014; Yamaguchi and coworkers 2015).

FREEHAND VS. GUIDED (S-CAIS) VS. NAVIGATED

To achieve the correct implant position, the initial drilling is of paramount importance. In the esthetic zone, pilot drilling must often start in the apical third of the palatal wall—not in the socket apex. In the posterior region, the drilling sequence usually starts in the interradicular septum (Figs 3a-d). Drilling in these areas is challenging, as the bur touches the wall at a flat angulation and may slide away. This is why freehand drilling may be difficult and can lead to an osteotomy in an inappropriate location (Buser and coworkers 2017).

Guided surgery using surgical guides (static computer-aided implant surgery, s-CAIS) based on preoperative surgical and prosthodontic planning has become a standard in contemporary implant surgery and may assist with implant insertion in the correct position (Happe and coworkers 2018).

Different workflows are possible with these guides:

- Guided pilot drilling but freehand final drilling and implant placement
- Fully guided drilling with freehand implant placement
- Fully guided drilling with guided implant placement using the guide

The accuracy of implant positioning increases through this series of workflows (Behneke and coworkers 2012). However, s-CAIS may result in errors up to 1.2 mm at the implant shoulder and 1.8 mm at the apex (Schneider and coworkers 2009; Tahmaseb and coworkers 2014; Schnutenhaus and coworkers 2018). Considering the anatomical width of single-tooth gaps and the recommended minimal distance of 1.5 mm (Grunder and coworkers 2005; Chappuis 2017) between the implant and the natural tooth, these inaccuracies cannot be disregarded, and the position of the implant should be double-checked during the surgery.

More recently, navigated surgery has also be used to guide the implant installation (Pellegrino and coworkers 2021). However, the risk of the bur sliding against the palatal wall remains high.

4.1.5 Socket Management

Immediate implant placement does not prevent horizontal and vertical bone loss after tooth extraction (Araújo and coworkers 2005; Araújo and coworkers 2006; Araújo and coworkers 2006). To limit this physiological bone remodeling, several studies demonstrated the application of alveolar ridge preservation. For immediate implants, as reported in recent consensus reports (Tonetti and coworkers 2019), it is recommended to fill the remaining socket with a bone grafting biomaterial that acts as a facial shield to obtain an adequate thickness of the facial bone after the expected remodeling of the facial plate (Chen and Buser 2009; Esposito and coworkers 2010) (Figs 4a-d and 5a-b).

A recent systematic review reported less horizontal facial bone resorption and less midfacial soft tissue recession when immediate implants were combined with socket grafting (Seyssens and coworkers 2022). However, when combined with immediate implant placement, this kind of socket management requires a recommended facial gap of at least 2 mm. To achieve this, current concepts rely on palatal positioning of the implant and the selection of implant diameters narrower than the socket. However, once the remaining part of the socket is filled with the bone substitute, the occlusal part of the socket should be closed to protect the biomaterial from infection.

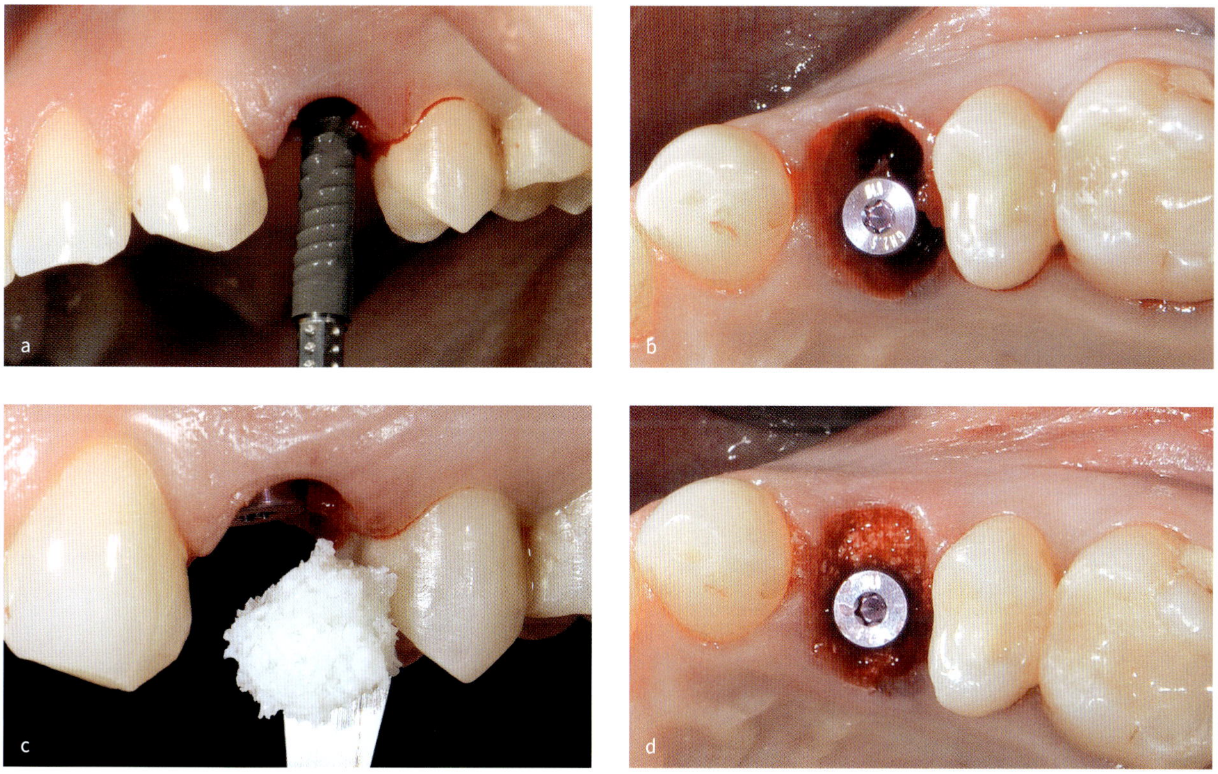

Figs 4a-d Immediate implant placement for the replacement of an upper premolar. The implant was positioned to leave enough space on the facial aspect to fill the remaining socket with deproteinized bovine bone mineral (DBBM).

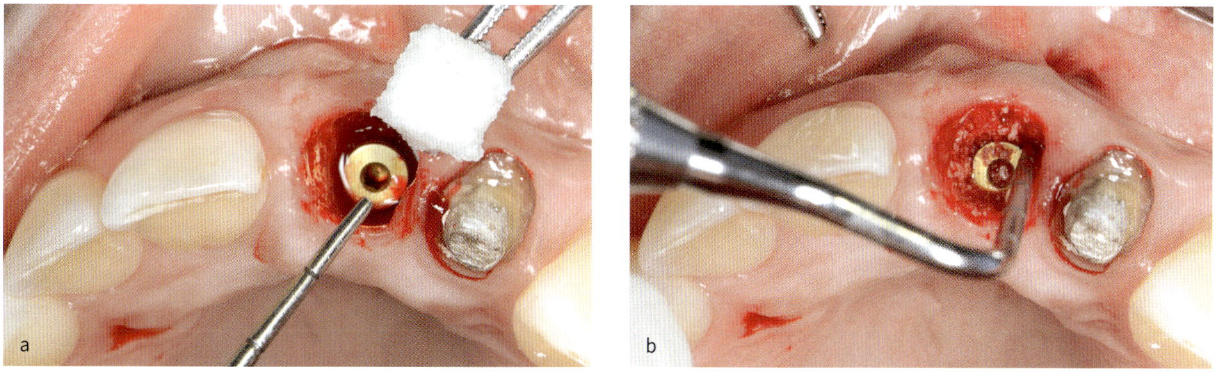

Figs 5a-b Socket grafting with a combination of DBBM and collagen biomaterial (Bio-Oss Collagen, Geistlich, Wolhusen, Switzerland) using a plugging instrument.

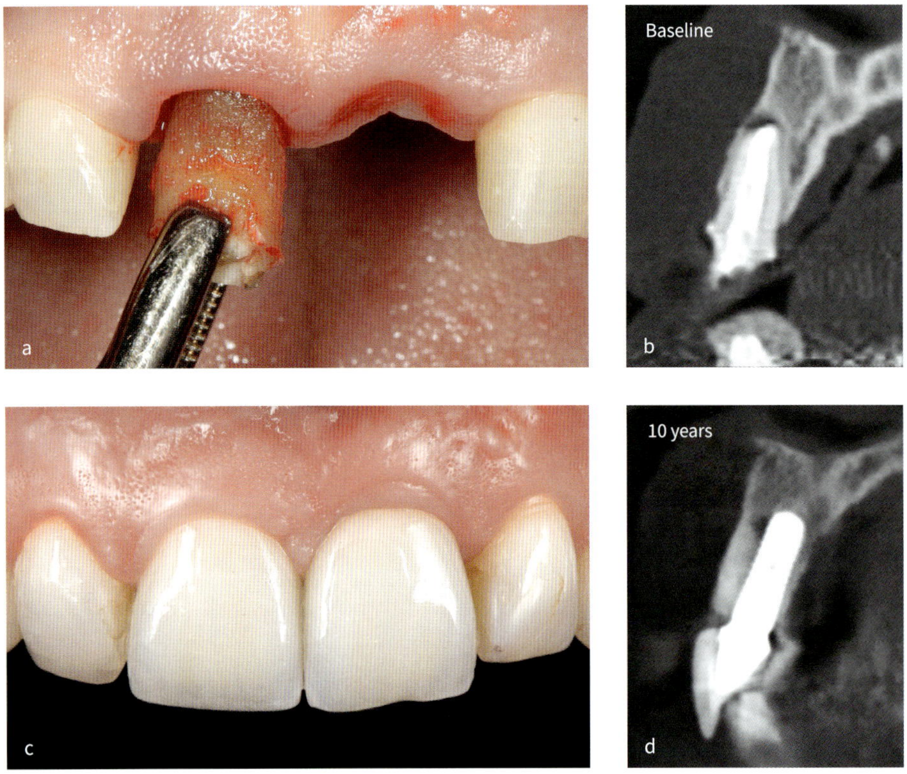

Figs 6a-d An immediate implant at site 11. The 10-year follow-up CBCT documents the dimensional stability of the alveolar ridge after socket grafting with a DBBM.

4.1.6 Biomaterial Selection

Animal studies (Araújo and coworkers 2011) and clinical trials (Chen and coworkers 2009; Tsuda and coworkers 2011; Tarnow and coworkers 2014) have shown that filling the gap between the implant and the facial bone plate with DBBM produces better volumetric stability of the facial tissues and less soft tissue recession. Although there is no consensus regarding the biomaterial selection, the use of a slowly resorbable material may result in better long-term 3D stability, as suggested by some authors (Tonetti and coworkers 2019) (Figs 6a-d)

When selecting a bone substitute biomaterial, it is important to consider their osteoconductive properties and their capacity to osseointegrate, commonly reported as the bone-to-material contact, which appears to be influenced by the surface characteristics of the biomaterial and the manufacturing process (Lambert and coworkers 2017; De Carvalho and coworkers 2019) (Figs 7a-l).

It is therefore important when selecting a space filling material to rely not only on the chemical composition or the origin of the material itself, but also on the biological performance reported in the literature. Beyond biocompatibility and osteoconductive performance, a slowly resorbable hydroxyapatite such as DBBM has often been used in clinical trials investigating immediate implants used in the esthetic zone and in the posterior region (Seyssens and coworkers 2022) to preserve the dimensions of the alveolar ridge.

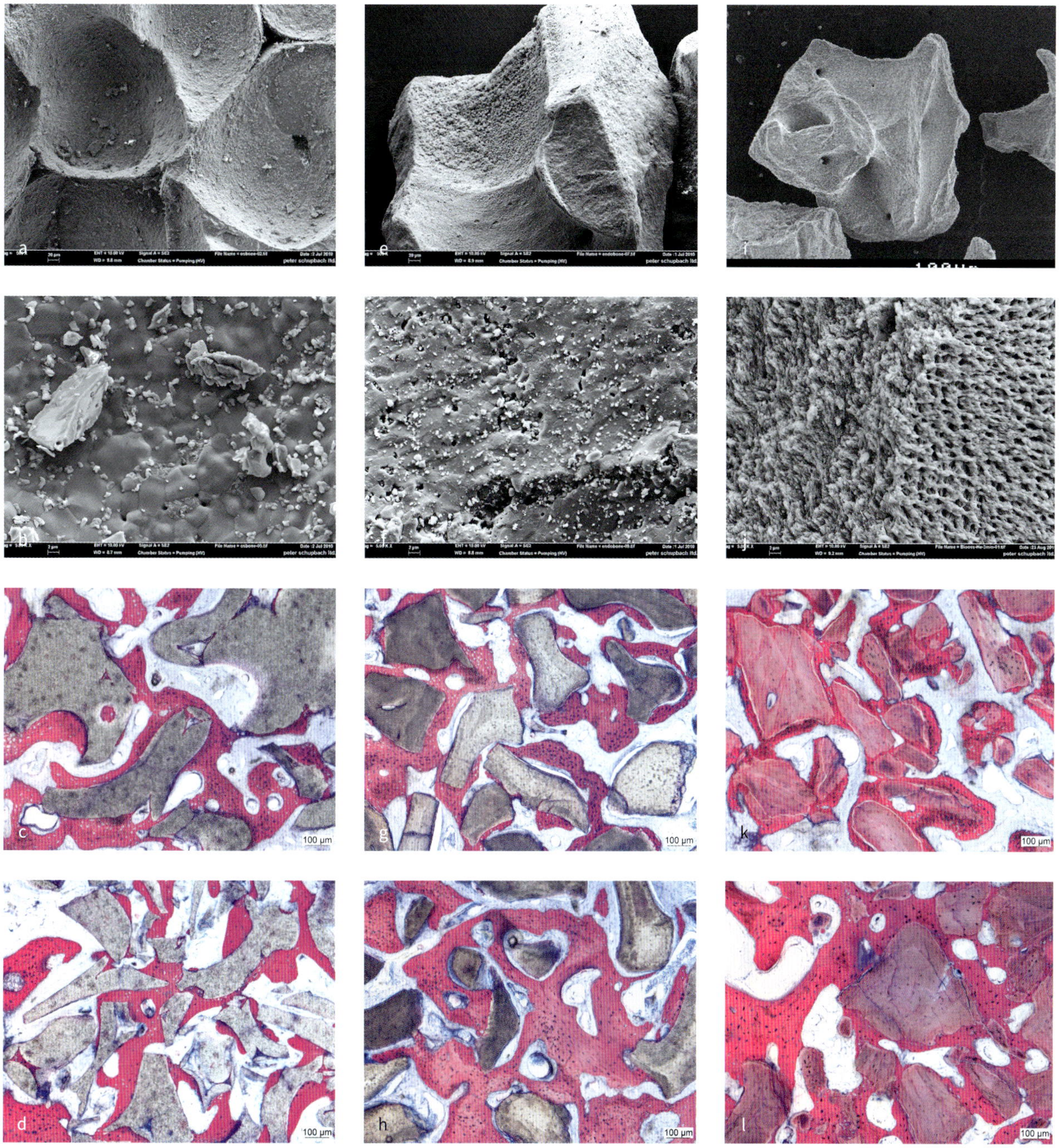

Figs 7a-l Scanning electron microscope images (×500 and ×5000) and microscopic 2D images of three hydroxyapatite- (HA-) based biomaterials—a synthetic HA sintered at a high temperature (Osbone; Curasan, Kleinostheim, Germany) (a-d), a bovine xenograft deproteinized at high temperature (Endobon; Biomet 3I, Warsaw, IN, USA) (e-h), and a bovine xenograft chemically deproteinized at low temperature (Bio-Oss; Geistlich) (i-l). The bone-to-material contact, which reflects the osteoconductivity of the materials, was observed to be higher on the HA, whose surface microtopography was preserved.

4.1.7 Connective Tissue Grafting and Alternatives

Long-term studies have demonstrated similar implant survival rates and peri-implant bone levels for both immediate and delayed implants (Sanz and coworkers 2015; Cosyn and coworkers 2016). However, typical complications with immediate placement are soft tissue related. Loss of the facial contour, soft tissue recession, or shine-through effects were often described with immediate implants (Buser and coworkers 2017). Nevertheless, soft tissue thickening with connective tissue grafts seems to prevent facial recession and improve the esthetic outcomes (Sanz-Martín and coworkers 2022).

As early as 2004, Bianchi and Sanfilippo (2004) reported that connective tissue grafts facial to immediate implants enhance peri-implant soft tissue quality and esthetic outcomes, This was recently confirmed in a systematic review (Seyssens and coworkers 2021). These techniques require surgical preparation of a full- or split-thickness pouch by tunneling the facial soft tissue to provide a bed for the soft tissue graft. An intrasulcular incision design provides access to the facial bone, and the facial soft tissue is tunneled with a microsurgical blade and or a microreleaser (Figs 8a-b and Figs 9a-d).

Soft tissue thickening is mainly indicated in cases with thin periodontal phenotypes or those presenting with an existing gingival recession. Soft tissue grafting was also considered to compensate for the expected post-extraction bone loss (Braut and coworkers 2011), especially in esthetic cases. However, in cases of a thin gingival phenotype. a split-thickness preparation of the thin facial soft tissue may result in perforation and compromised blood supply; therefore, a full-thickness flap design without any releasing incisions may be preferred. Clinical studies showed favorable outcomes of this technique (Grunder 2011; Tsuda and coworkers 2011); an animal study comparing immediate implant with (test) and without (control) a subepithelial connective tissue graft showed similar peri-implant bone remodeling; the peri-implant mucosa, however, was significantly thicker and more coronally positioned in the test group (Caneva and coworkers 2013).

Alternatively, the connective tissue graft may not involve a pouch and may rely on the transgingival vascular bed (Mankoo 2007). This technique allows a thickening of the soft tissue in the most critical area (Chen and Buser 2009); however, adequate removal of the junctional and sulcular epithelium together with proper graft stabilization are key aspects for graft integration (Figs 10a-f). This technique allows the harvesting of a smaller CTG, for example from the tuberosity, if available. Peri-implant soft tissue optimization represents a strategic step for immediate implants, especially in the esthetic zone. CTGs can be harvested in different manners and from different sites (Figs 11a-e).

There are now many alternatives to autologous connective tissue grafts. These biomaterials consist of xenogeneic collagen derivatives and acellular collagen matrixes (ADM), proved to thicken the oral mucosa (Thoma and coworkers 2016; Cairo and coworkers 2017; Thoma and coworkers 2017; Fischer and coworkers 2019) with some studies suggesting that the results are not significantly different from those for connective tissue grafts (Lissek and coworkers 2020).

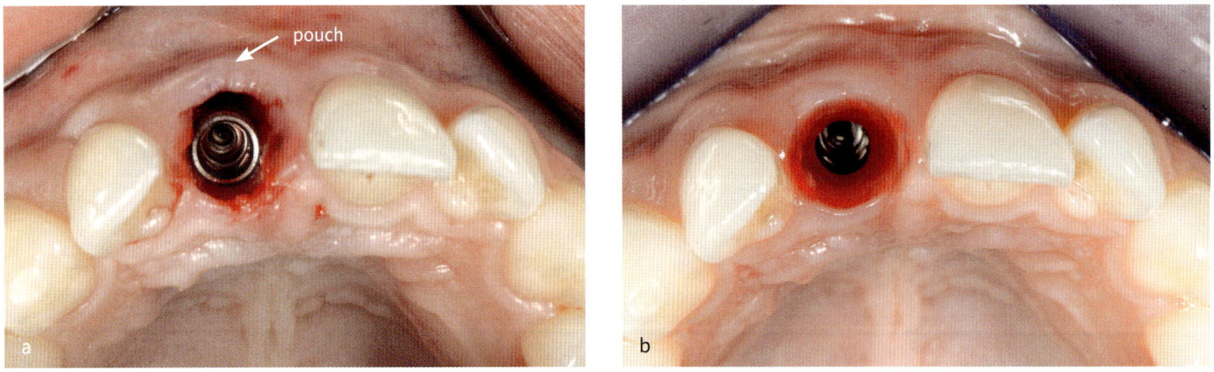

Figs 8a-b Example of a transfer from periodontal tissues to peri-implant tissues. Immediate implant placement combined with a CTG. A split-thickness pouch (a) created to insert the graft harvested from the palate.

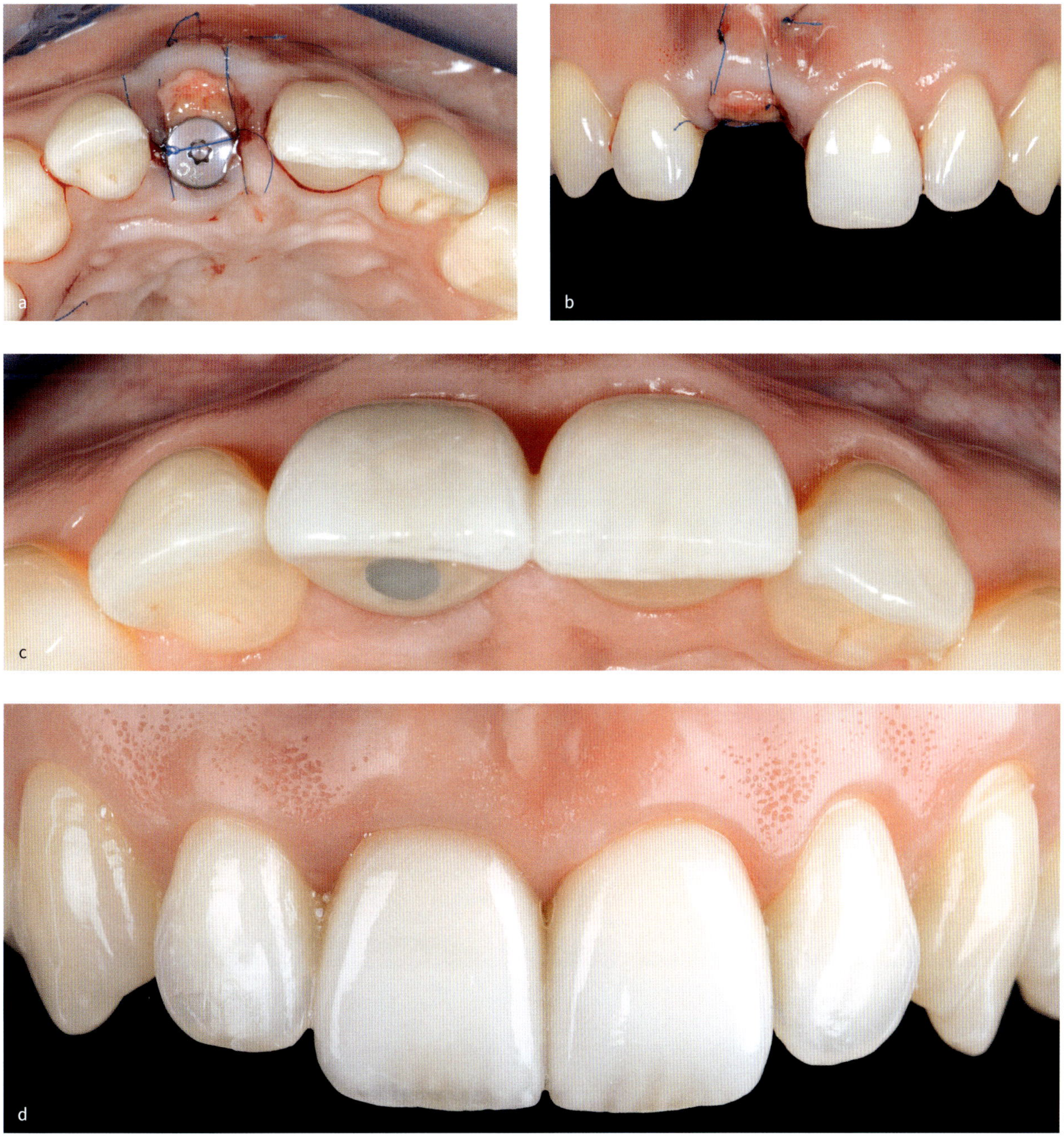

Figs 9a-d Another example of a transfer from periodontal tissues to peri-implant tissues. Immediate implant placement combined with a CTG.

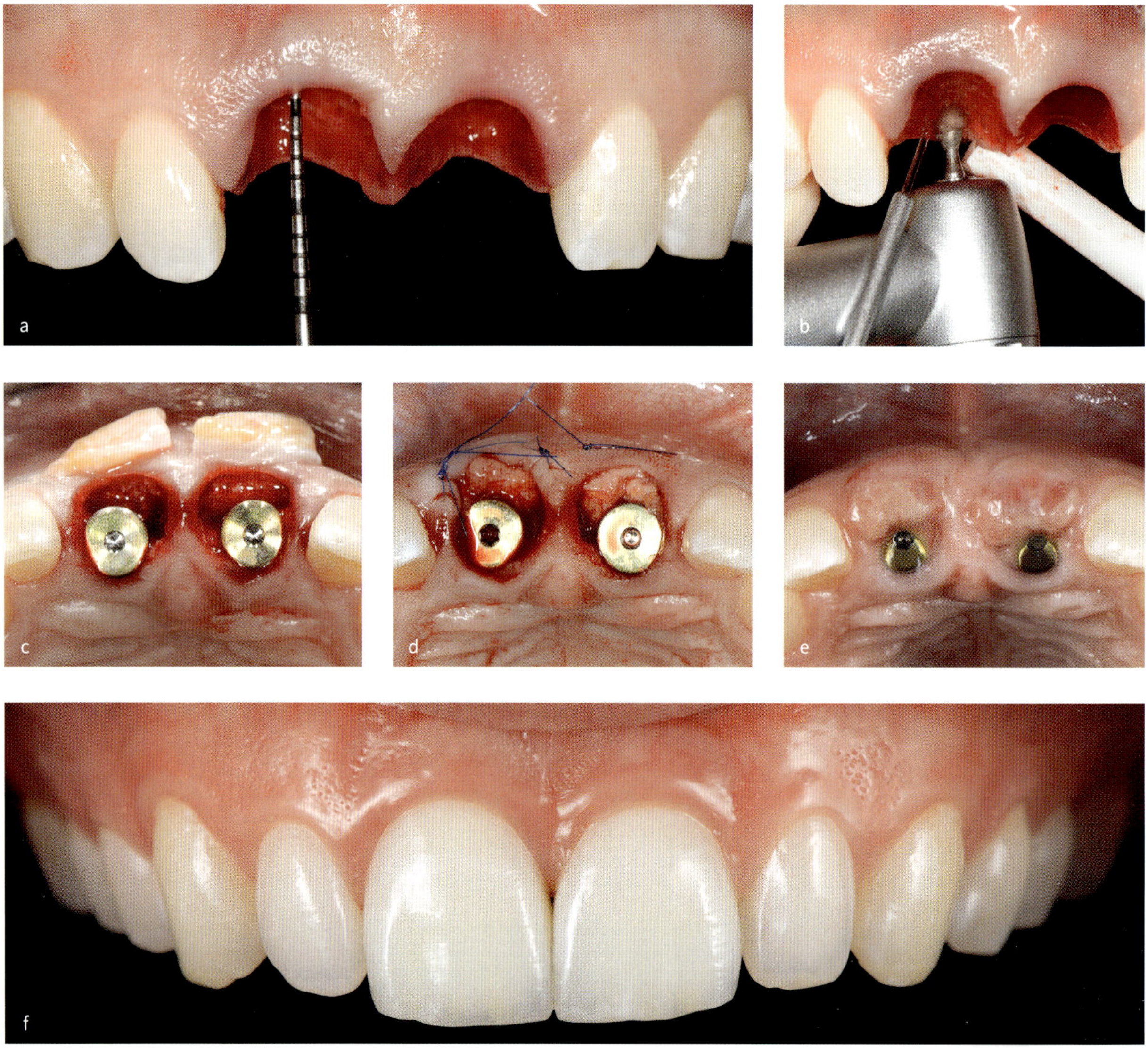

Figs 10a-f Immediate implants combined to a pouch-free CTG harvested from the palatal area and inserted transmucosally, between the healing abutment and the labial mucosa. The deepithelialization of the sulcular and junctional epithelia facilitated the vascularization of the graft.

Recent studies comparing CTG and ADM reported similar results in terms of clinical and esthetic outcomes over a one year follow-up (Happe and coworkers 2022a; Happe and coworkers 2022b), with ADM presenting significantly less postoperative morbidity (Happe and coworkers 2022a). The main advantage of these materials is the absence of a second surgical harvesting site, thereby limiting postoperative morbidity (Figs 12a-h).

However, according to a recent systematic review, soft tissue augmentation procedures are efficacious on soft tissue thickening and, in particular, CTG demonstrated a gain in soft tissue thickness when compared to no graft or soft tissue substitutes (Valles and coworkers 2022). Consequently, the consensus meeting of expert concluded that connective tissue graft remains the standard of care in terms of increasing mucosa thickness (Jung and coworkers 2022).

Finally, some authors have suggested occluding the transmucosal part of the socket with socket grafting material such as xenografts (Chu and coworkers 2012). Although the scientific evidence is rather limited, this may represent an alternative treatment approach especially in cases with favorable soft tissue phenotypes or in the posterior region (Figs 13a-h and 14a-h).

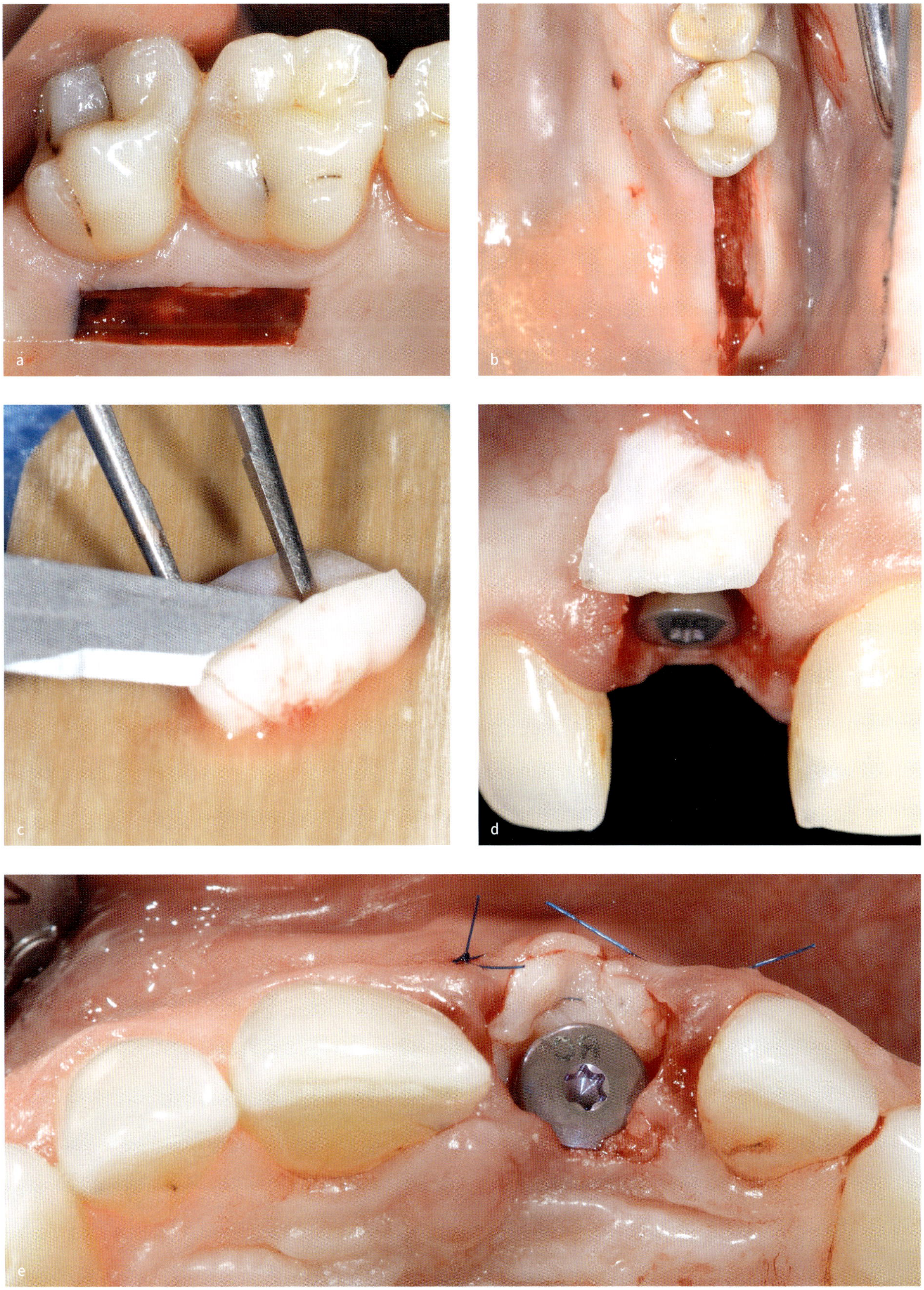

Figs 11a-e CTG harvested from the palatal area (a) and tuberosity (b). Removal of the epithelium (c). CTG before (d) and after (e) insertion.

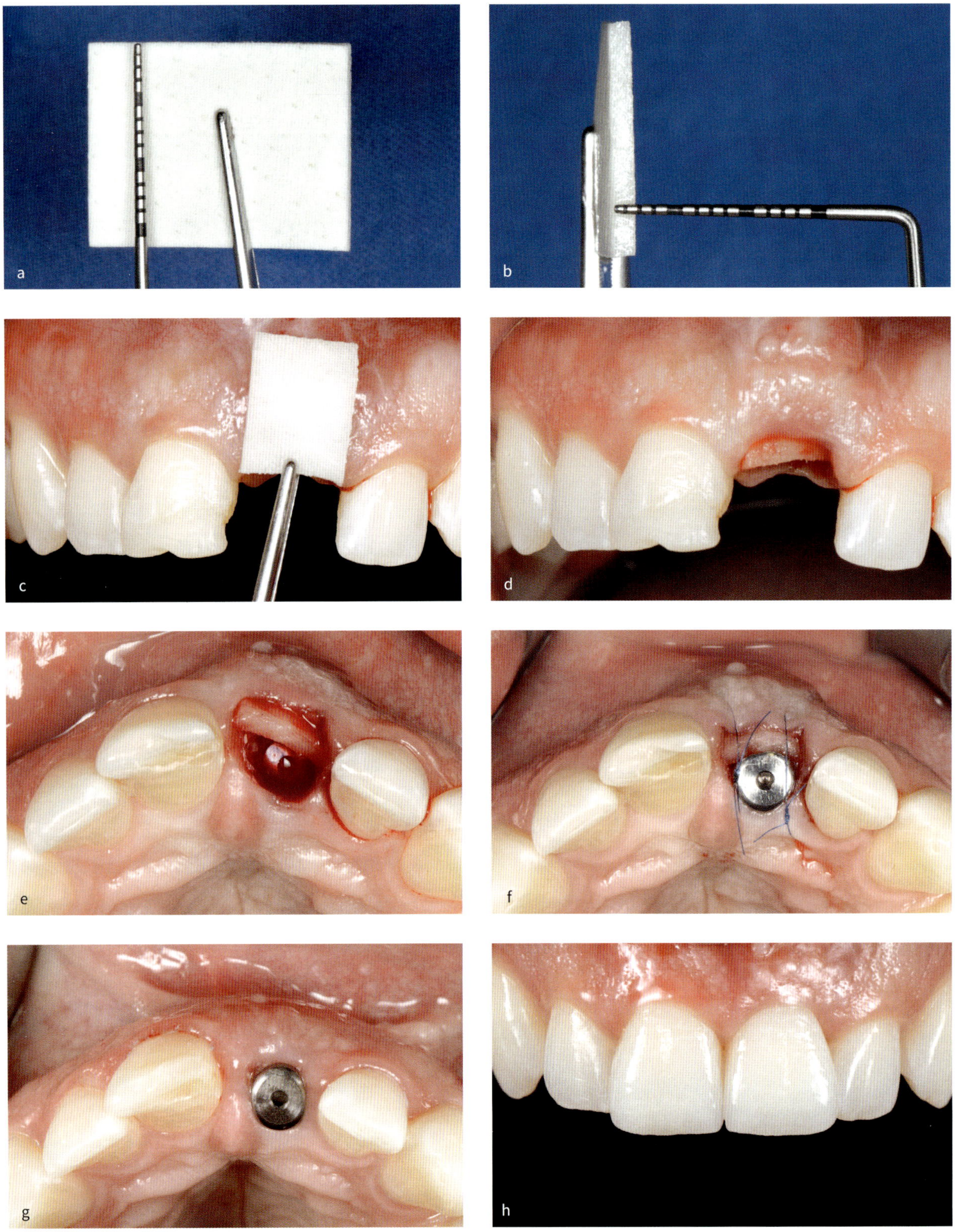

Figs 12a-h Acellular dermal matrix (Botiss, Berlin. Germany) (a-b). Implant in place and socket filled with DBBM and insertion of the dermal matrix (c-e). Sutures (f). Healing at 3 months (g). Final result at 1 year (h).

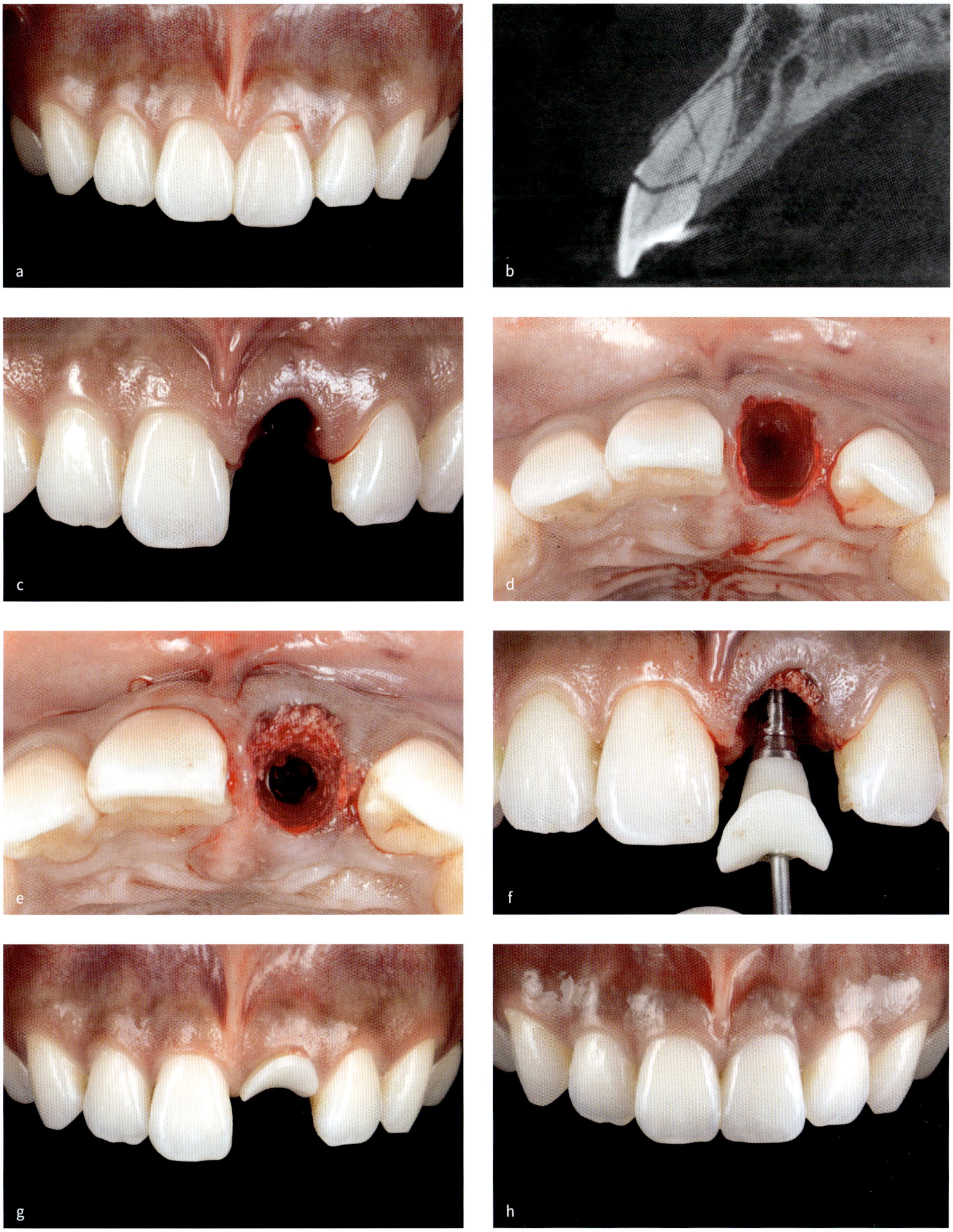

Figs 13a-h Immediate implant placement to replace a fractured maxillary central incisor (a-d) and delayed loading (type 1C). Grafting of the facial gap with deproteinized bovine bone mineral using the dual-zone technique (e), with the biomaterial material extending up to the mucosal margin. Concave socket-sealing custom healing abutment to contain the material and provide support to the mucosa (f). Removal of the custom healing abutment at three months (g). Final crown made of veneered zirconia. Clinical outcome at two years (h). (Images courtesy of Dr. Simon Doliveux.)

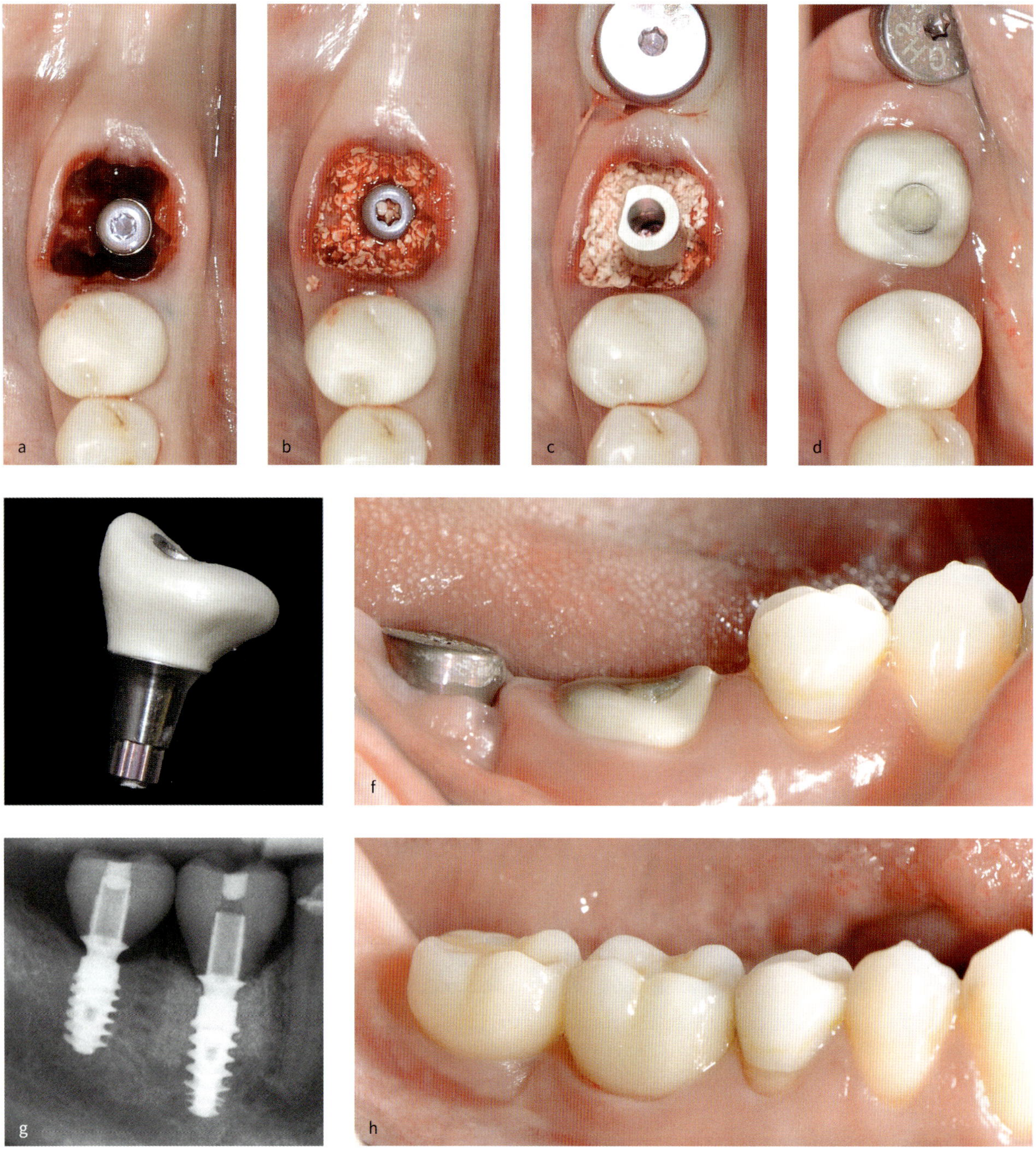

Figs 14a-h Immediate implant placement (type 1C) to replace a first molar and delayed implant placement (type 4C) to replace the second molar (a-d). A dual-zone technique using a socket-sealing custom healing abutment. PEEK anatomical abutment fabricated using a CAD/CAM system and placed within the same day (e-f). Final crowns made of lithium disilicate placed after three months. Clinical and radiographic outcomes after one year (g-h).

4.1.8 Alternative Socket Management: the Socket-Shield Technique

Socket grafting is commonly carried out with the intention of minimizing the loss of bundle bone. It is often combined with connective tissue grafting designed to compensate for post-extraction bone remodeling. The socket-shield technique, initially described by Hürzeler and coworkers (2010), was suggested as an alternative immediate placement protocol to preserve the facial bone plate, the alveolar crest volume, and consequently the esthetic outcomes (Bäumer and coworkers 2017).

From a biological point of view, the socket-shield technique relies on a partial extraction therapy: a tooth fragment on the facial side in the marginal area of the socket is left in place to maintain the periodontal complex, including the bundle bone. Implant osseointegration using the socket-shield technique was demonstrated both in preclinical and human models (Hürzeler and coworkers 2010; Schwimer and coworkers 2018). More recently, clinical prospective and retrospective studies emphasized the potential interest of this technique to maintain the alveolar crest and suggest superior esthetic outcomes when compared to more conventional immediate placement protocols involving socket and soft tissue grafting (Bäumer and coworkers 2017; Bramanti and coworkers 2018).

Several authors consider this technique to be a very promising approach for implants in the esthetic zone. At the same time, though, related studies also mention a lack of available long-term evidence, the occurrence of complications, and a limited range of indications (Blaschke and Schwass 2020; Ogawa and coworkers 2022). Indeed, the socket-shield technique can only be applied in the absence of pathologies such as periodontal disease or facial root fractures or cracks, which significantly reduces the indications for this technique.

A retrospective clinical study by Gluckman and coworkers (2018) highlights a complication rate close to 20% up to four years, associated with exposure of the shield either during the initial healing phase or subsequent to final restoration. According to the inventors of the technique, such complications may be related to the continuing facial growth of the anterior maxilla; they have proposed addressing the anterocaudal movement of the dentin shield by locking the shield to the implant in the most apical or proximal regions, thereby blocking any migration linked to ongoing facial growth (Staehler and coworkers 2020).

Although the biological concept of the socket-shield technique may appear to be efficient in preserving the peri-implant hard tissue dimensions, the procedure has a certain level of complexity and may be highly technique-sensitive. Hence, the surgeon should be experienced and trained in that technique. Additionally, long-term results remain scarce, and well-designed clinical studies with long-term follow-up periods are required before routine clinical practice and general treatment recommendations can be given (Figs 15a-h).

When considering immediate implant placement—especially combined with socket grafting—the occlusal part of the socket should be sealed to protect the biomaterial from infection.

A coronally advanced flap of the peri-implant soft tissues is an option that involves displacement of the mucogingival line and that may therefore jeopardize the esthetic result. Most often, the socket is sealed with a connective tissue graft or a provisional crown, or with an anatomical healing cap (Kan and coworkers 2009; Tarnow and coworkers 2014; Finelle and coworkers 2019). Clinical research has shown that the transmucosal healing of implants—commonly for immediate implants in the esthetic zone when combined with socket management—displays results similar to those seen with submerged healing (Sanz and coworkers 2015). A provisional crown or a custom healing abutment can also be used for socket closure and to support the architecture of the surrounding tissue.

4.1.9 Postoperative Drug Administration and Instructions

As for all implant procedures, the patient will be provided with pain killers and anti-inflammatory medications (NSAIDs) preoperatively and on the days following the surgery (Moore and Hersh 2013). In the absence of evidence to the contrary, the prescription of antibiotics can be a matter for discussion, and their use might not be necessary , particularly in light of the increasing need for rigorous antimicrobial stewardship. However, in case of preoperative local infection, prophylactic antibiotics might be prescribed depending on the clinical needs. The application of bone or soft tissue substitute and of course the patient general condition may also justify the use of antibiotics.

Patients are also instructed to avoid brushing at the surgical site until the sutures are removed and to use an antiseptic mouth rinse three times a day.

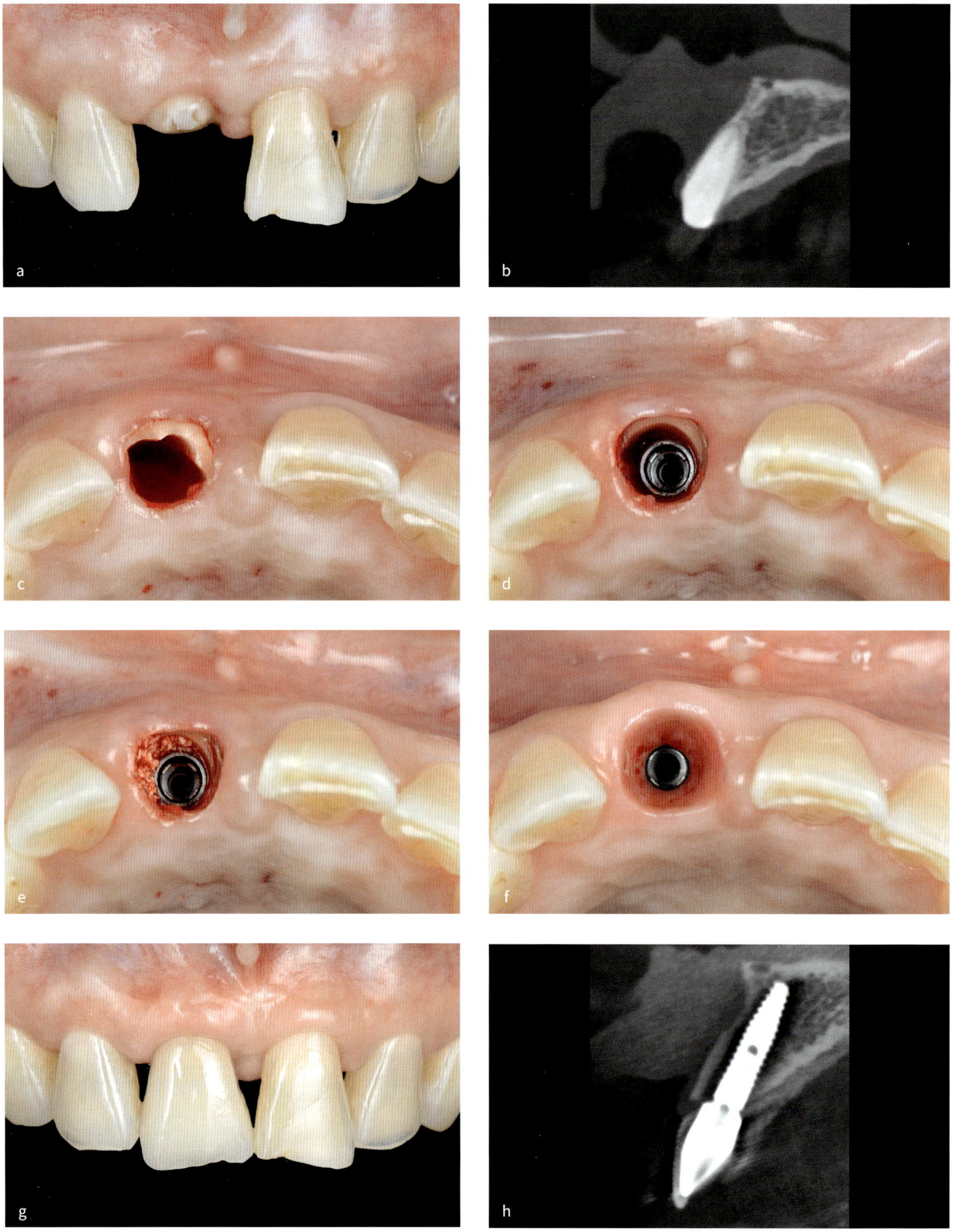

Figs 15a-h Replacing a central incisor with the socket-shield technique. Baseline situation (a-b). Partial extraction (c). Implant placement (d). Filling of the remaining socket with DBBM (e). Occlusal view at six months (f). Clinical (g) and CBCT (h) outcomes after one year. (Images courtesy of Dr. Prannai Nakapaksin.)

4.2 Immediate Restoration

To achieve the desired esthetic outcomes, a key aspect of a flapless immediate implant is to use a well-constructed and well-designed immediate provisional prosthesis for soft tissue support. The immediate provisional may be in the form of a removable prosthesis, a fixed conventional or bonded bridge, or an implant-supported prosthesis.

A removable prosthesis is often the most cost-effective and simple solution. However, due to compromises in esthetics, phonetics, and comfort, this is often the patient's least desired option. Case reports demonstrate how the soft tissues can be supported with a removable partial denture following immediate implant placement (Kan and coworkers 2001). However, as the mucosal support is difficult to control and can lead to hypercompression of the surrounding soft tissue, this is also commonly the biologically least desirable option.

A fixed tooth-supported prosthesis can provide ideal soft tissue support through an ovate pontic carefully extended into the socket to predictably maintain the soft tissue architecture (Bakshi and coworkers 2018). This option is available if the adjacent teeth are scheduled for fixed restorations or if the occlusion is favorable and sufficient enamel is present on the adjacent teeth for a bonded fixed provisional restoration (Figs 16 to 22).

A fixed implant-supported provisional is one of the most desirable interim options; however, the intraoperative criteria for immediate loading of an immediate implant must be met to minimize the risk of implant failure. Several studies have demonstrated superior esthetic outcomes where type 1A protocols were utilized compared to type 1C protocols with standard cylindrical healing abutments (Block and coworkers 2009; De Rouck and coworkers 2009).

Although clinically documented, the studies of type 1A placement reviewed have more heterogeneous outcomes than conventional loading protocols (Gallucci and coworkers 2018). Strict inclusion and exclusion criteria should therefore be applied (Morton and coworkers 2014). The preoperative criteria for case selection for the type 1A protocol of immediate implant placement and loading are reviewed in detail in Chapter 3. The upcoming sections will outline the basis for the intraoperative criteria required to determine the suitability of an immediately placed implant for immediate loading, as well as the clinical techniques to perform this.

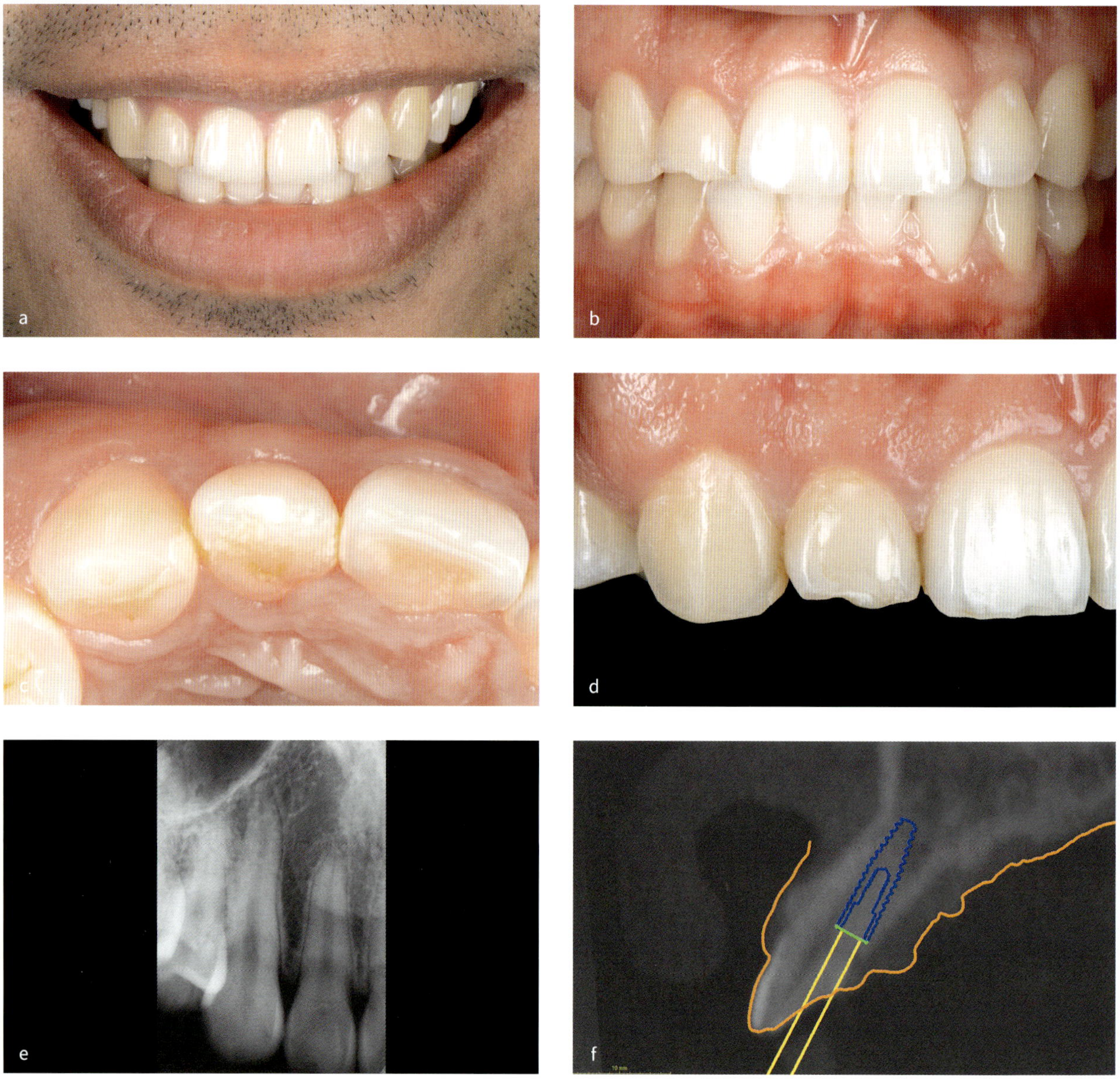

Figs 16a-f A maxillary right lateral incisor with an undisplaced horizontal crown/root fracture horizontal due to trauma scheduled for replacement with an immediate implant and a bonded fixed provisional restoration.

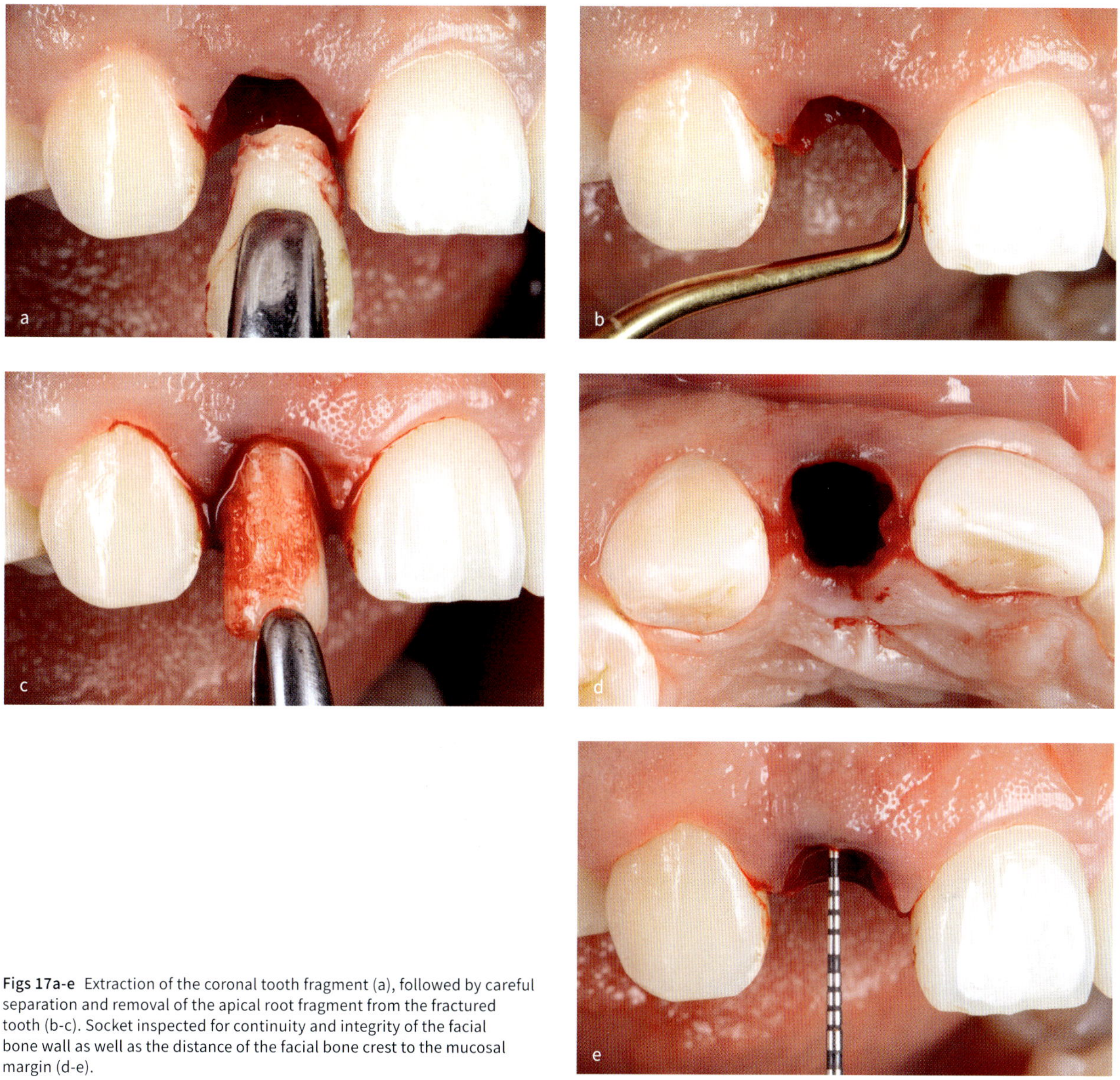

Figs 17a-e Extraction of the coronal tooth fragment (a), followed by careful separation and removal of the apical root fragment from the fractured tooth (b-c). Socket inspected for continuity and integrity of the facial bone wall as well as the distance of the facial bone crest to the mucosal margin (d-e).

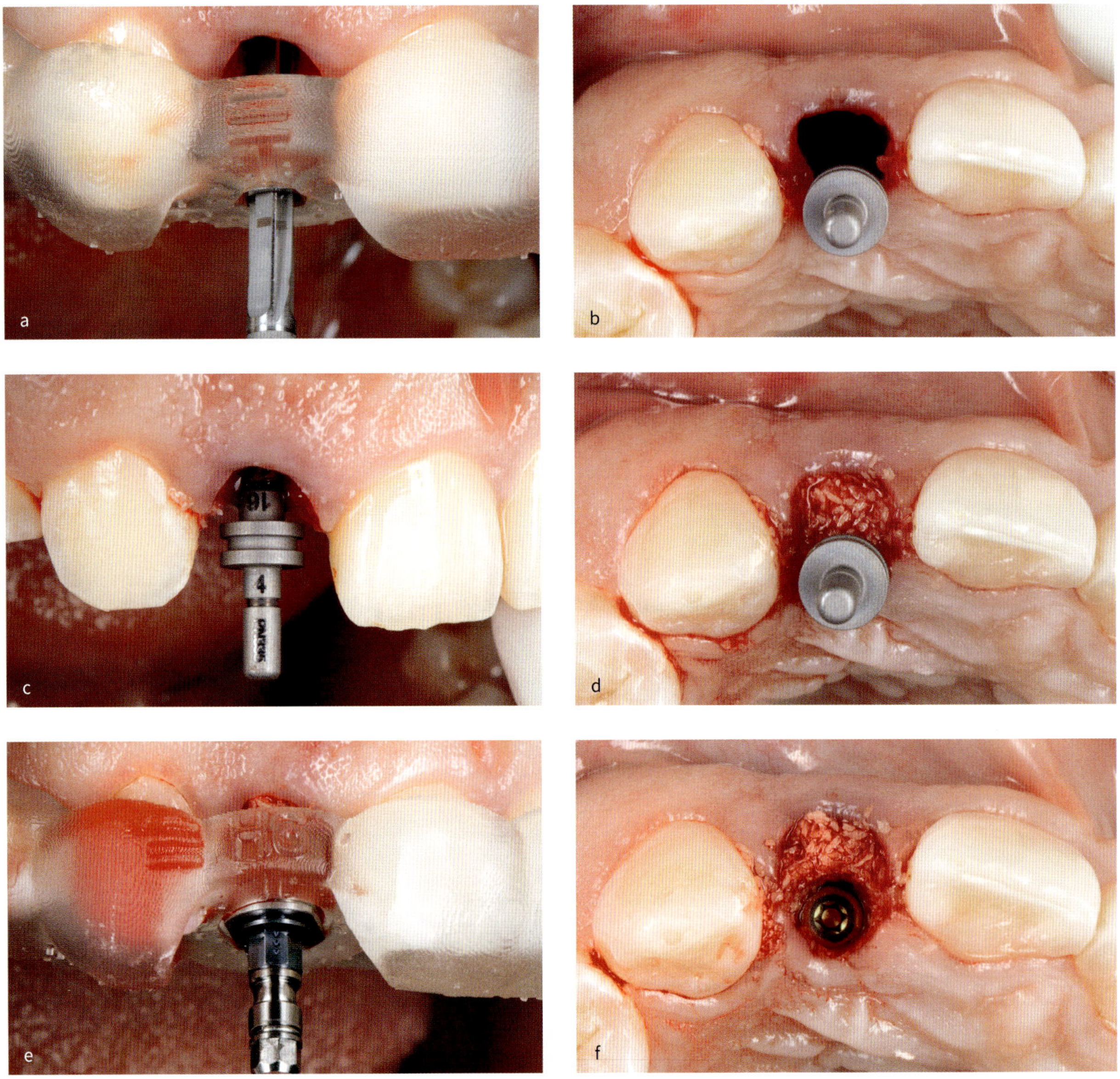

Fig 18a-f S-CAIS utilized for preparation of the implant osteotomy with verification of the osteotomy position (a-c), followed by placement of bone biomaterials (d) and subsequent immediate implant placement into the extraction socket (e-f).

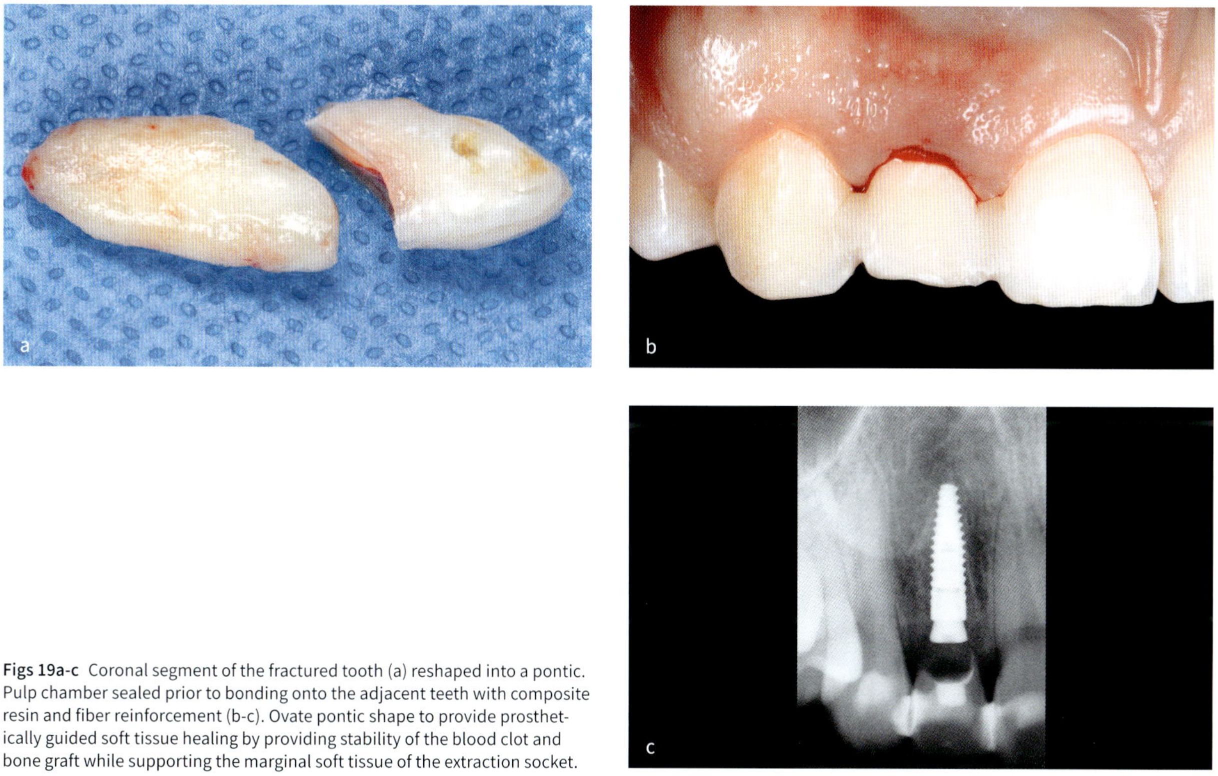

Figs 19a-c Coronal segment of the fractured tooth (a) reshaped into a pontic. Pulp chamber sealed prior to bonding onto the adjacent teeth with composite resin and fiber reinforcement (b-c). Ovate pontic shape to provide prosthetically guided soft tissue healing by providing stability of the blood clot and bone graft while supporting the marginal soft tissue of the extraction socket.

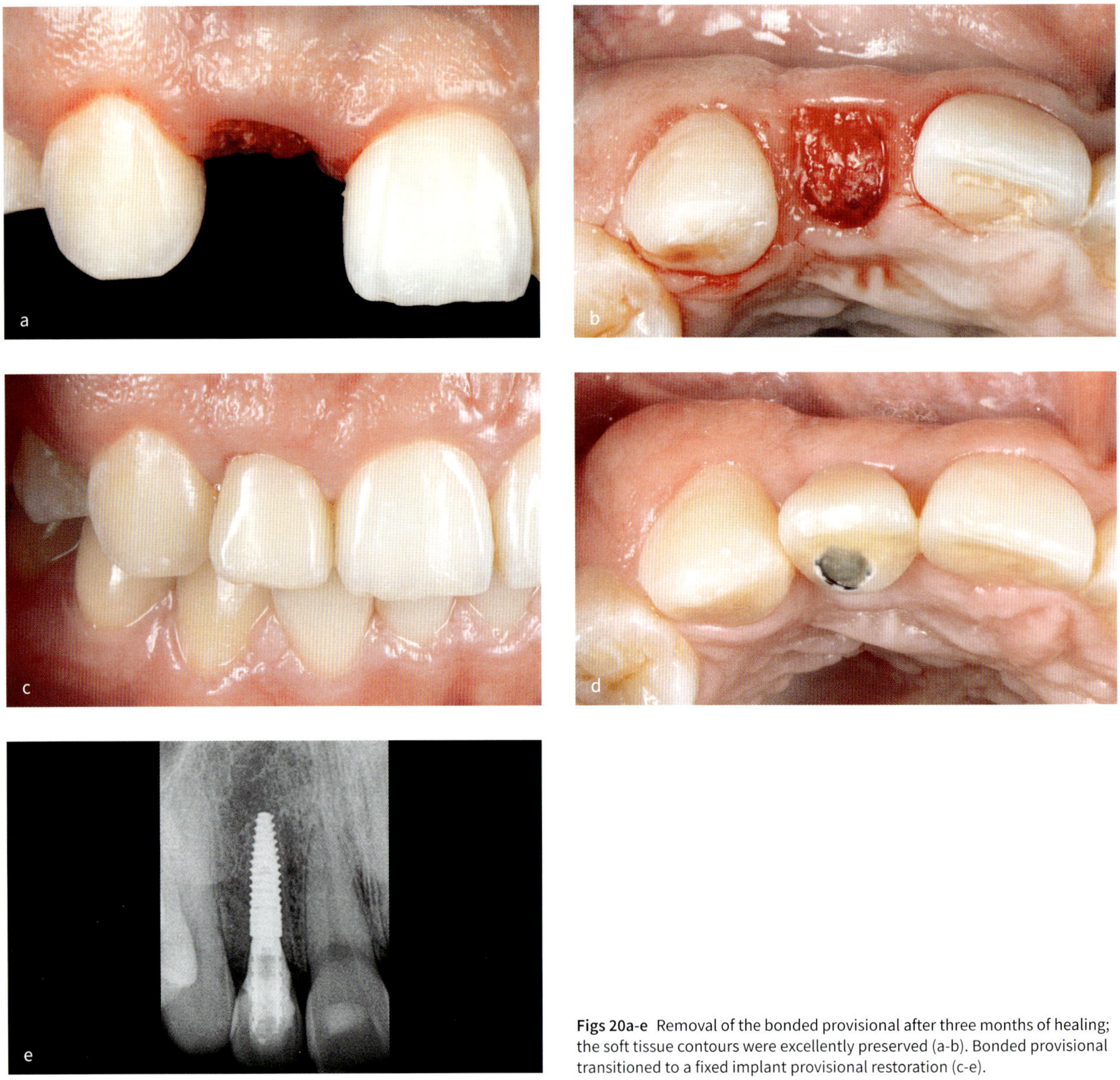

Figs 20a-e Removal of the bonded provisional after three months of healing; the soft tissue contours were excellently preserved (a-b). Bonded provisional transitioned to a fixed implant provisional restoration (c-e).

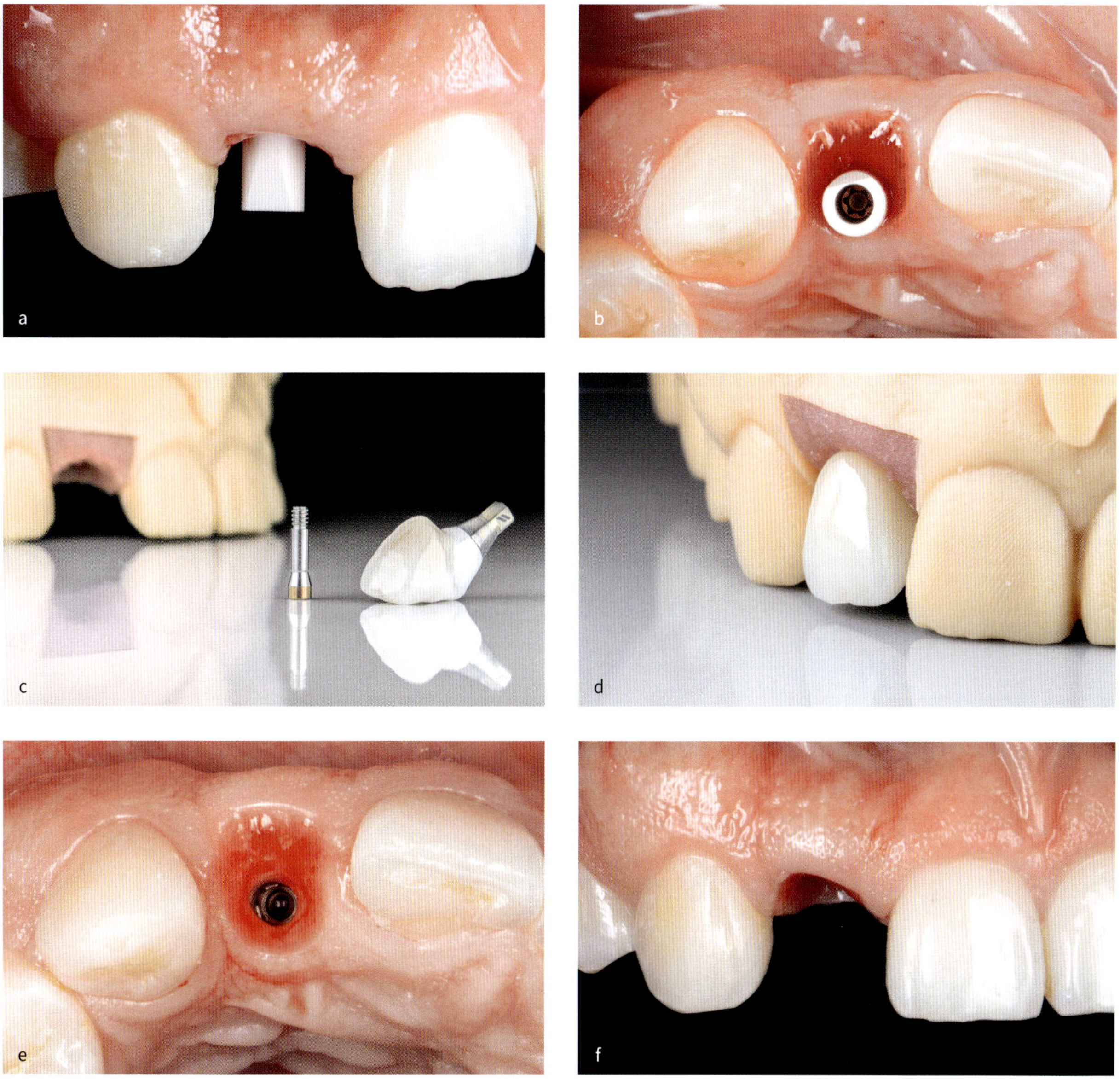

Figs 21a-f Digital intraoral implant impressions (a-b) for the fabrication of a definitive layered zirconia crown on a titanium base abutment (c-d). Soft tissue contours and volume prior to restoration delivery (e-f) showing an excellent profile, health and volume as developed by the bonded provisional and subsequent fixed implant-supported provisional restoration.

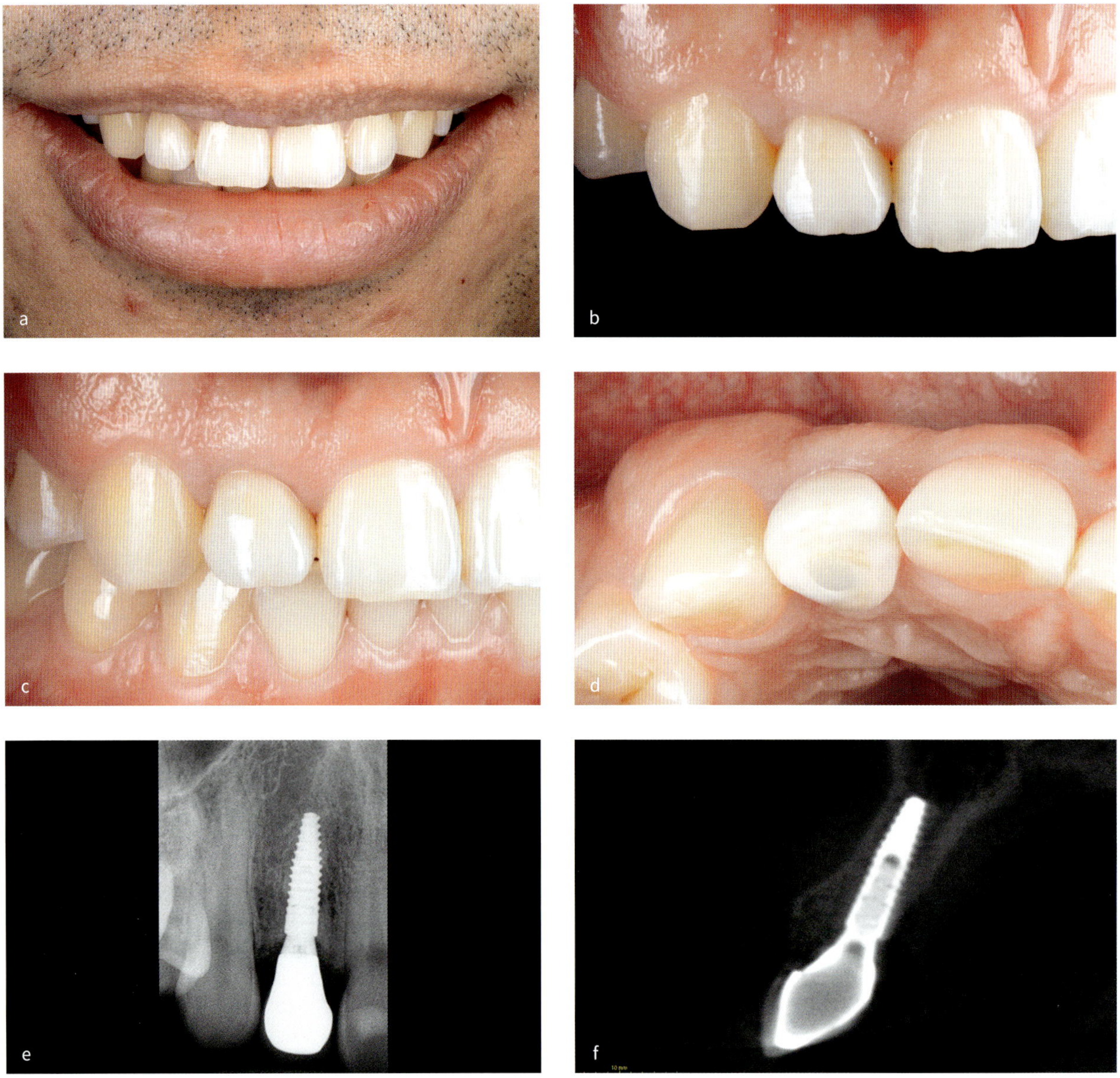

Figs 22a-f The 18-month follow-up with excellent soft and hard tissue volume and health around the implant.

4.2.1 Clinical Criteria for Immediate Loading and Restoration

If, based on the patient's wishes and preoperative planning, type 1A immediate implant placement and loading is selected, treatment goals will include the provision of a fixed implant-supported provisional restoration. For a predictable outcome and overall success, however, each treatment step needs to be assessed individually to ensure that the intraoperative clinical conditions are met. Any procedural complications identified may require measures to achieve the clinical conditions required; alternatively, the treatment plan may need to be modified to a different implant placement and loading protocol.

That intraoperative modifications of the prescribed treatment protocol may be needed is something that should be discussed with the patient at the outset to obtain his or her valid consent and to avoid accusations of treatment failure, should it be decided to use a more predictable treatment approach based on intraoperative clinical findings. Such intraoperative changes to the prescribed implant treatment protocol form the basis of the "intention-to-treat" concept in clinical trials (Newell 1992; Heritier and coworkers 2003; Gallucci and coworkers 2018). It provides patients and clinicians with guidance as to the likelihood of intraoperative conditions being unsuitable where, preoperatively, a type 1A protocol was indicated.

Once it is confirmed that the implant has been correctly inserted and positioned, an assessment should be made as to whether the necessary intraoperative conditions, outlined in Table 2 of Chapter 3, have been met before proceeding with immediate restoration of the implant. The key criterion for successful osseointegration is the resistance of the implant to micromovement during the healing phase (Chang and coworkers 2010). It will depend on the anticipated forces and their directions on the restoration during the healing period, as well as the direct mechanical connection of the implant to the bone immediately after insertion and throughout the healing period. Micromovements at the implant-to-bone interface during healing can result in resorption and fibrous encapsulation; larger forces may even dislodge the implant as a result of fractures of the bone surrounding the osteotomy (Lioubavina-Hack and coworkers 2006; Javed and Romanos 2010; Monje and coworkers 2019).

Currently, there is no scientifically validated measurement method to accurately determine the ability of an immediately placed implant to resist occlusal loading or masticatory forces (Norton 2011). Historically, implant insertion torque has been the most frequently reported criteria for determining the suitability of an implant for immediate loading (Monje and coworkers 2019). Insertion torque measures the resistance of the implant to rotational forces and depends on the rotational friction between the implant and the osteotomy. It is not a direct measurement of the stability of an implant (Norton 2013).

There are instances where high insertion torque and rotational friction can be achieved, yet the ability of the implant to resist lateral tipping forces may be compromised. During immediate placement, the insertion torque should be evaluated. Based on criteria reported in clinical studies, the implant should resist 25 to 45 Ncm of rotational torque, depending on the implant design, to be considered for immediate loading (Wöhrle 1998; Lee and coworkers 2009; Falco and coworkers 2018; Gallucci and coworkers 2018). A low insertion torque may be indicative of insufficient resistance to masticatory and occlusal loading forces if implants are immediate loaded during the healing period (Ottoni and coworkers 2005).

Peak insertion torque and rotational friction are somewhat correlated with the compression of bone during implant insertion (Wilson and coworkers 2016; Ikar and coworkers 2020). Excessive insertion torques are not recommended, as hypercompression of the bone can also lead to necrosis and resorption (Stavropoulos and coworkers 2016; Monje and coworkers 2019). The insertion torque should also take into consideration the implant design and size. Achieving 35 Ncm of insertion torque on a narrow-diameter implant will likely require significantly more lateral compression of the bone than the same insertion torque on a wide-diameter implant (Norton 2013). Similarly, the presence and design of threads on implants will influence insertion torques. However, it is unclear how this simultaneously affects bone compression or resistance to lateral loading of the implant (González-Martín and coworkers 2012).

Resonance frequency analysis may also be performed as an adjunctive or alternative clinical tool for making decisions about immediate loading (Meredith and coworkers 1996). it provides information about the stiffness of the surrounding bone and bone-to-implant contact. Clinical studies that have implemented this tool reported an implant stability quotient (ISQ) value of greater than 70, which is considered suitable for immediate loading (Chen and coworkers 2019).

Given the absence of a direct correlation between the available clinical measures of insertion torque and the results of resonance frequency analysis with the resistance to loading of an immediately placed implant, any values should be interpreted based on clinical modifiers such as implant length, implant diameter, implant design, bone density, and the proportion of the implant in contact with surrounding circumferential bone. As immediate implants are placed within an extraction socket that will aim to maintain a facial gap of 2 mm, the effective implant length in contact with circumferential bone contact may be limited unless there is significant bone apical to the socket and a longer implant can be placed. With modern implant designs and under-preparation of the osteotomy, it may be possible to achieve 35 Ncm of insertion torque with only 1 to 2 mm of the apical portion of the implant actually engaging bone. In this situation, despite meeting the criteria for 35 Ncm of insertion torque and resistance to rotation, immediate loading should be approached with caution.

4.2.2 Prosthetically Guided Soft Tissue Healing

One of the objectives in modern post-extraction implant placement is to provide an environment conducive to prosthetically guided soft tissue healing (Schubert and coworkers 2019). This is achieved by adequately supporting the mucosal margin and sealing the fresh extraction socket following minimally traumatic extraction using a flapless approach. This can be achieved with a customized healing abutment, immediate provisional restoration, or an ovate pontic. This aims at preserving the pre-extraction soft tissue contours throughout the treatment rather than attempting to recontour the tissue following early or late implant placement, where the papilla and soft tissue contours need to be restored (Al-Harbi and Edgin 2007).

Prosthetically sealing the socket also provides a means for containing the blood clot and any biomaterials while minimizing direct exposure to saliva and oral fluids in the initial stages of healing (Alexopoulou and coworkers 2021; Finelle and coworkers 2021). To highlight the effect of the prosthesis on healing, clinical studies have shown that sealing a fresh extraction socket with an ovate pontic only, without any other form of socket management, can be as effective as a socket graft in maintaining the blood clot and reducing resultant changes in the dimensions of the alveolar ridge (Bakshi and coworkers 2018; Song and coworkers 2022).

Both custom healing abutments and provisional restorations should feature emergence profiles that are undercontoured in the subcritical zone to allow for maximum volume of bone, biomaterial, or soft tissue graft material in this area, while the critical zone should extend to and be in contact with the former gingival margin and papillae.

The provisional restoration must provide mechanical support for the supracrestal gingiva and a mechanical barrier function to prevent movement of the graft (Harvey 2007). The materials and prosthetic design of the provisional restoration also need to be biologically tailored to promote wound healing and tissue stability.

A provisional restoration can also provide a surface for adhesion of the marginal soft tissue during the initial stages of healing. Soft tissue adhesion to biocompatible restorative materials such as titanium, gold, ceramics, acrylic resin, composite resin, and other dental materials is documented in the literature, provided that these materials exhibit clean and smooth surfaces (Abrahamsson and coworkers 1998; Linkevicius and Apse 2008; Welander and coworkers 2008; Linkevicius and Vaitelis 2015; Saito and coworkers 2016). Soft tissue adhesion may create a biological barrier, protecting the underlying tissues during healing.

The use of the coronal segment of the extracted tooth as a provisional has also been shown to provide favorable biological conditions for healing. This provides a shape that precisely fits the extraction socket and promotes reattachment for the supracrestal connective tissue fibers to the dentin/cementum root surface (Margeas 2006; Steigmann and coworkers 2007; Trimpou and coworkers 2010).

Given the potential advantages, it seems fundamental to fully understand the proper design and shape of the emergence profile to optimize the healing process and to contribute adequate soft tissue support.

4.2.3 Contours of the Emergence Profile

The emergence profile of the immediate provisional restoration is a crucial factor for optimizing the esthetic and biological potential of prosthetically guided healing. Two areas within the transmucosal zone have been defined based on the response of the peri-implant mucosal tissues to modifications of the abutment or crown contours (Su and coworkers 2010): the critical and subcritical contours (Fig 23). The critical contour is the most superficial area; it will influence the location of the mucosal margin and zenith. The subcritical contour corresponds to the deeper area and influences the peri-implant soft tissue support and, consequently, the shade of the gingiva. These two areas are linked, as the apical or coronal displacement of the critical contour will influence the length of the subcritical contour.

The main objectives of temporary restorations for immediate implants, besides patient comfort and esthetics during healing, are as follows (González-Martín and coworkers 2020):

- *Maintaining the existing soft tissue architecture.* Providing support to the circumferential soft tissue margin and papillae. The current rationale is based on the idea that the temporary restoration will support the soft tissue contours, thus avoiding collapse of the facial and interproximal tissues. Immediate placement and restoration are generally indicated in cases where the existing architecture is adequate or shows only minor discrepancies. An immediate implant could still be considered, in conjunction with regenerative techniques, if a large defect associated with a hopeless tooth is present, but an immediate implant-supported restoration may be risky and difficult to manage, leading to suboptimal results.
- ***Avoiding soft and hard tissue compression.*** Following the same surgical principle of avoiding facial and interproximal compression forces to the bony housing when planning the implant placement, the soft tissues should not be compressed by the restoration.

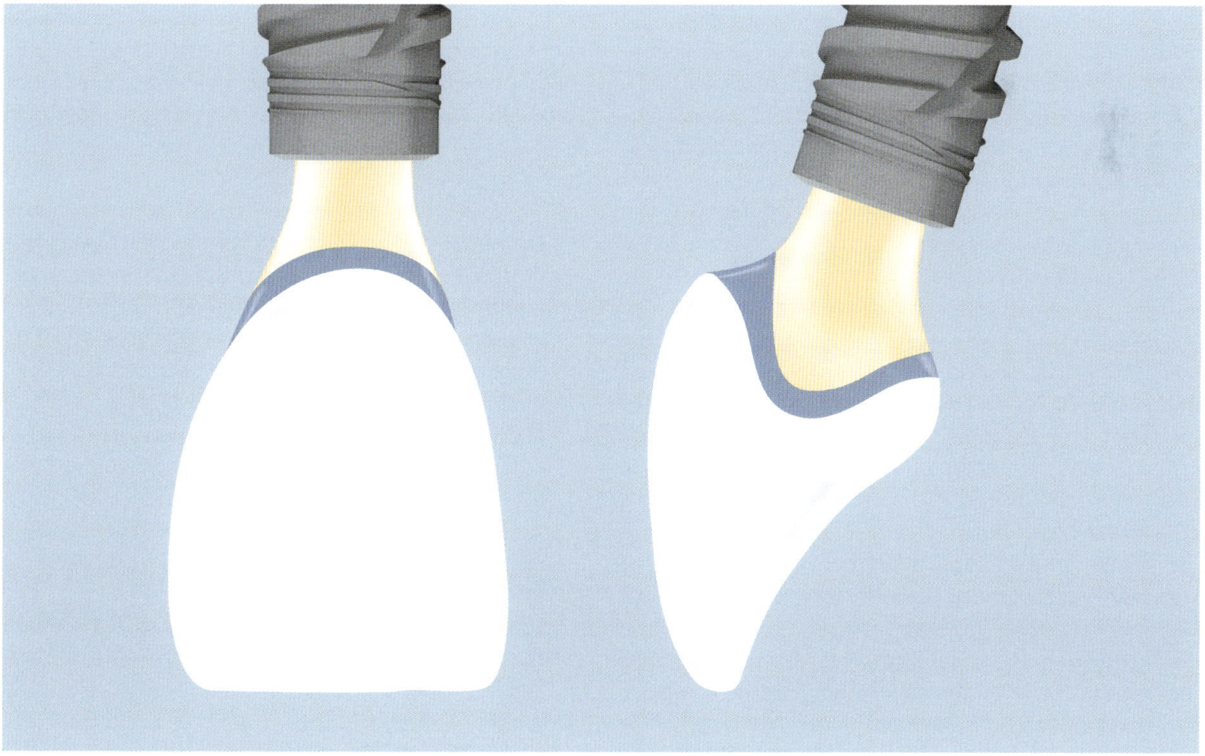

Fig 23 The emergence profile is divided into two zones: the subcritical zone outlined in orange, which should be narrow and convex to maximize the amount of biomaterial and tissue volume, and the critical contour outlined in blue, which is convex and provides support to the peri-implant soft tissue.

- *Providing space for the regenerative process.* The space created between the surface of the restoration and the supracrestal gingival complex should permit a gentle seal of the extraction socket to minimize salivary contamination and potential loss of the blood clot or grafting material. It can lead to the formation of a stable blood clot alone or in combination with a soft tissue graft or bone substitutes. Failure to achieve a stable coagulum or inability to maintain the regenerative space may result in soft tissue collapse and insufficient volume.

To accomplish the desired soft tissue stability and architecture, the transmucosal zone of the immediate provisional restoration should be shaped according to the following guidelines (González-Martín and coworkers 2020):

- A critical contour supporting the existing gingival margin and papillary height. Two variants are feasible: (1) The provisional outline maintains the facial, interproximal, and palatal existing outline. (2) The original soft tissue outline is maintained palatally and interproximally but is facially reduced by 0.5 to 1 mm to favor a slight coronal shift of the gingival margin after healing. This is especially applicable where the tooth shows some shallow gingival recession preoperatively.
- A subcritical contour as concave as possible to allow space for the coagulum and grafting material to stabilize and potentially reconstruct the bony ridge. Overcontoured restorations will result in thinning of the soft tissue with compromised vascularity and may lead to future apical migration of the marginal mucosa. Undercontoured restorations without support of the marginal soft tissues will result in collapse of the soft tissue into the socket as the collagen fibers contract.
- A smooth, polished, and biocompatible surface will help create a gentle transition and minimize contamination and inflammation during healing.

The restoration must seat passively and completely to ensure that adequate screw preload can be maintained throughout the healing process. This will minimize micromovements and the risk of screw loosening, which could result in movement of the provisional restoration. Movement of the provisional restoration will cause an inflammatory response within the transition zone and surrounding biological compartment and may compromise the regenerative potential of bone at the crest of the implant that is crucial for long-term peri-implant health and esthetics. This issue has been reported as being a result of subcrestal implant placement relative to the proximal bone peaks, where the flare in many of provisional abutments would contact the bone and prevent complete seating of the restoration (Schoenbaum and coworkers 2012). This should be carefully assessed both clinically and radiographically and the abutments modified to ensure there is no direct contact with the bone.

4.2.4 Occlusal Considerations

Any provisional restoration attached to immediately placed implants should be considered immediate loading, as it is inevitable for the restoration to be loaded during function even in the complete absence of occlusal contacts. However, a distinction can be made between immediate loading with direct occlusal contact, as required in immediately loaded full-arch restorations, and immediate loading without direct occlusal contact, which is often termed "immediate restoration" in partially edentulous situations.

For immediate single-tooth replacements, the occlusion should be carefully adjusted to remove all contacts in maximum intercuspation and any lateral excursive movements of the mandible. For anterior tooth replacements, this may result in an esthetic compromise if the incisal edge has to be shortened to remove protrusive or lateral excursive contacts. It will, however, help protect the restoration from occlusal loads during function or parafunction. Dietary instructions should recommend eating a soft diet and avoiding chewing directly on the restoration in order to minimize the transmission of forces to the restoration.

4.2.5 Fabrication Techniques

Techniques for fabricating an immediate provisional restoration can be divided into direct and indirect techniques. Access to and availability of dental laboratory support, the skills of the clinician, and workflow efficiency should all be considered when deciding on the best possible approach. The following principles should be observed for all fabrication techniques:

- The surgical site should be always protected to minimize the risk of contamination of the implant surface, extraction socket, or bone substitute materials. This is achieved by careful and judicious use of minimal amounts of restorative materials intraorally to index the position of the implant or provisional shell crown. Additionally, if preferred, a small piece of sterile rubber dam or PTFE tape can be placed around the temporary abutment as a barrier to prevent restorative materials from entering the socket. The fabrication and adjustment of the provisional restoration should take place extraorally at chairside or in a dental laboratory.
- The provisional abutment or restoration should not be in contact with any part of the bony socket walls, as this will impede the seating of the restoration and lead to early screw loosening. If the implant is placed slightly subcrestally relative to the facial bone, the palatal bone crest is often positioned further coronally than the facial crest in maxillary anterior sites, so impingement of the palatal bone with the provisional prosthesis is a particular risk.

- The emergence profile of the provisional restoration should be contoured to maximize the gain in soft tissue thickness while providing adequate support to the mucosal margin and papillae to promote prosthetically guided soft tissue healing.
- The restoration should seal the entire socket at the level of the mucosal margin to prevent any movement or loss of bone substitute material or connective tissue graft.
- The restoration surface should be highly polished and free of porosity to minimize plaque accumulation and bacterial adhesion while promoting soft tissue healing and fibroblast attachment. The material selected is a key factor when making the provisional.
- The restoration should be completely free of occlusal contacts. In particular, contacts in mandibular excursive movements must be eliminated.
- The proximal contacts should be very light to minimize force transmission from adjacent tooth movement.
- Direct screw retained access is recommended for the provisional restoration, regardless of the position of the access hole.

INDIRECT FABRICATION: ANALOG METHOD WITH INTRAOPERATIVE IMPLANT INDEX

Once the implant has been placed, its position can be intraoperatively recorded and transferred to a preoperative diagnostic cast to for the purpose of fabricating the provisional restoration in a dental laboratory setting. This technique has several advantages, including a minimized risk of contamination of the surgical site during restorative procedures and reduced chair time, which may provide increased time efficiency for the clinician.

The clinical and laboratory steps for the fabrication of a provisional restoration for a maxillary second premolar are illustrated in Figures 24 to 29. The intraoperative implant index is fabricated by capturing the position of the immediately placed implant relative to the adjacent teeth. For this purpose, an open-tray impression coping can be used together with a small amount of rigid impression silicone or restorative material covering the occlusal surfaces of the adjacent teeth. The preoperative stone cast is modified by creating a socket at the site of the extracted tooth while preserving the contours of the gingival margin. This will allow the technician to exactly copy the shape of the extracted tooth at the cervical aspect of the provisional (critical contour), providing ideal support to the soft tissue. The intraoperative surgical index is then used to transfer an implant analog to the modified preoperative cast. Once the implant position has been transferred to the modified master cast, fabrication of the provisional crown can be completed using conventional techniques.

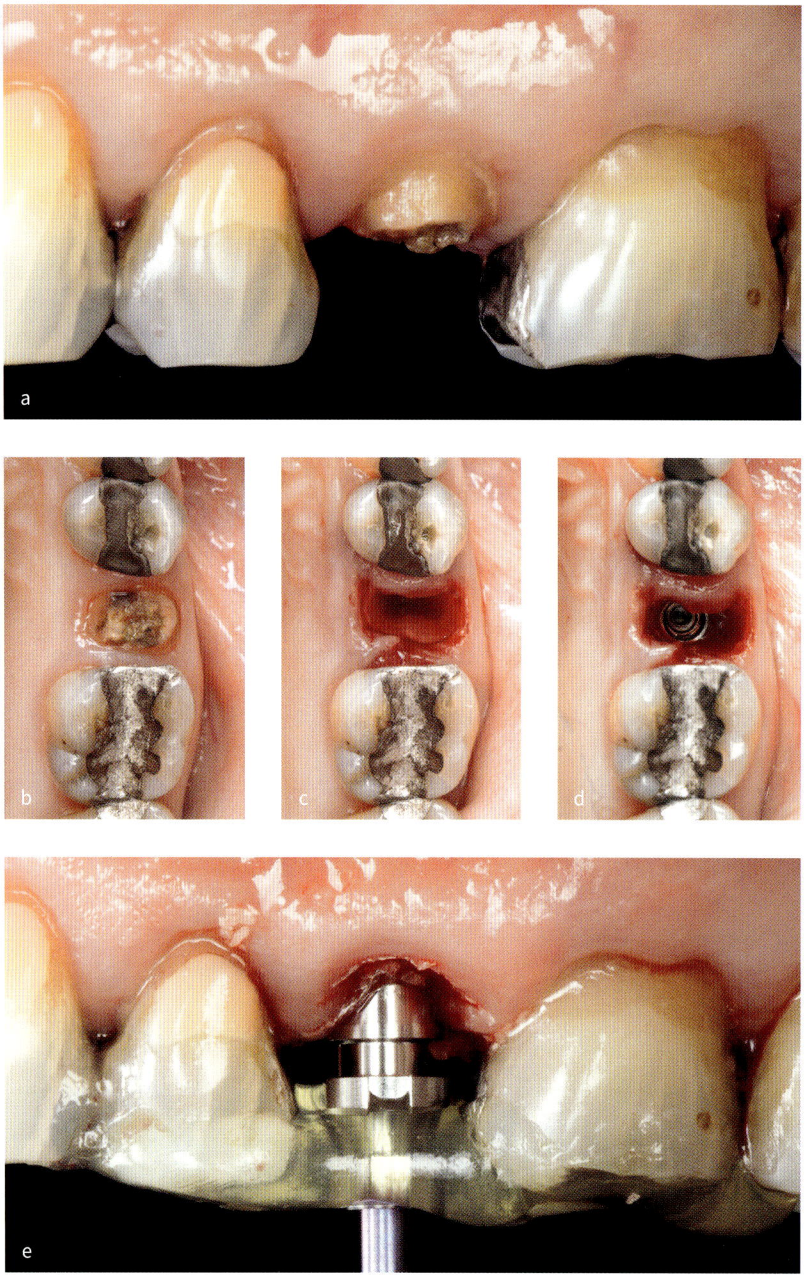

Figs 24 a-e Fractured maxillary second premolar extracted (a-d) and replaced by an immediate implant (e). Implant position captured with an open-tray impression coping to the occlusal surfaces of the adjacent teeth with a light-curing resin (Triad Gel, Dentsply Sirona, York, PA, USA).

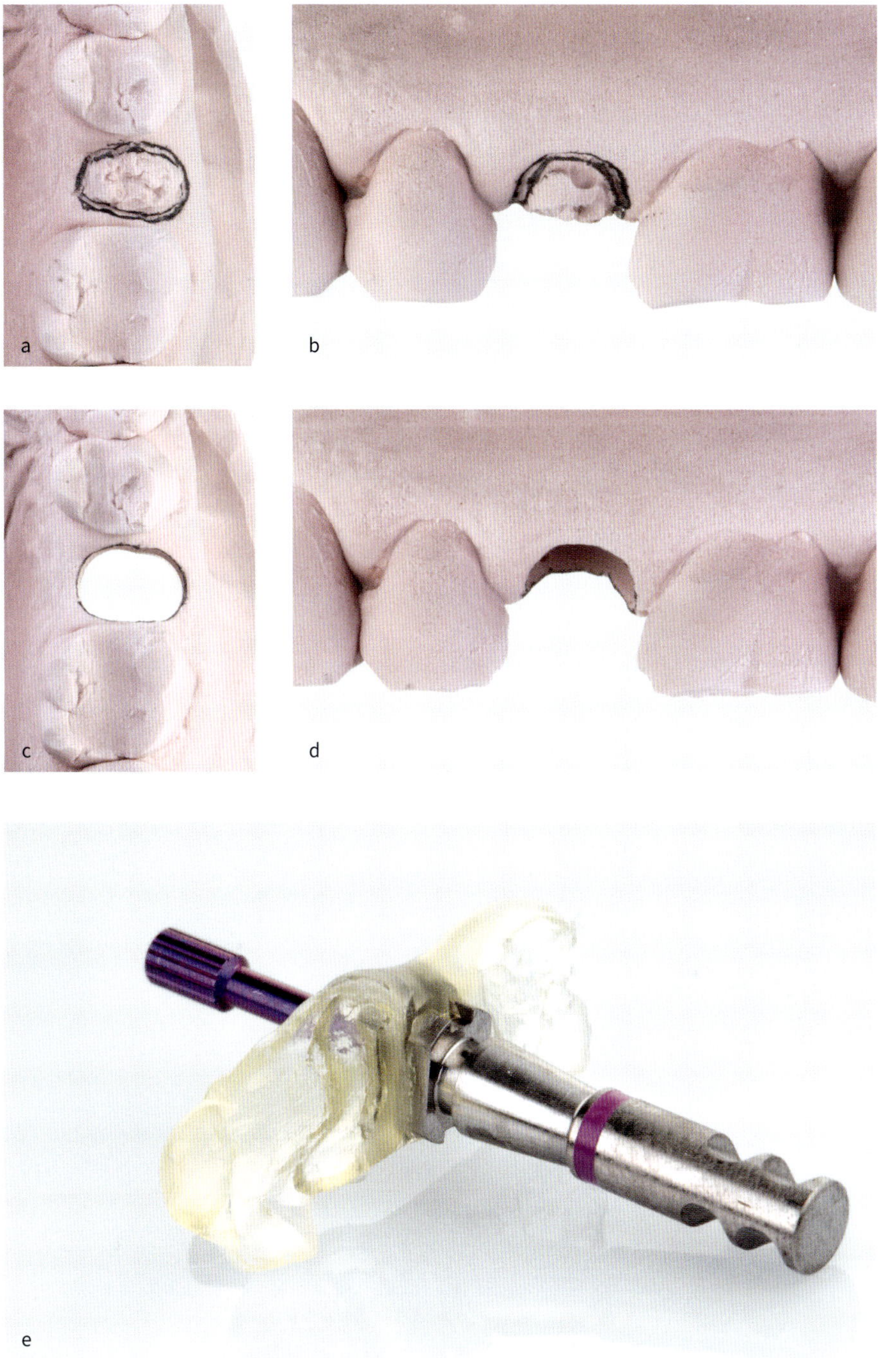

Figs 25a-j Extracted tooth, outlined and carefully removed from the preoperative stone cast, creating a hole that preserved the gingival margin position of the extracted tooth and exited through the base (a-d). Implant analog attached to the intraoperative implant index and seated on the cast (e-f) with the analog passively entering the hole (g). Dental stone poured into the hole around the analog to secure it to the preoperative cast (h-j).

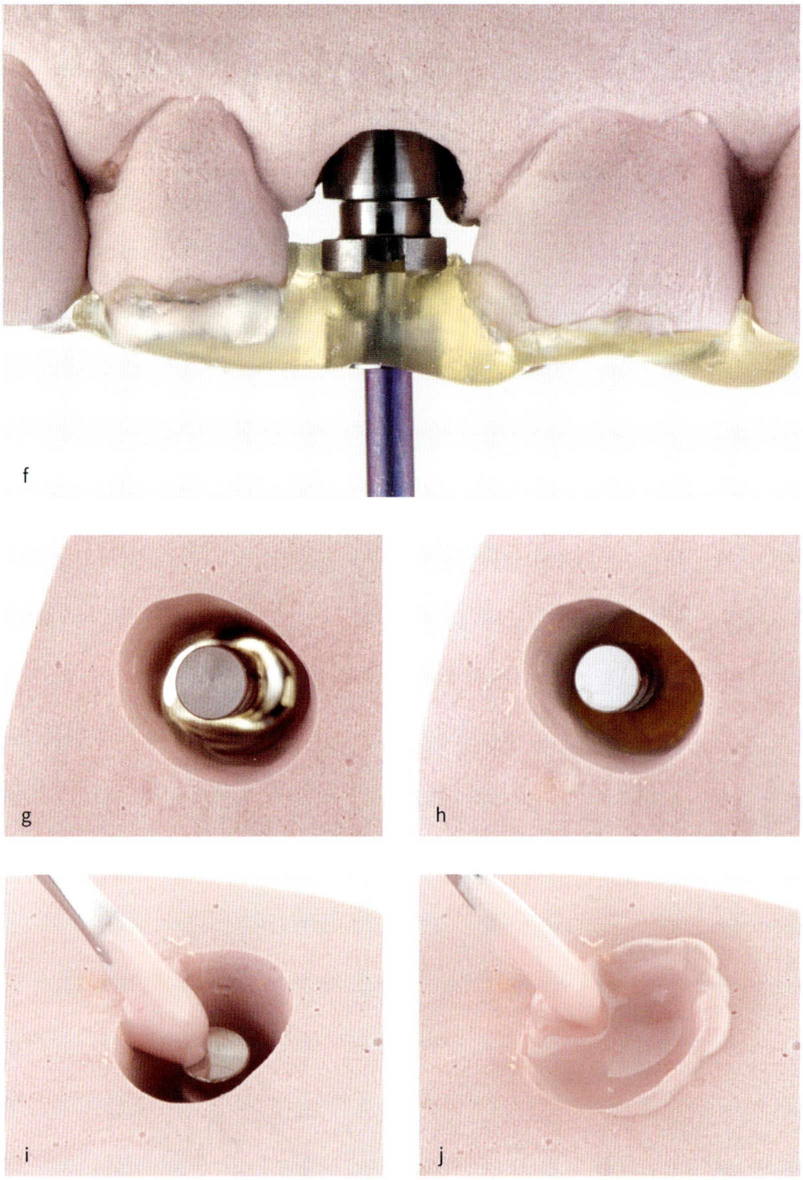

Figs 25a-j (continued)

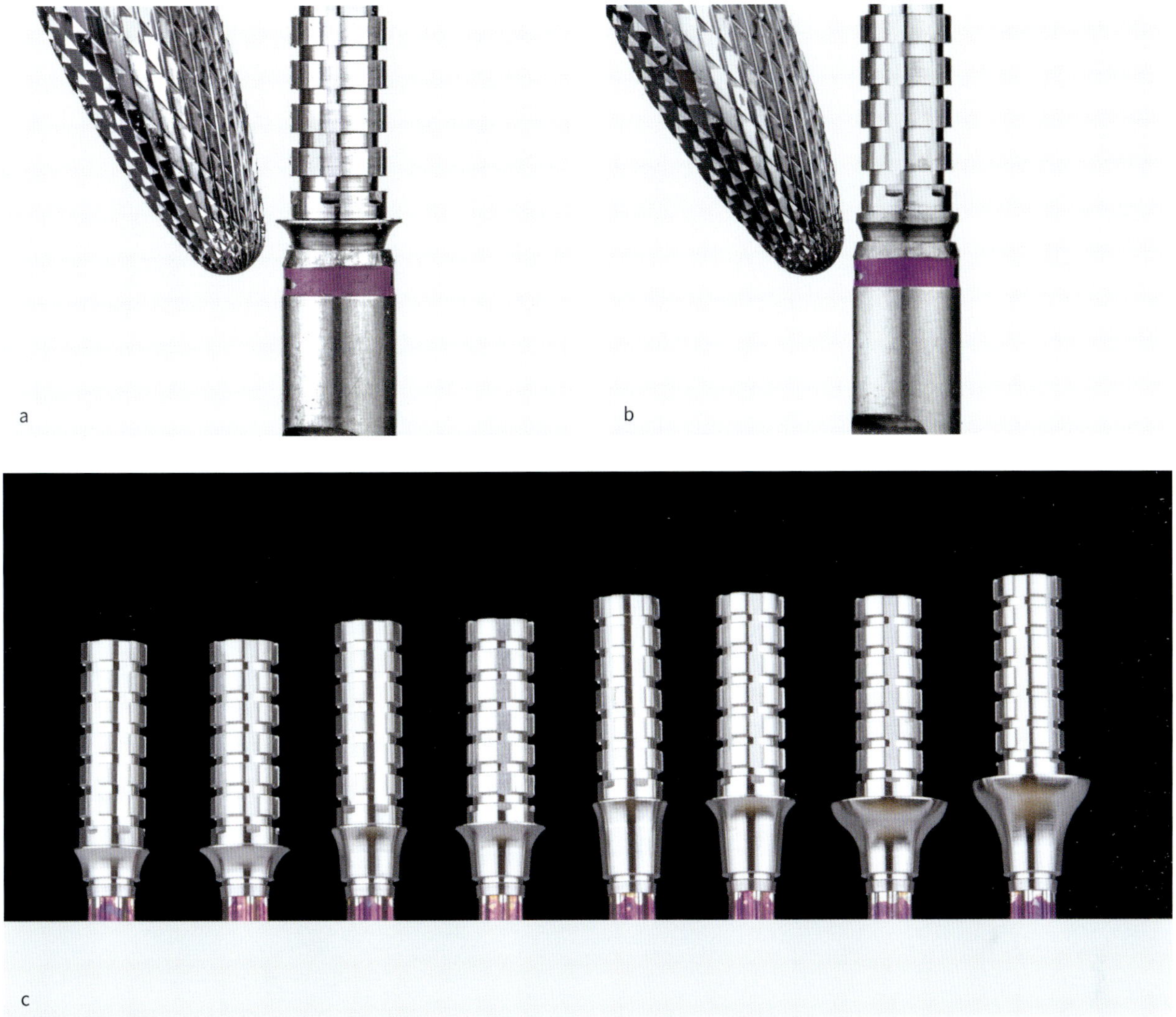

Figs 26a-c Modification of the provisional titanium abutment to remove the widening of the first 1–2 mm of the emergence profile at risk of contacting the bone and preventing seating of the restoration (a-b). Abutment inserted into a laboratory analog and held in an analog holder to prevent damage to the implant-abutment connection and hands of the operator. Modern titanium provisional abutment designs with varying gingival collar heights and diameters, which, when selected appropriately, can provide the ideal biological, mechanical, and esthetic outcome without modification of the initial emergence profile (c).

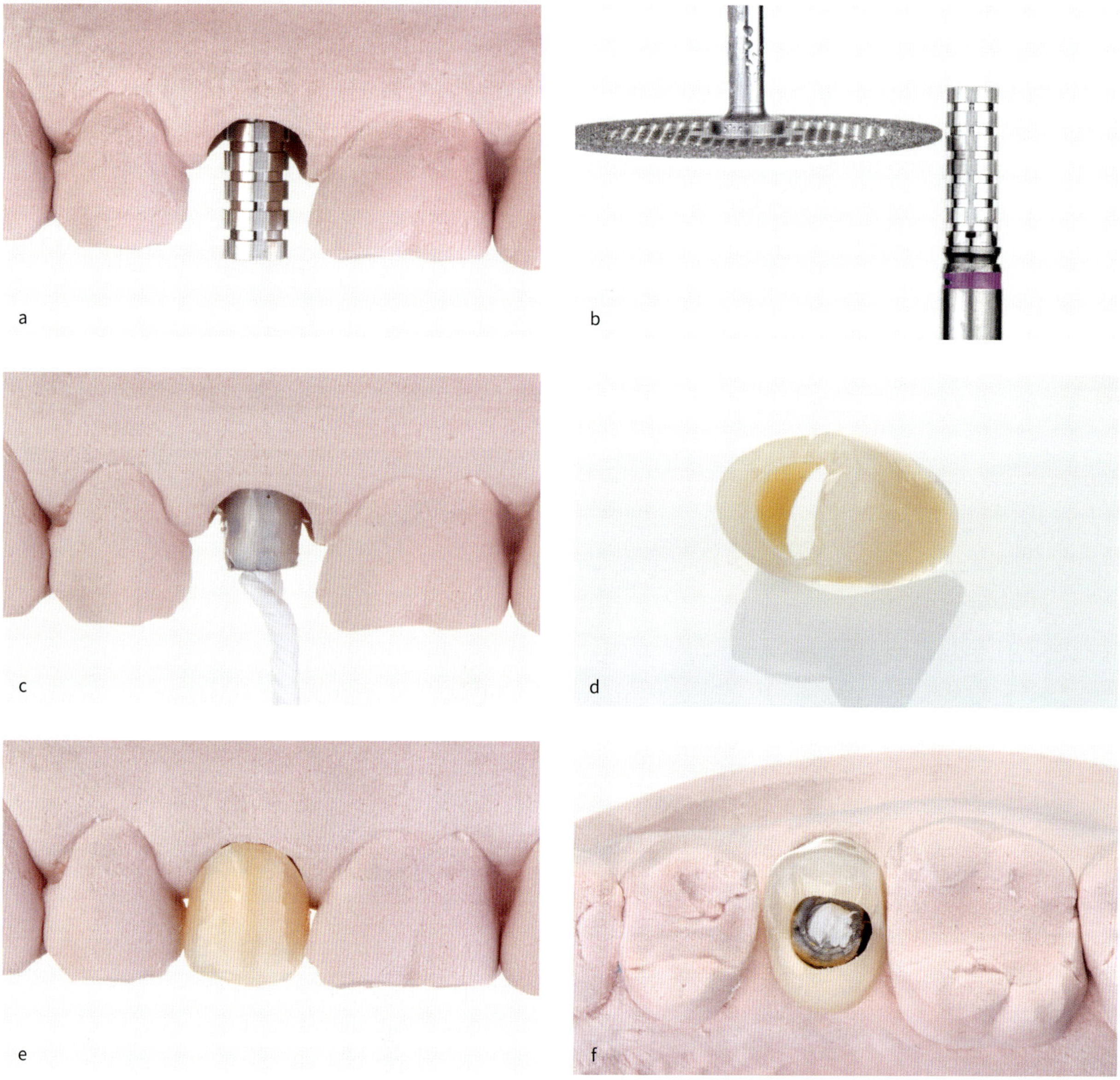

Figs 27a-f Adjustment of the height of the titanium provisional abutment with a diamond disk (a-b).Opaquer used to block out the grayness of the titanium; PTFE tape is inserted into the screw access hole to protect the screw during fabrication (c). A hollowed-out denture tooth adjusted to fit over the provisional abutment and to conform to the gingival margin of the extracted tooth (d-f). Flowable composite or acrylic resin applied between the abutment and denture tooth to connect the shell to the provisional abutment.

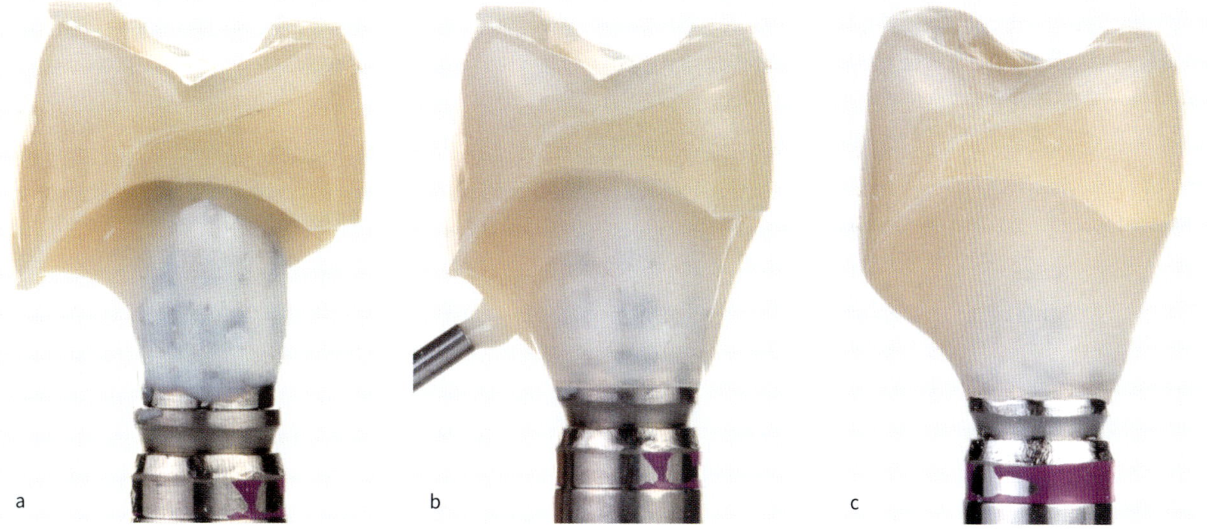

Figs 28a-c Once removed from the cast, additional material was added to recreate the desired emergence profile and fill any voids between the denture tooth and abutment. Undercontoured first 1–2 mm of the provisional to avoid contact with bone and to maximize the soft tissue volume.

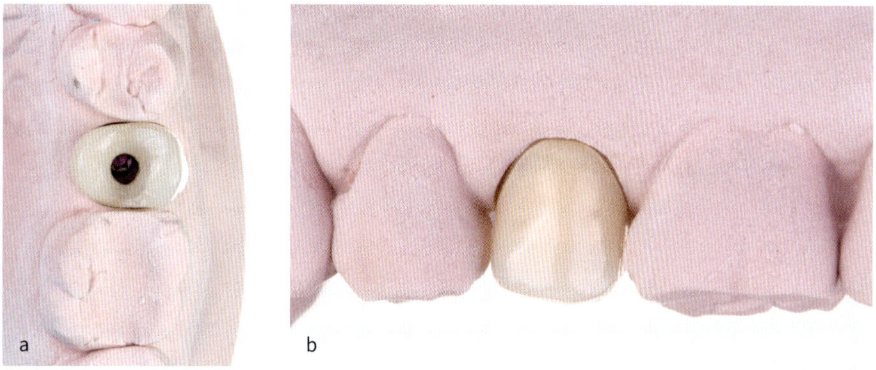

Figs 29a-b Completed provisional seated onto the cast, with the gingival margin of the extracted tooth closely approximating the contours of the restoration. This will provide a mechanical barrier to prevent loss of the graft material while supporting the pre-extraction soft tissue architecture.

INDIRECT FABRICATION: DIGITAL METHOD WITH INTRAOPERATIVE DIGITAL IMPLANT IMPRESSION

As an alternative to conventional techniques, digital impressions and pathways can be utilized to fabricate a CAD/CAM provisional restoration as illustrated in Figures 30 to 32. Preoperative intraoral surface scans can be combined with an intraoperative scan of the implant position to design a restoration whose contours match the gingival margin of the extracted tooth. Digital workflows in immediate loading provide advantages, as no impression materials or restorative materials need to be utilized in the surgical field and procedures can be performed very efficiently.

Digital intraoral surface scanners that utilize powder or liquid coatings to optimize the reflectance of the tissue should be avoided, as this would contaminate the surgical site; however, many highly accurate powderless scanners are commercially available.

The workflow commences with the acquisition of preoperative scans of the maxilla, mandible, and a buccal bite scan. The tooth to be extracted can then be trimmed from the digital impression to prepare for the intraoperative scan. The scan should ideally capture a small portion of the internal aspect of the socket at the level of the former gingival margin to guide the technician on forming the emergence profile and location of the critical contour zone. Following acquisition of the scans, socket management should be performed with grafting of the gap and any required soft tissue augmentation, if not already done prior to digital impressions. The surgical site should be protected with a narrow healing abutment and pressure with gauze while the restoration is being fabricated.

The scans are then loaded into the CAD software, where the crown contours and emergence profile are established and the design is finalized. A milled or 3D-printed polymethylmethacrylate provisional crown with a titanium-base abutment can then made and cemented to the titanium abutment extraorally with resin cement prior to delivery.

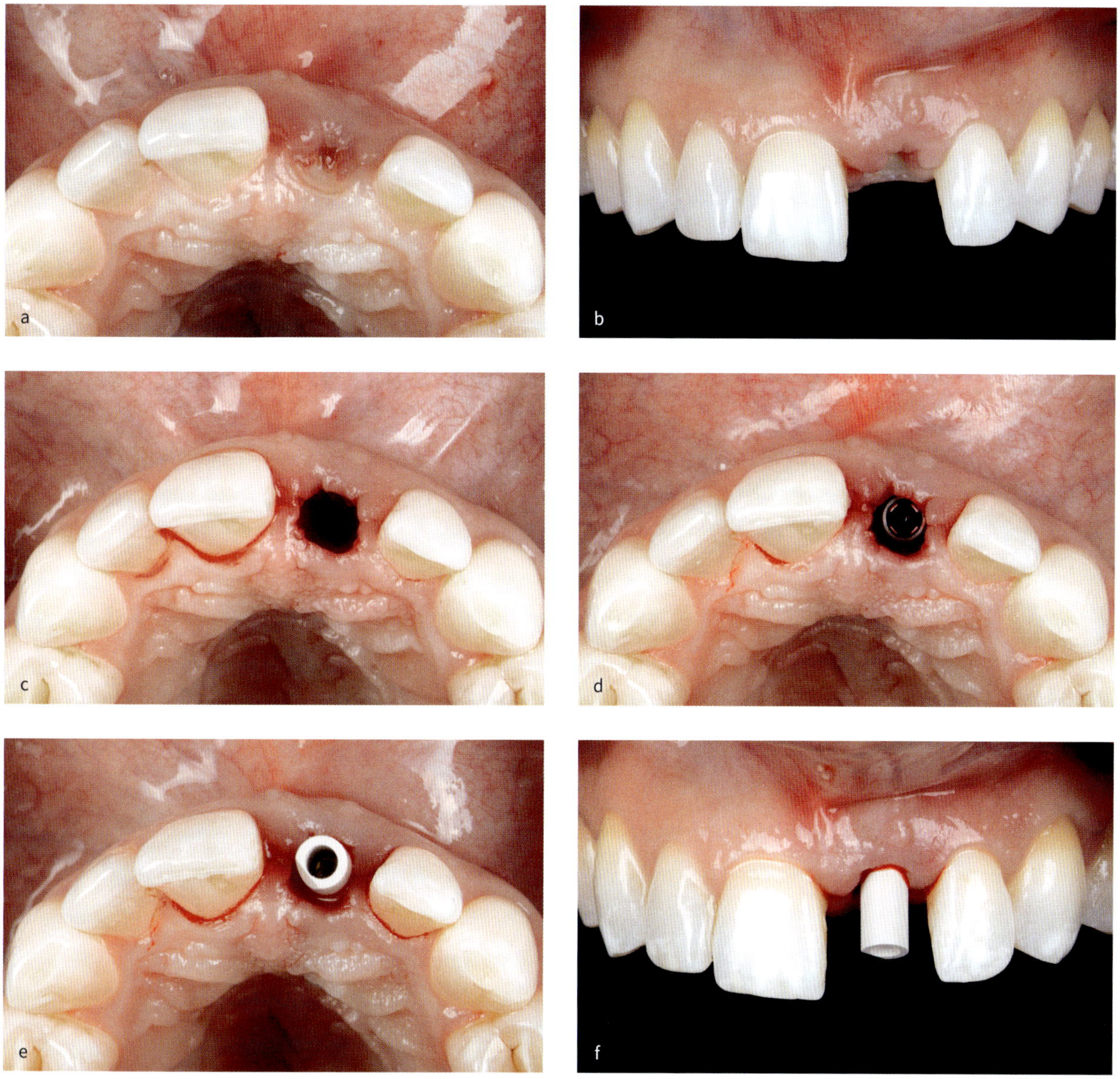

Figs 30a-f Extraction of a fractured maxillary left central incisor and immediate implant placement with simultaneous socket grafting using deproteinized bovine bone matrix and a subepithelial connective tissue graft (a-d). Digital intraoral scans at the time of surgery with a scan body attached to the immediately placed implant to capture the implant position relative to the adjacent teeth and soft tissues (e-f).

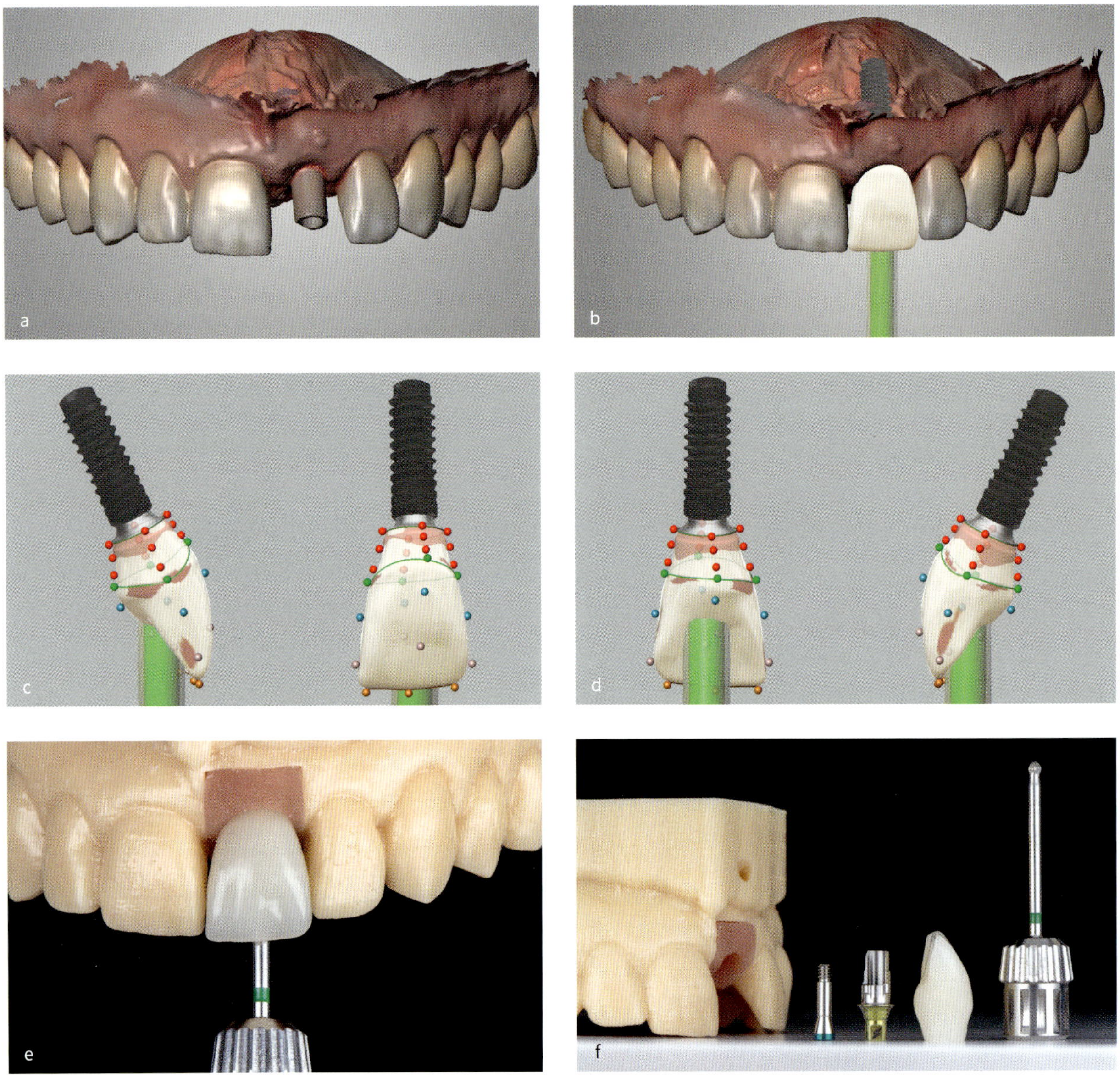

Figs 31a-f An immediate provisional crown on a titanium-base abutment with an angulated screw channel designed in CAD software based on the intraoperative digital scans. The emergence profile matches the gingival margin of the pre-extraction tooth.

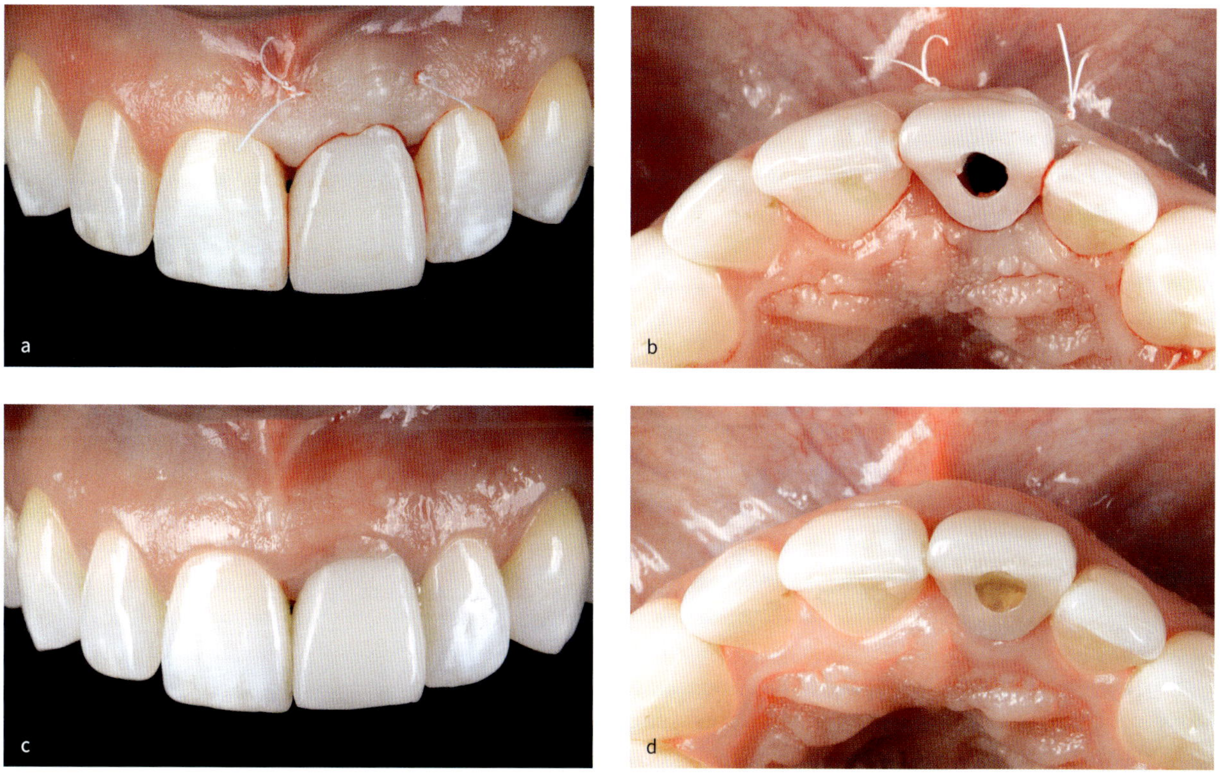

Figs 32a-d Digitally fabricated, immediately loaded restoration delivered on the same day, with the occlusion slightly relieved (a-b). Suture removal three weeks later, with adequate support of the marginal mucosa and papillae visible as provided by the interim restoration (c-d). (Images courtesy of Dr Armand Putra.)

DIRECT FABRICATION

Direct chairside fabrication of an implant-supported provisional restoration can also be used to provide the patient with an immediate tooth replacement after tooth extraction. However, this approach requires refined clinical skills and increases chair time.

Because restorative materials (e.g., free monomers and resin materials) are applied directly into a fresh wound site, care must be taken to ensure that these materials do not directly contact the implant or bone graft materials, which may have a detrimental effect in the healing response. For this purpose, two different chairside protocols may be utilized:

Direct fabrication, prefabricated restoration attached to provisional abutment, customization of the submucosal area (Figs 33 to 37). The first step is the selection of an appropriate provisional abutment for the immediate restoration. Titanium provisional abutments are recommended due to their durability and lower risk of technical complications, which could be detrimental to socket healing. An abutment with an appropriate gingival height and narrow emergence profile should be selected where possible, or if required, the prefabricated provisional abutment should be modified, including a reduction in height and width as appropriate, particularly at the most apical aspect of the abutment, as the platform of immediate implants is typically located slightly subcrestally, and contact of the abutment with the crestal bone would prevent it from seating fully (Schoenbaum and coworkers 2012). An opaquing agent may be applied to the abutment to prevent graying of the provisional, which may be critical in sites of high esthetic priority.

Following modification and insertion of the abutment, the internal fixation screw is then finger tightened, and the chimney of the abutment is obturated, for example with polytetrafluoroethylene (PTFE) tape. Additionally, a protective barrier (e.g., a small piece of sterile rubber dam or PTFE tape) should be applied over the exposed socket and bone-graft material.

An external crown form comprising either a custom shell crown, a hollowed denture tooth, or the extracted tooth crown, is then modified to fit around the temporary abutment. A custom crown form can be indirectly fabricated using preoperative impressions with digital or analog methods. A positioning index supported by the incisal edges of adjacent teeth can also be added to the prefabricated crown form to allow precise repositioning as part of the intraoral pick-up procedure.

A small bead of acrylic or flowable composite is then used to join the crown form to the coronal aspect of the abutment. After retrieving the provisional restorative elements from the mouth, the remaining gaps between the crown and abutment are then filled, and the emergence profile is shaped and polished while the provisional restoration is held in a laboratory analog holder. The surface of the submucosal segment of the restoration must be polished extensively.

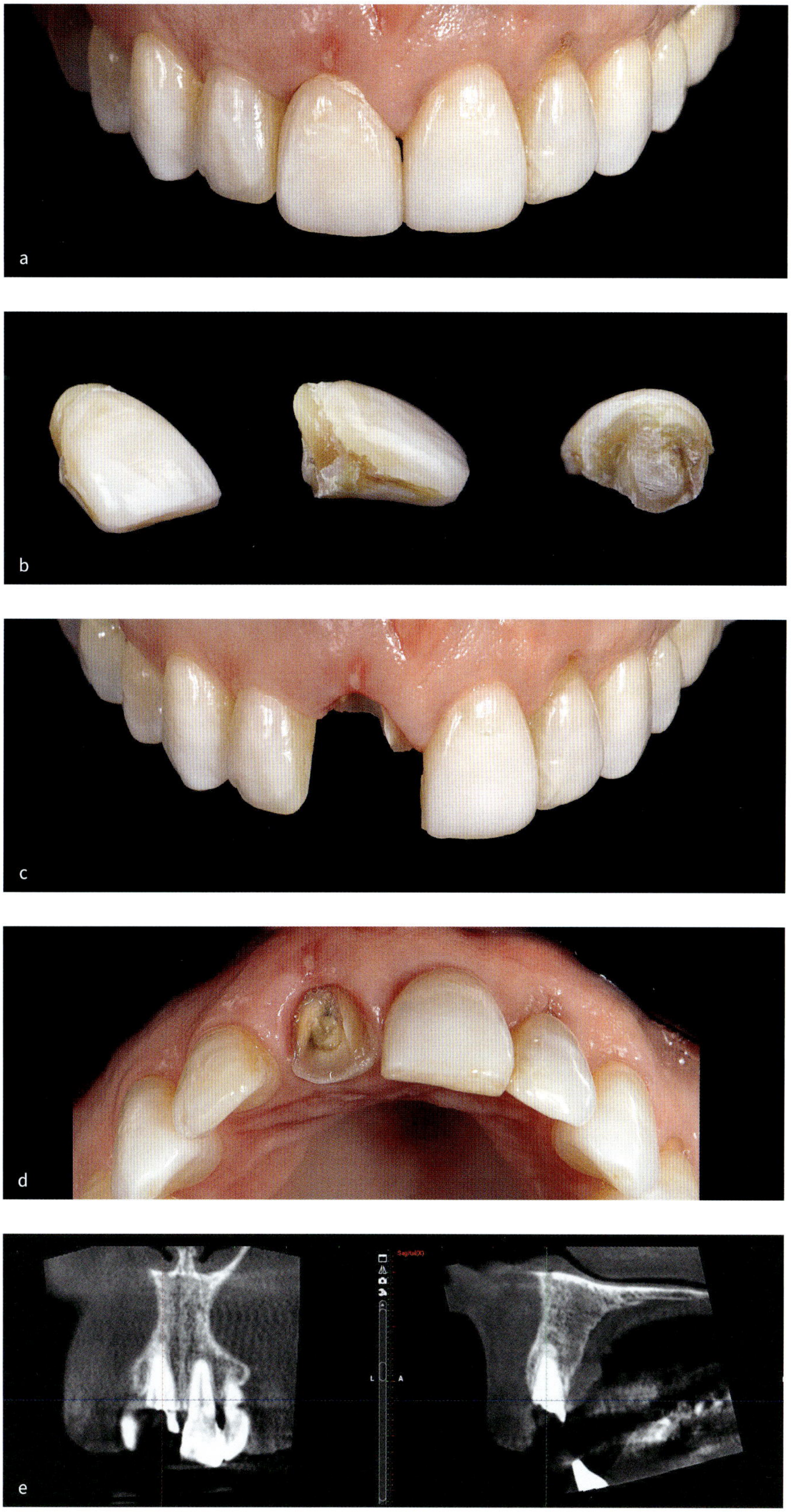

Figs 33a-e Maxillary right central incisor with a horizontal fracture, deemed unrestorable (a-d). CBCT evaluation showing favorable facial, apical, and palatal bone (e). Replacement of the tooth with a type 1A immediate implant placement and immediate loading was planned.

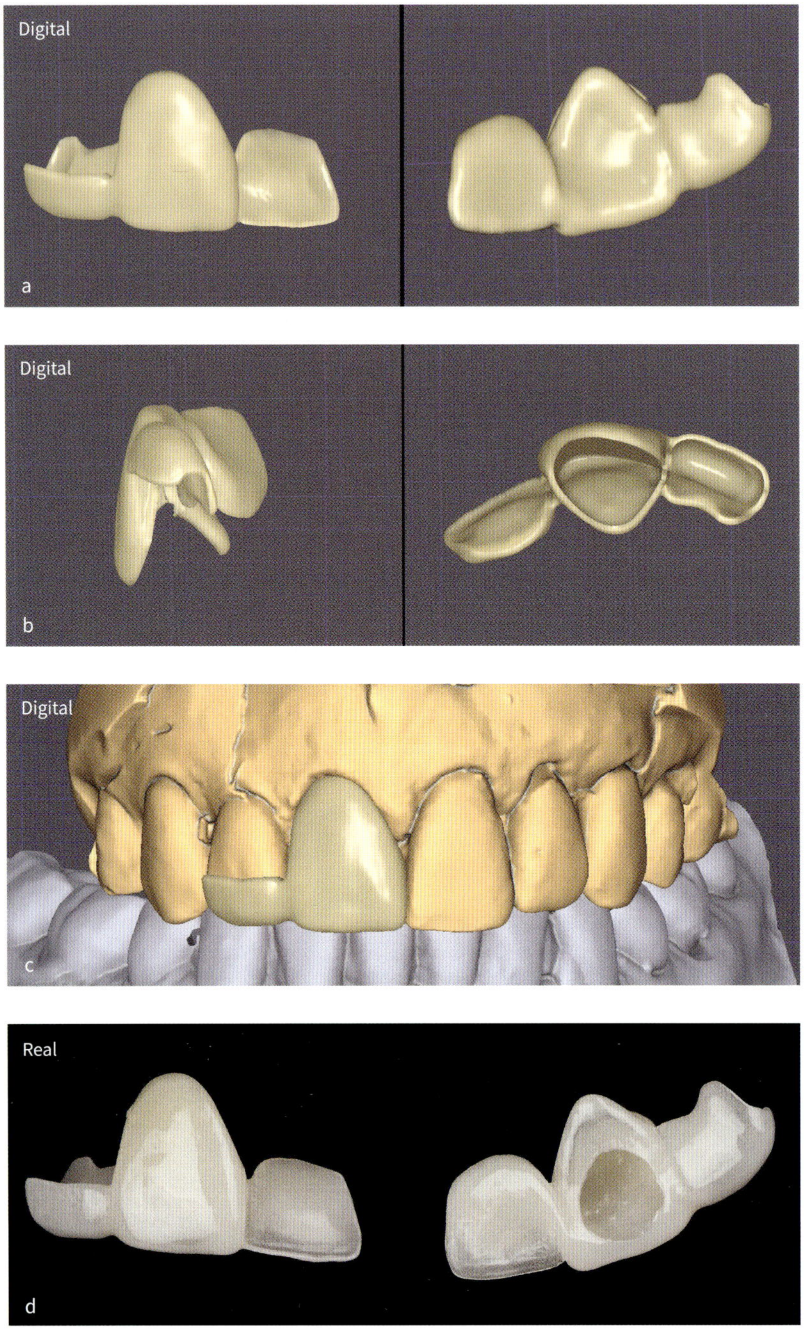

Figs 34a-d Digital design of a custom shell temporary for tooth 11 incorporating seating guides on teeth 11 and 21 to assist in positioning the shell during intraoral pick.up (a-b). Shell crown closely following the gingival margin to allow for adequate mucosal support (c). Shell temporary milled or 3D printed and manually polished prior to the surgical appointment.

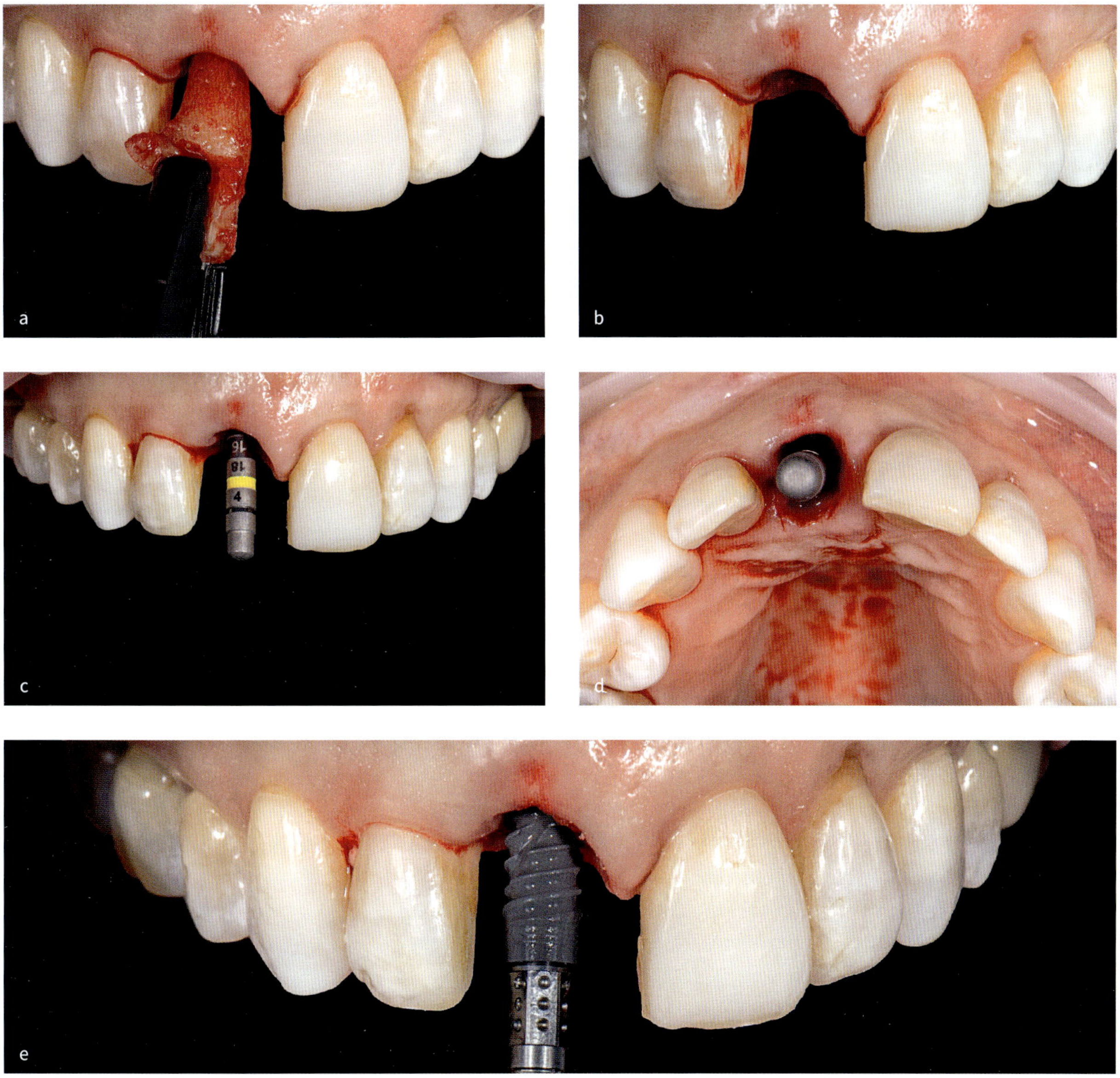

Figs 35a-e Surgical procedures for a type 1A protocol, including extraction of the root (a), socket evaluation and debridement (b), osteotomy preparation (c-d), and implant placement (e), followed by grafting gap with deproteinized bovine bone matrix.

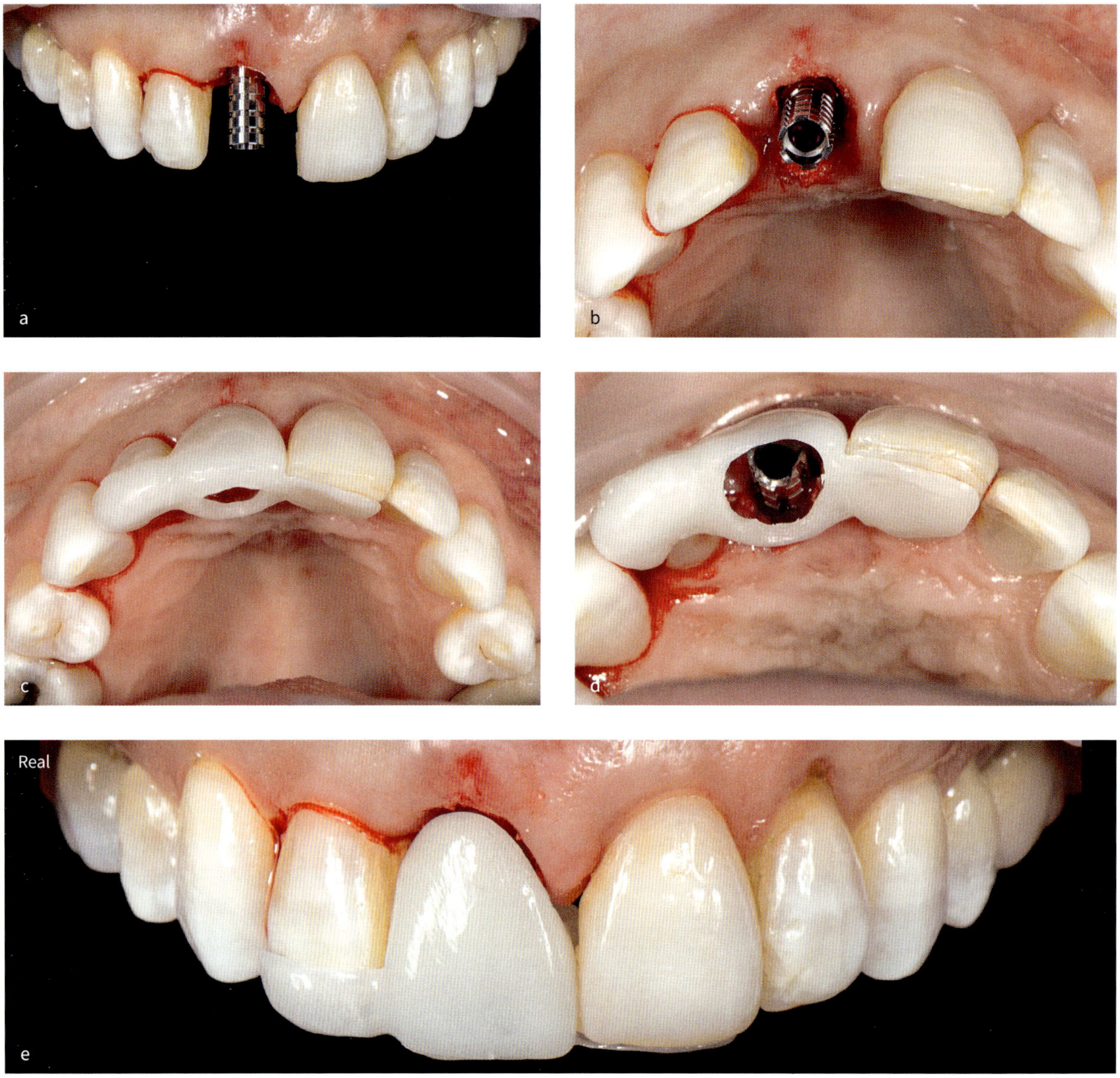

Figs 36a-e Titanium provisional abutment following implant placement (a-b). Custom shell temporary seated for intraoral spot pick-up with flowable composite or acrylic resin (c-e).

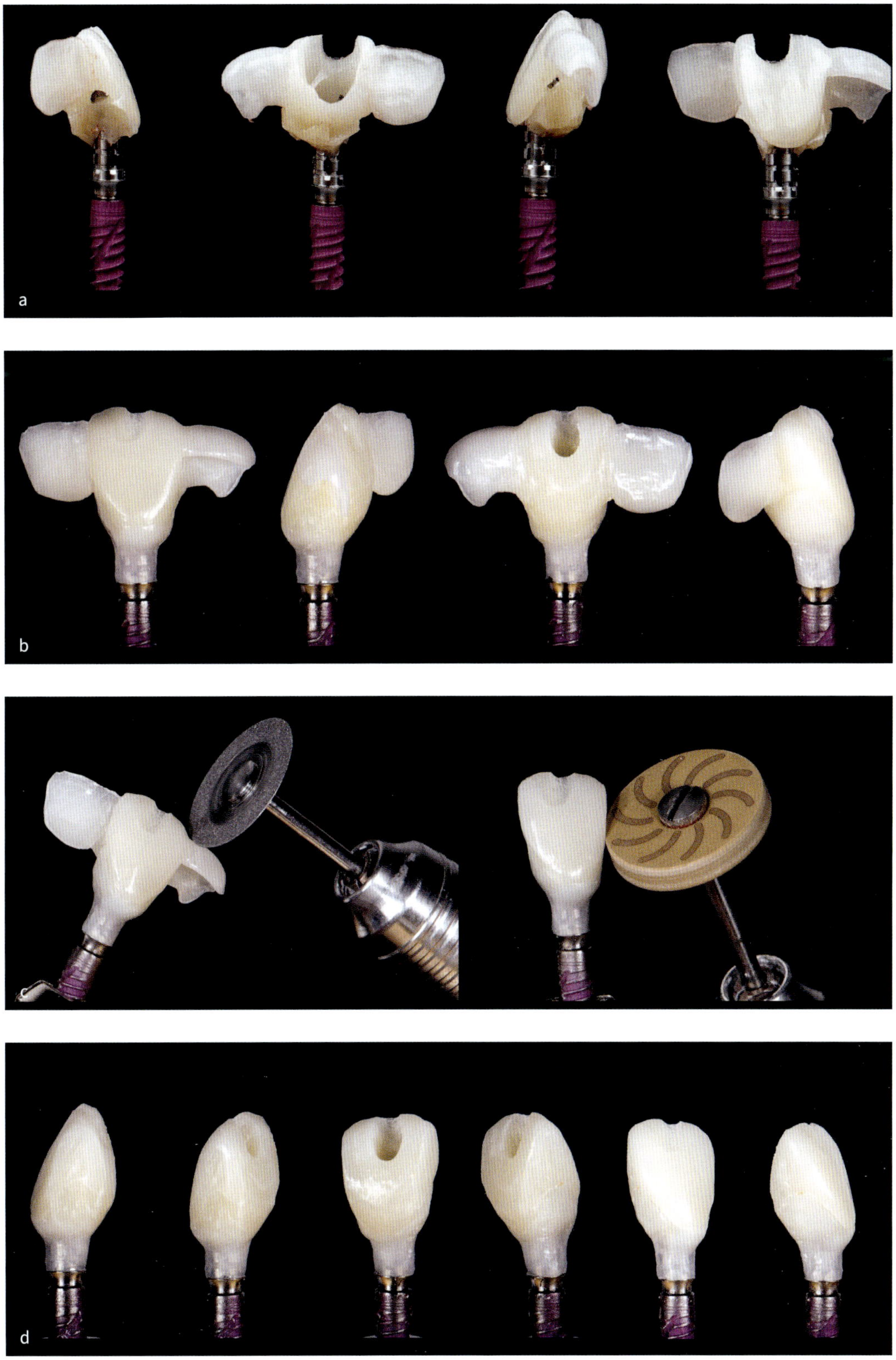

Figs 37a-d The abutment and shell temporary removed from the implant (a) with addition of acrylic resin or flowable composite to complete the connection between the abutment and shell temporary, as well as developing an adequate emergence. Shell temporary wings removed (c) and the completed provisional carefully shaped and polished with the aid of a laboratory analog (c-d).

Direct fabrication, customized submucosal profile, fully contoured crown (Figs 38 to 41). The main advantage of this option is that it avoids of the risk of infiltration of the restorative material at the surgical site during fabrication.

The first step involves obtaining a study model to capture the critical contour dimensions of the existing tooth, particularly the buccolingual and mesiodistal dimensions of the socket orifice. It is also critical to determine the distance between the mucosal margin and the planned position of the implant platform using CBCT imaging. With that information, flowable composite is added to a provisional abutment extraorally to create a tentative but close configuration of the submucosal profile. The subcritical contour must be as concave as possible on the facial and interproximal regions. The surface of the submucosal segment of the restoration must be polished extensively.

After immediate implant placement, the customized temporary abutment is carefully inserted to determine whether any minor adjustments are necessary for proper seating. The abutment must be modified meticulously to recreate a critical contour that properly supports the existing facial mucosal margin and papillae, and a subcritical contour as concave as possible to create sufficient space for the coagulum and graft material to ensure an optimal healing outcome.

When the submucosal contour of the provisional restoration meets the desired objectives, the next step is to make the crown portion using a previously fabricated silicone key. Commercialized temporary shells can alternatively be used to aid the fabrication of the submucosal profile. However, contour refinements will usually be necessary.

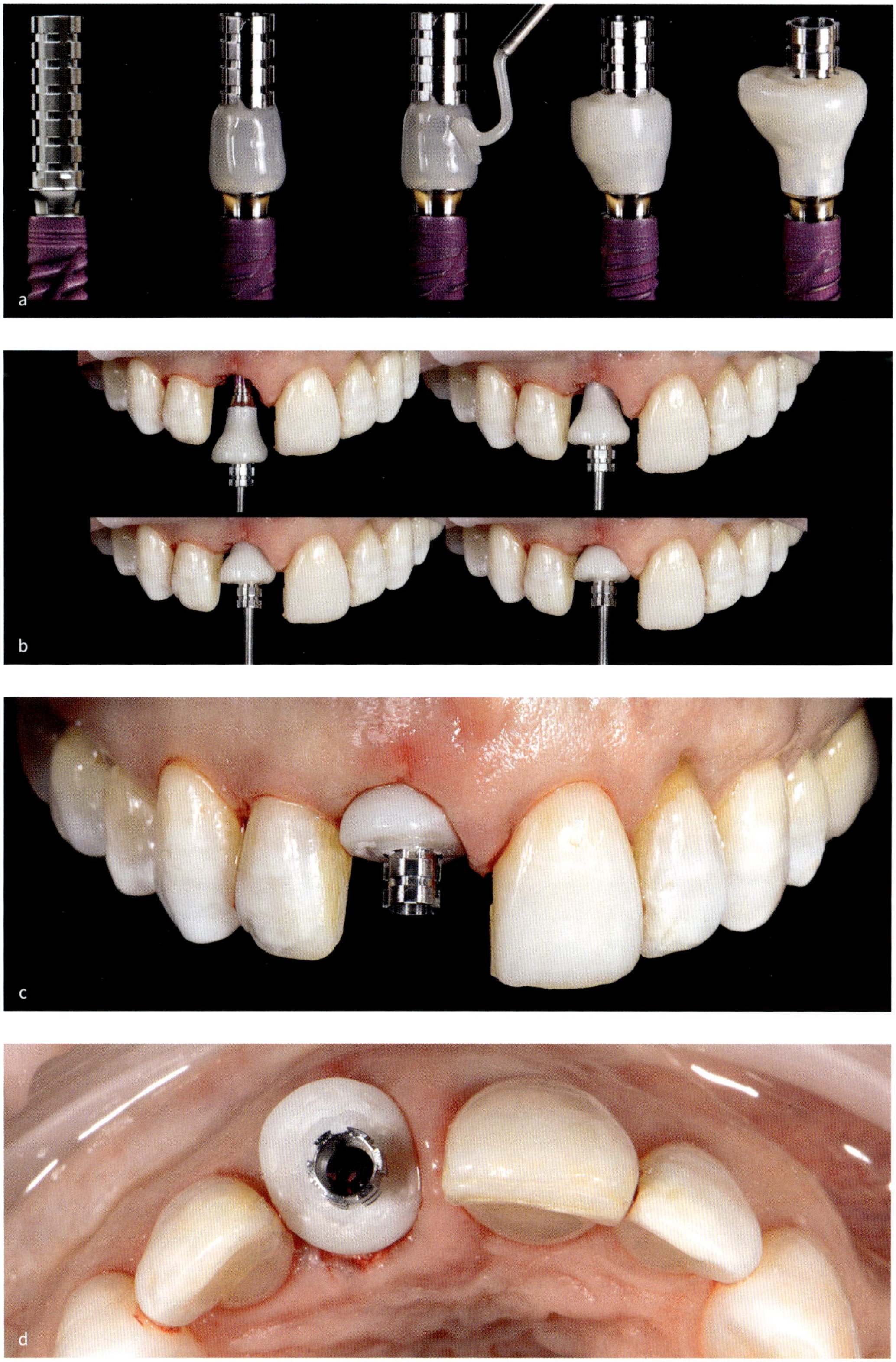

Figs 38a-d Creation of the emergence profile of the provisional restoration to conform to the marginal gingival contours of the extracted tooth using flowable composite (a-b). The socket sealed with the emergence profile aspect of the provisional restoration, which provides a barrier for the direct fabrication of the crown (c-d).

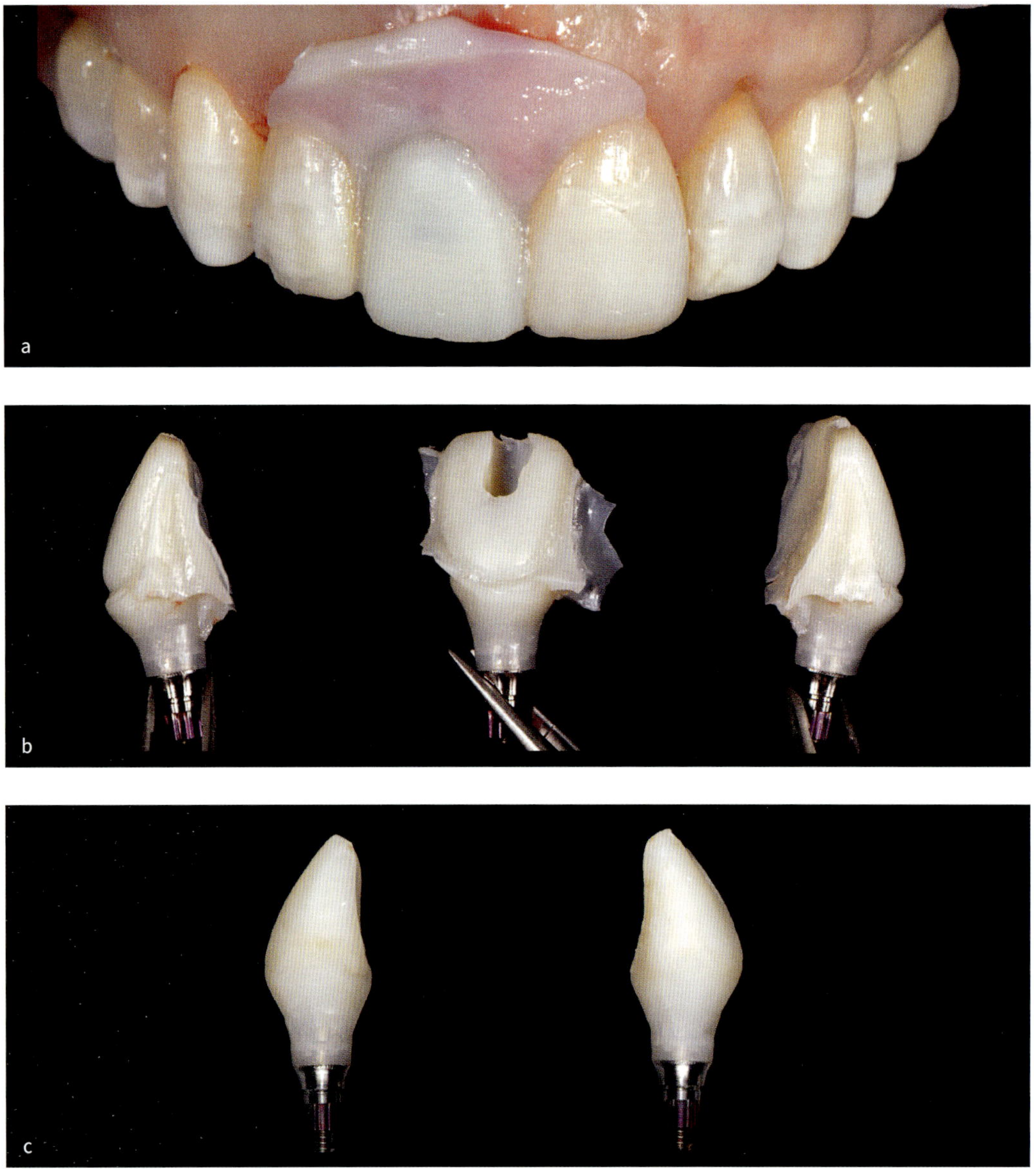

Figs 39a-c External matrix on a diagnostic wax-up used to create a direct provisional with bisacryl composite or acrylic resin (a-b). The socket must be sealed prior to this step; the screw access hole and undercuts must be blocked out. Restoration trimmed and polished extraorally to create the final restorative contours (c).

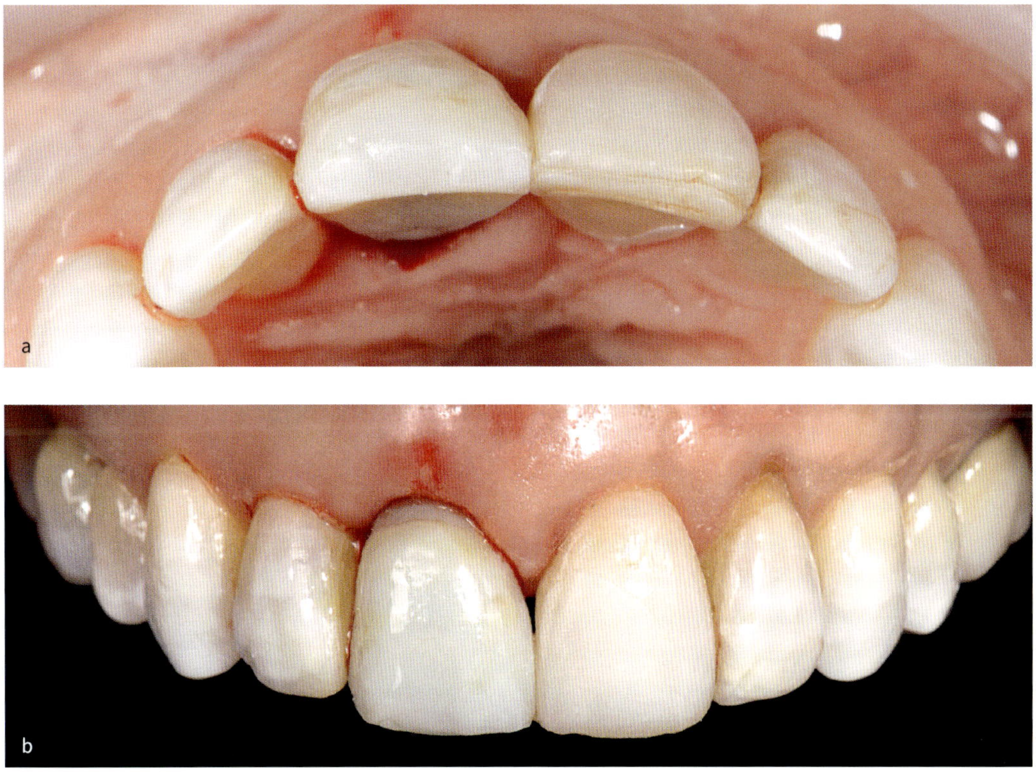

Figs 40a-b Immediate provisional delivered on the day of extraction and implant placement, demonstrating adequate support to the marginal mucosa and sealing of the socket.

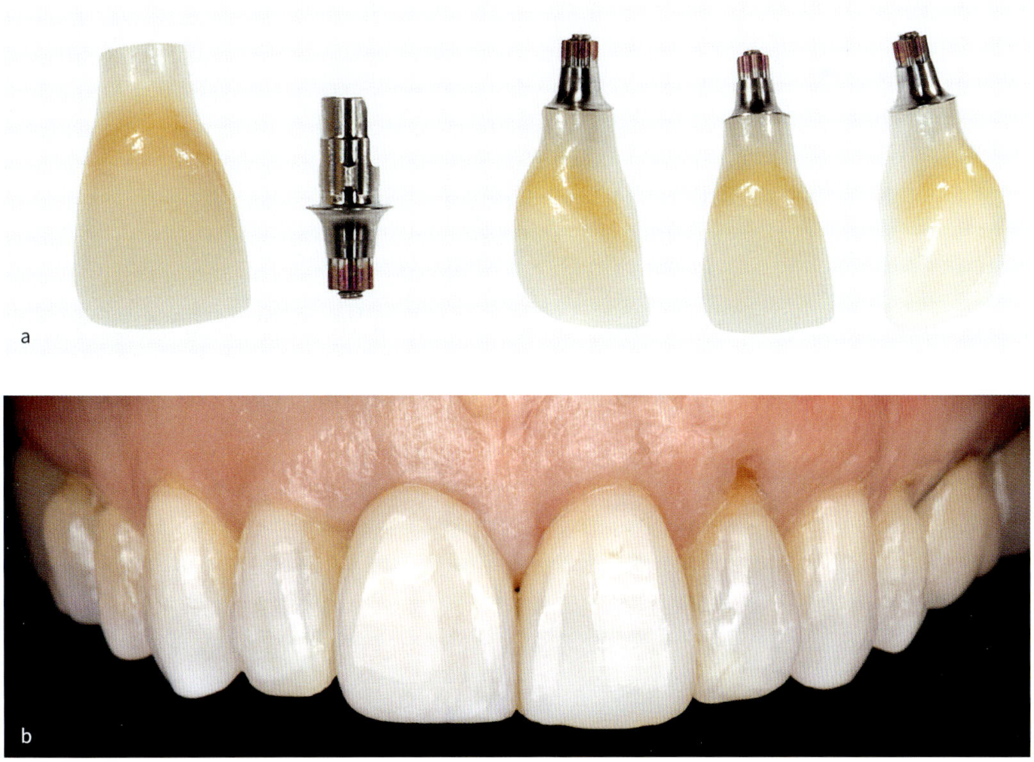

Figs 41a-b Definitive restoration fabricated after six months of healing using a titanium-base abutment and layered zirconia (a). Final restoration demonstrating an excellent esthetic outcome and peri-implant soft tissue health (b).

DIGITALLY PREFABRICATED CUSTOM PROVISIONAL

With a fully digital approach complete with virtual implant planning and guided implant surgery, a provisional restoration can be fabricated to completion based on the virtually planned implant position, as shown in Figures 42 and 43. This requires a highly accurate workflow, and there should not be any need to modify the planned implant position intraoperatively. Any slight modification or deviation of the implant position from the planned position will result in a provisional restoration that will need to be extensively modified or cannot be utilized at all (Hamilton and coworkers 2022). Advantages include a significant reduction of the time between the implant placement and the delivery of the restoration. This also reduces the risk of contamination of the surgical site.

The digital pathway also allows for the prefabrication of a digitally designed custom healing abutment that copies the shape of the existing tooth root at the level of the free gingival margin if a type 1C protocol is chosen, or the intraoperative criteria for immediate loading are not met. The CAD implant restoration contour can also be assessed relative to the bone anatomy visible in the CBCT to ensure that bone impingement is avoided.

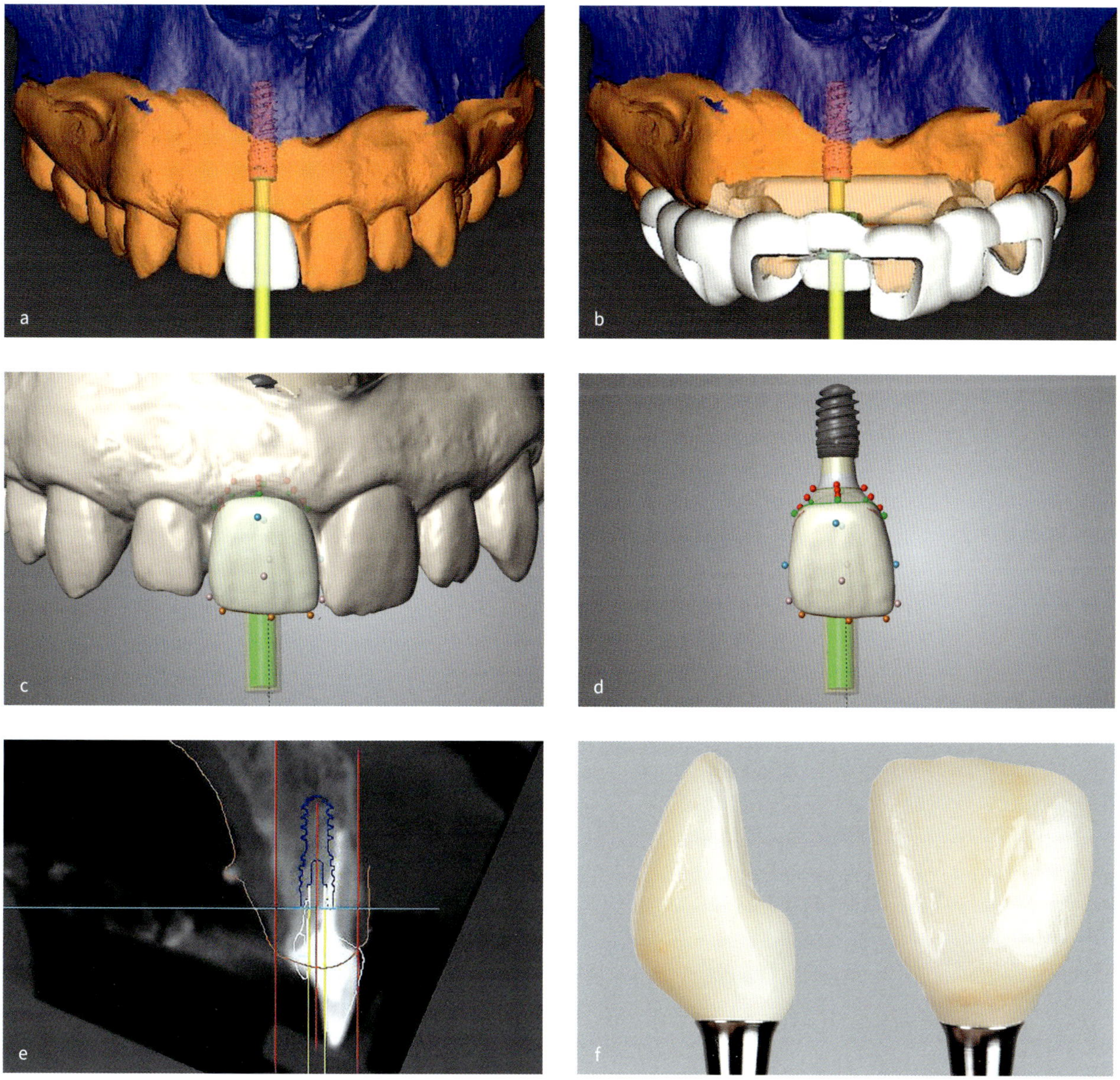

Figs 42a-f Digital fabrication of a custom implant-supported provisional crown based on the virtually planned implant position (a). Contours of the restoration guiding the restoratively driven implant position (b). Emergence profile designed in the CAD software, with the critical contour made to match the gingival outline of the tooth planned for extraction (c-d). Design of the restoration transferred to the virtual implant planning software to visualize any areas of potential bone impingement (e). Restoration milled in PMMA and cemented extraorally onto the titanium base abutment for the surgical appointment (f).

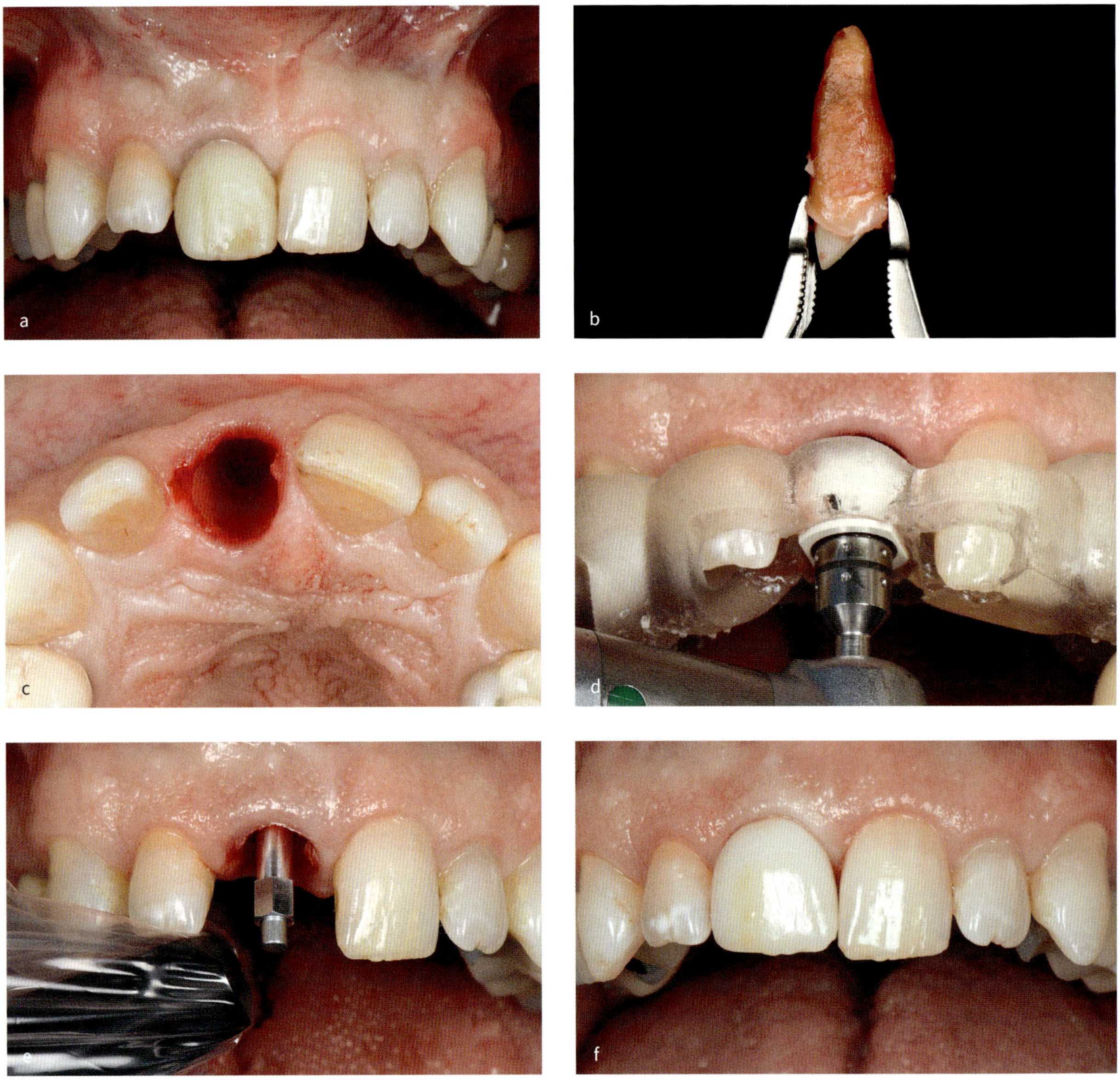

Figs 43a-f Tooth extracted on the day of the surgery (a-c). Implant placed following a fully guided surgical protocol (d). If the intraoperative criteria for immediate loading are met (e), the custom prefabricated provisional can be inserted (f). (Images courtesy of Dr Luiz Gonzaga.)

4.2.6 Restoration Insertion

Delivery of the restoration begins with careful removal of the healing abutment placed for the duration of the fabrication process to prevent graft material from entering the implant/abutment connection. The provisional restoration is carefully inserted and a radiograph taken to verify complete seating. The abutment screw of the provisional restoration is tightened according to the manufacturer's specifications for the provisional abutment selected and the access hole is closed with PTFE tape and a provisional plastic restorative material (Figs 44a-b and 45a-c).

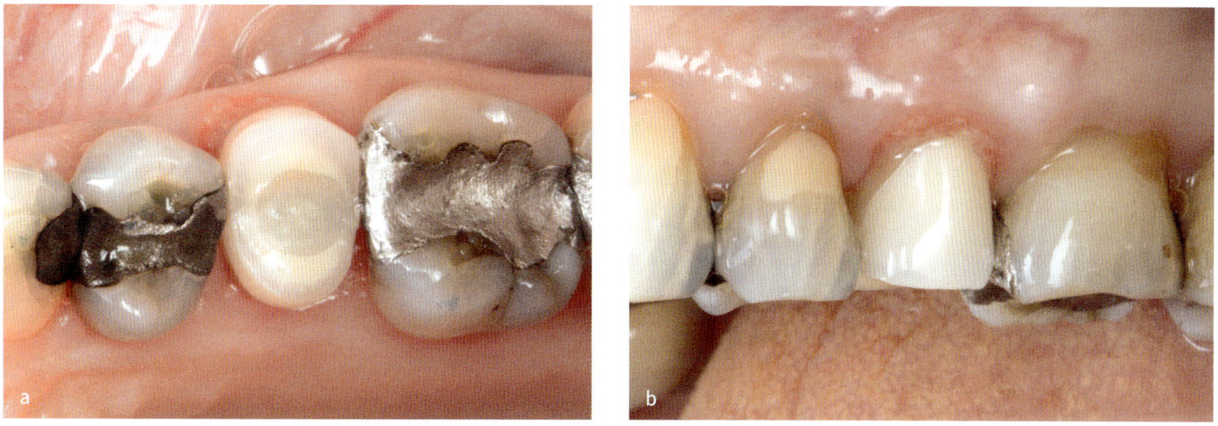

Figs 44a-b Immediate provisional crown two weeks after immediate implant placement and loading.

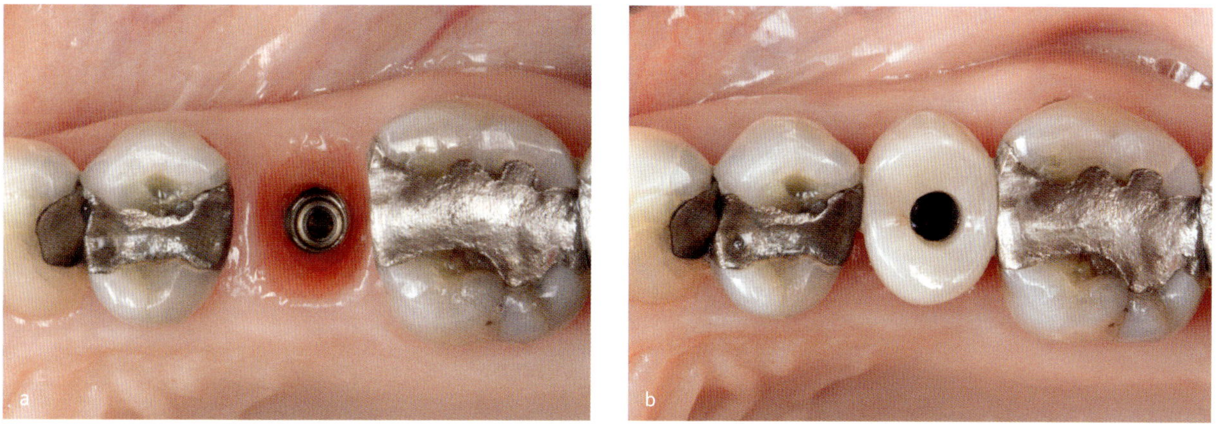

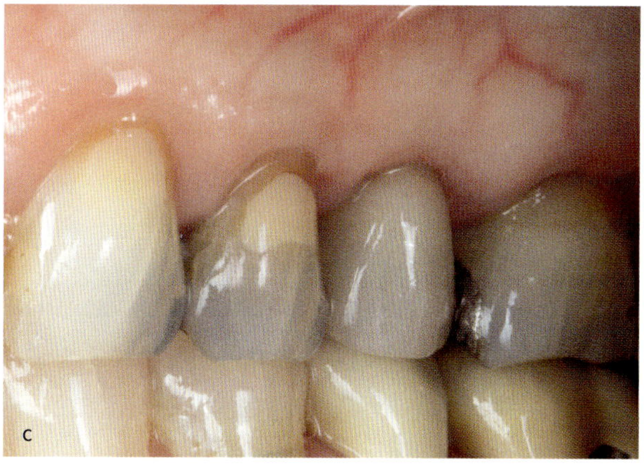

Figs 45a-c Final restoration and soft tissue contours nine months later.

4.2.7 Alternatives to Immediate Loading

In situations where indications for immediate loading are not present, or the intraoperative criteria for immediate loading are not met following immediate implant placement, the type 1C protocol is indicated. In this situation a customized healing abutment, or an appropriately shaped fixed pontic can be utilized to provide the same biological objectives as an immediate provisional restoration (Finelle and Lee 2017, Perez, Caiazzo and coworkers 2019, Alexopoulou, Lambert and coworkers 2021, Finelle, Popelut and coworkers 2021, Lilet, Desiron and coworkers 2022).

This technique is exemplified by the case of a maxillary left central incisor (tooth 21) that required extraction where adequate implant insertion torque was not achieved intraoperatively (Figs 46 to 56). Although the aim was for flapless immediate implant placement and immediate loading (type 1A), it was necessary to have a contingency plan in place in case of intraoperative complications that would preclude a type 1A protocol, such as damage to the facial bone plate necessitating flap elevation, or lack of sufficient initial stability for immediate loading.

The digital workflow in this case allowed for the prior construction of a custom healing abutment that could be used in conjunction with a removable provisional prosthesis as a back-up plan. The custom healing abutment provided ideal support for the supracrestal gingivae and contained the bone graft with the custom healing abutment following immediate implant placement.

Although this approach can be used in anterior sites, the technique is most beneficial in the posterior regions where the risk increases and the benefits of immediate loading are not as evident.

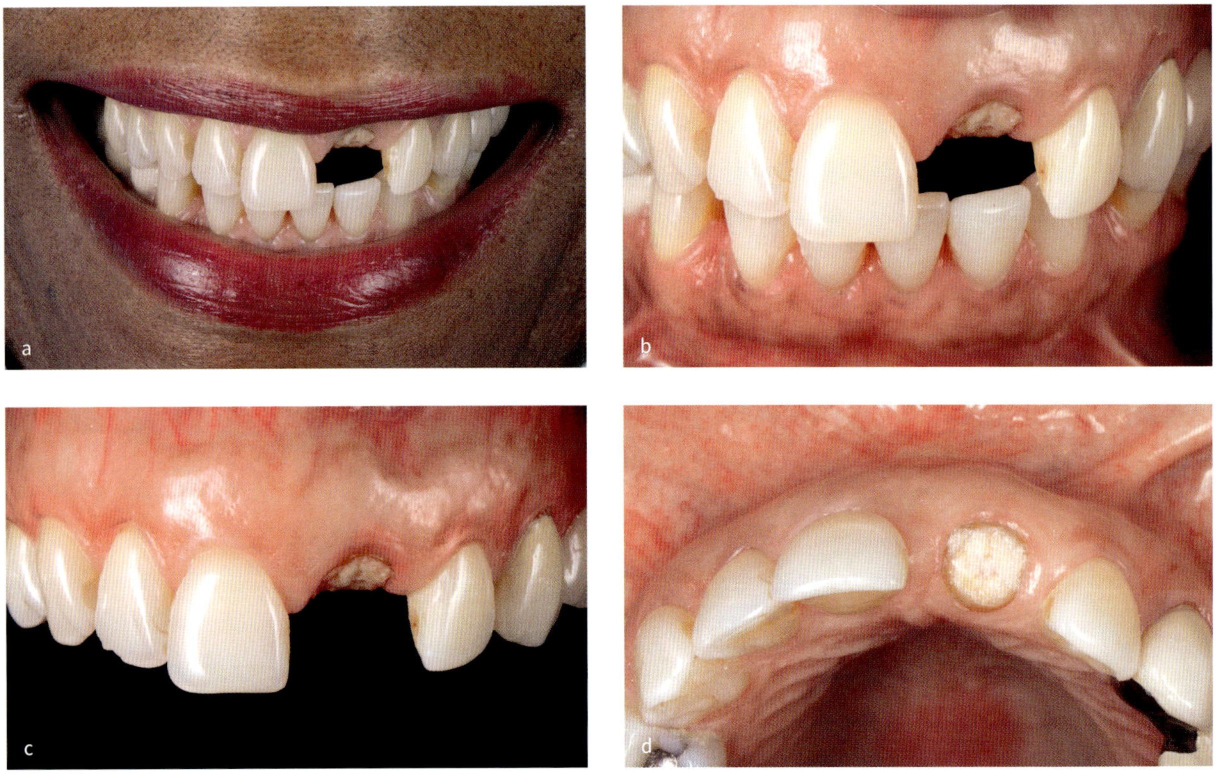

Figs 46a-d Preoperative clinical situation of tooth 21 in a patient with a medium-high smile line, thick gingival phenotype, and satisfactory gingival architecture.

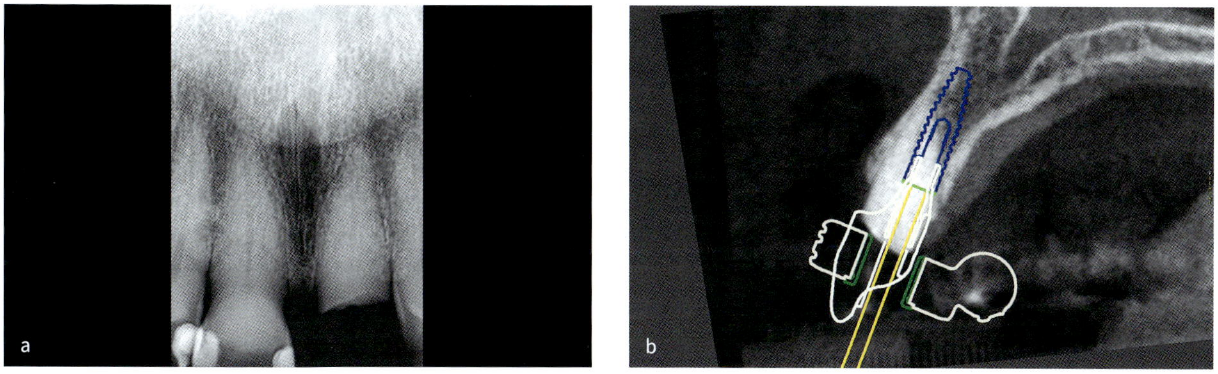

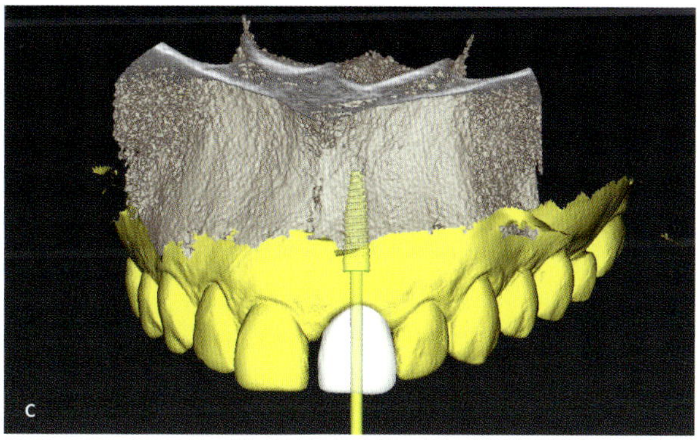

Figs 47a-c Radiographic evaluation with a periapical radiograph and a CBCT demonstrating a thick facial bone wall and adequate apical and palatal bone for primary stability.

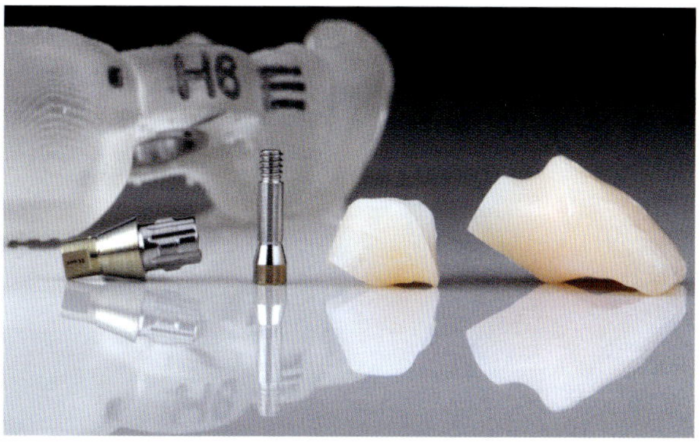

Fig 48 3D-printed surgical template, provisional crown, and custom healing abutment designed and manufactured based on the virtually planned implant position.

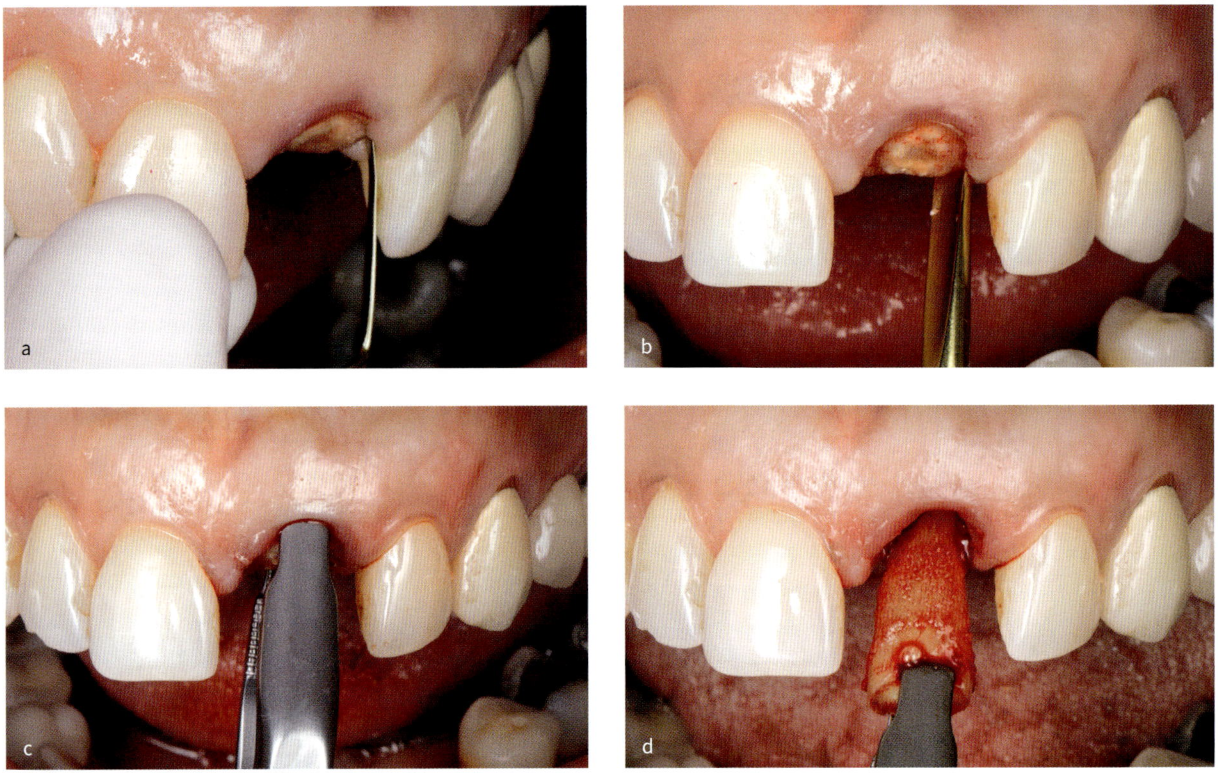

Figs 49a-d Minimally traumatic extraction of the root.

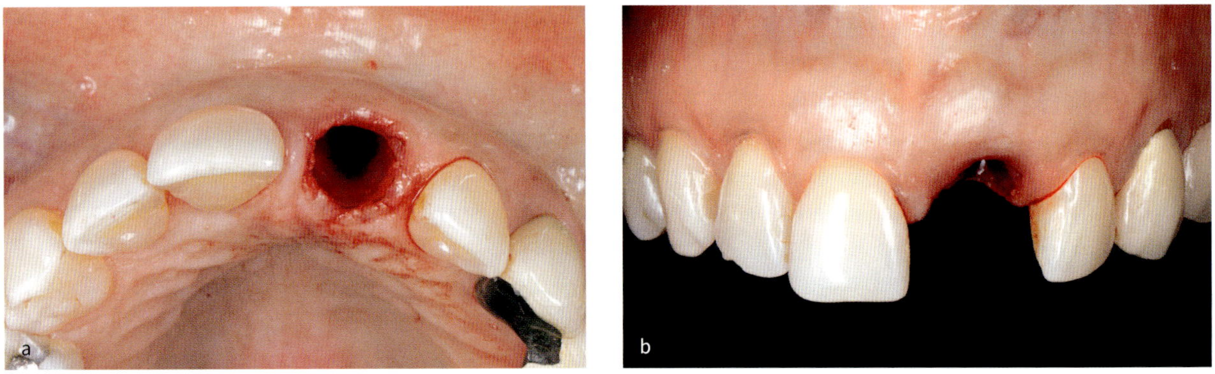

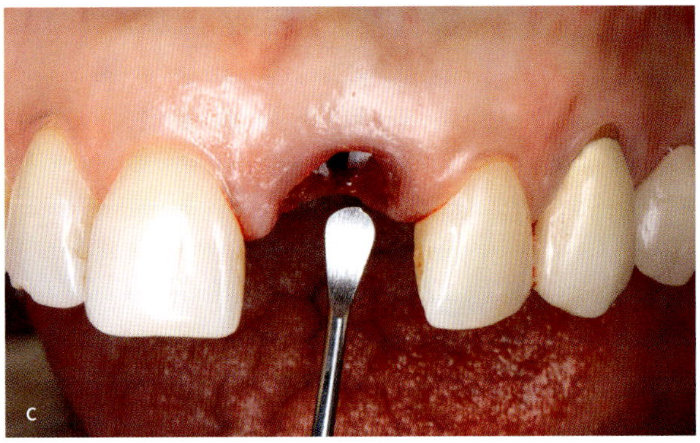

Figs 50a-c Socket walls and soft tissue intact and debrided with a curette to remove any remaining periodontal ligament.

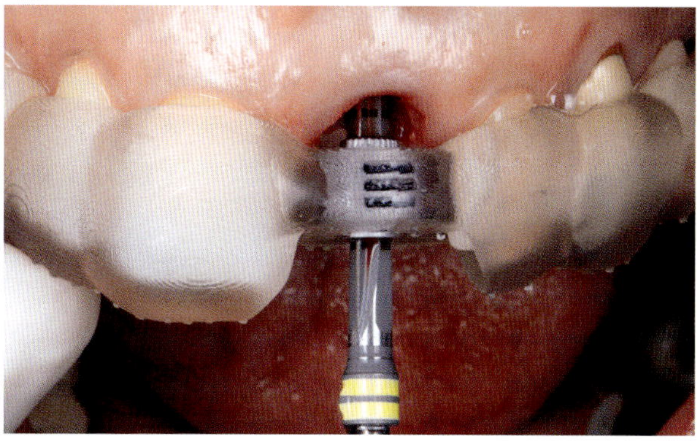

Fig 51 Guided osteotomy preparation.

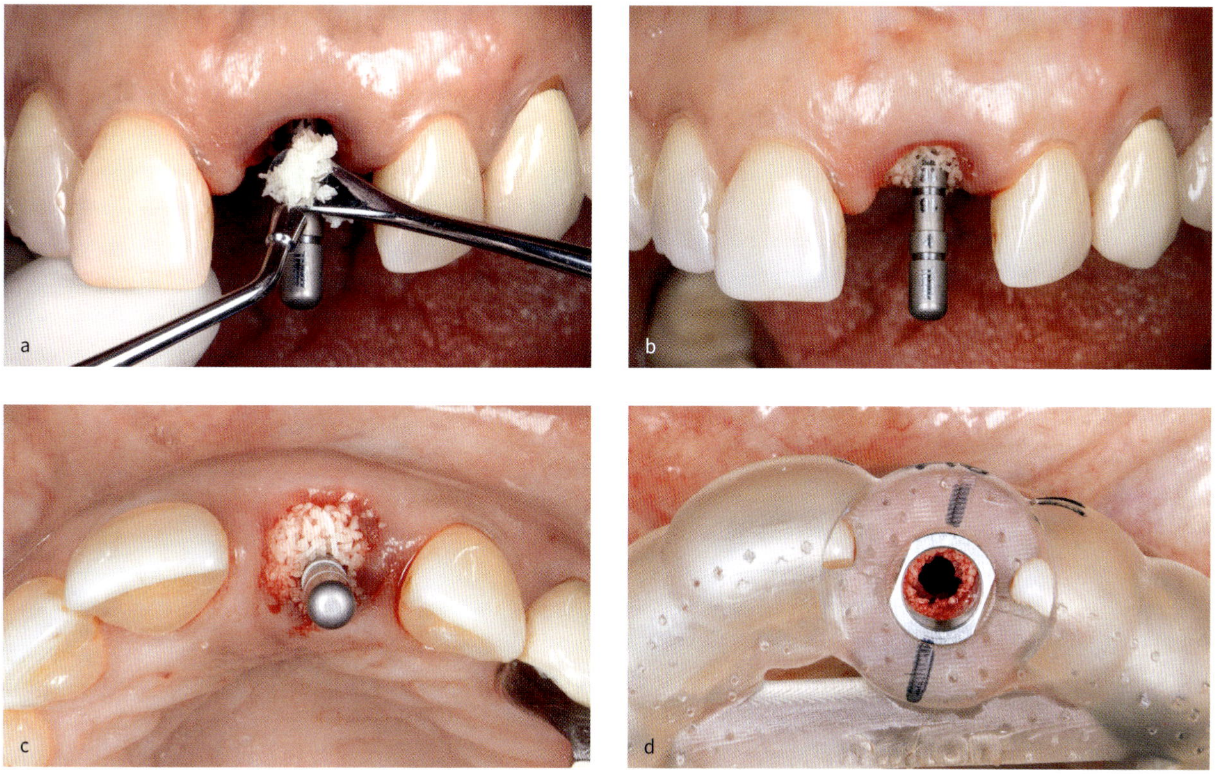

Figs 52a-d Placement of cortical freeze-dried bone allograft with a positioning indicator in place.

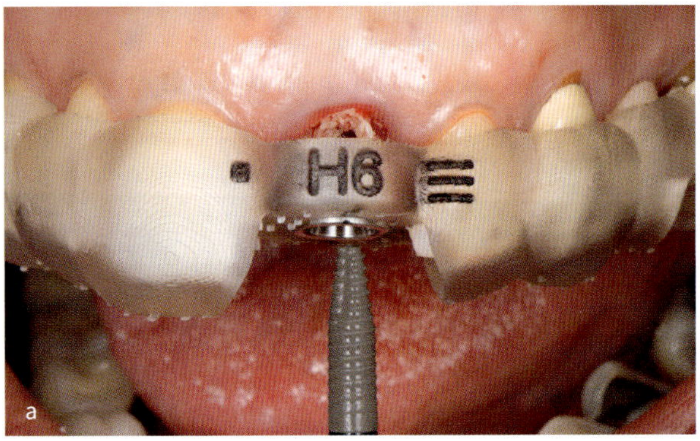

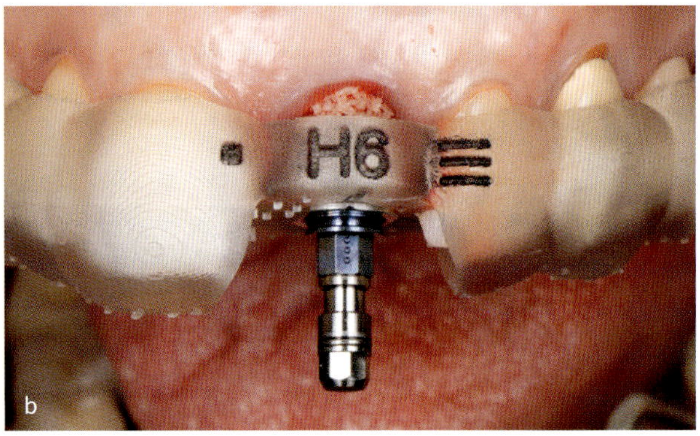

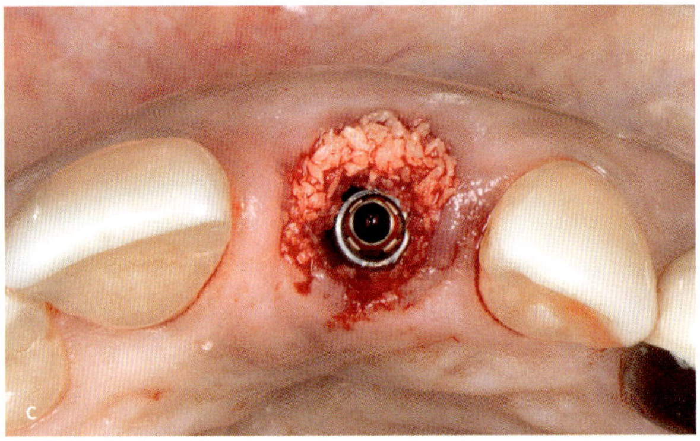

Figs 53a-c Guided implant placement and evaluation. Primary stability was achieved; however, an intraoperative insertion torque adequate for immediate loading was not. It was decided to switch to a type 1C treatment protocol (immediate implant placement and conventional loading).

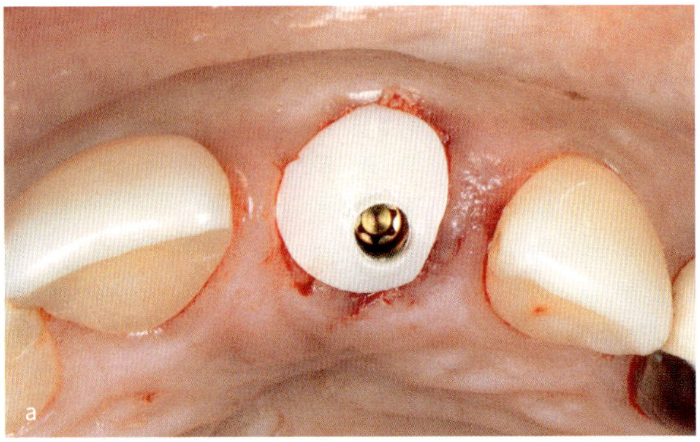

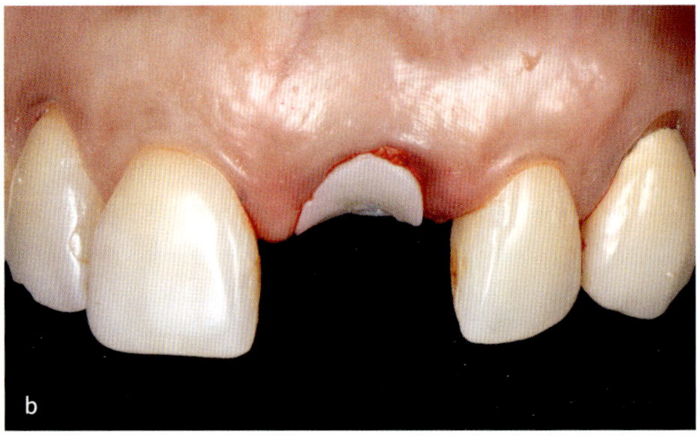

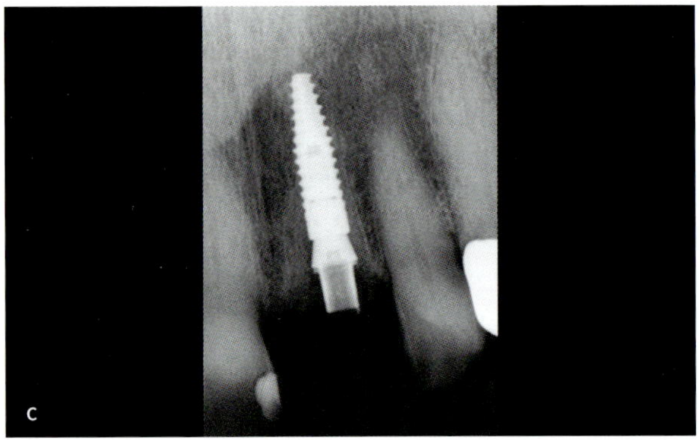

Figs 54a-c Insertion of the digitally prefabricated custom healing abutment and radiographic evaluation of complete seating.

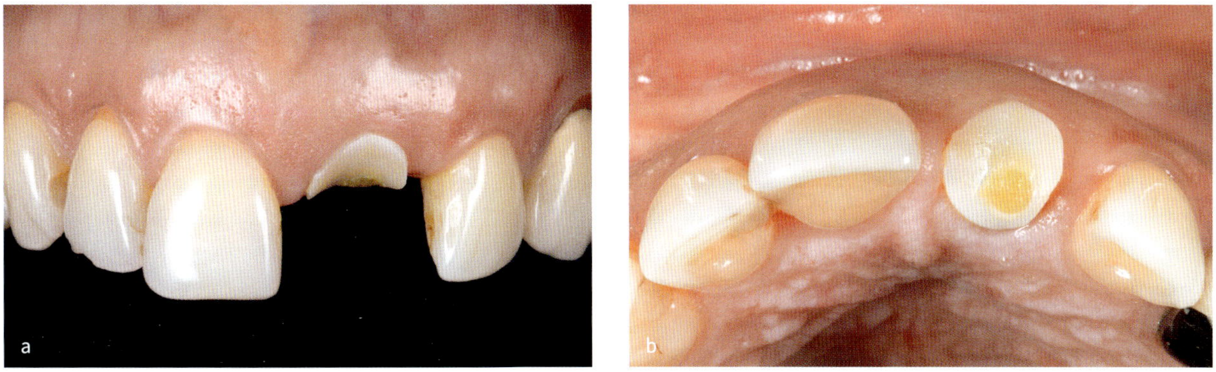

Figs 55a-b Eight week follow-up. Excellent soft tissue healing around the custom healing abutment.

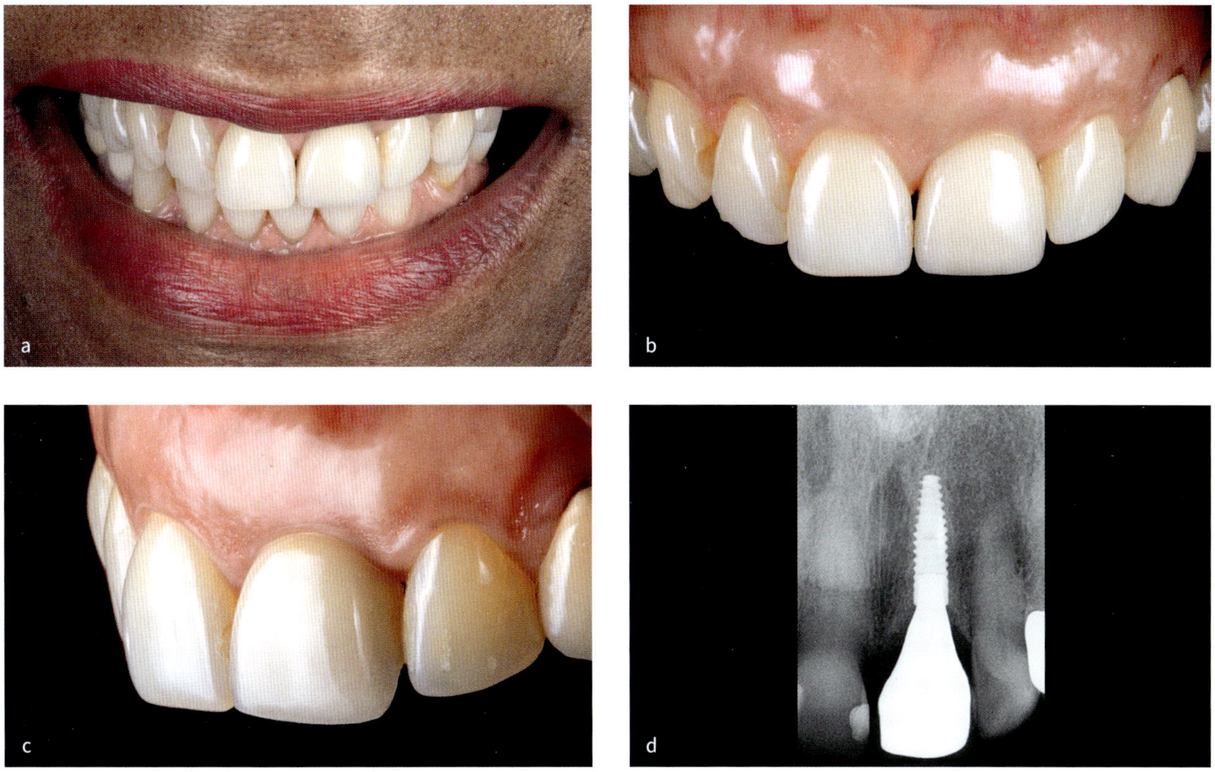

Figs 56a-d Twelve-month follow-up. No visible changes to the alveolar ridge contours, mucosal margin position or papillae, or marginal bone levels.

5 Clinical Case Presentations

5.1 Immediate Implant Placement and Immediate Provisionalization with a Prefabricated-Shell Provisional Crown

A. Happe

A healthy 31-year-old female patient presented with a failing maxillary left lateral incisor crown (Figs 1 to 3). The crown regularly loosened, and the remaining tooth was neither restorable nor rational to treat (Fig 4). The patient had a high smile line, a medium soft tissue biotype with a compromised mesial papilla (shorter than the contralateral one), and a horizontal scar in the buccal soft tissue as a result of past periapical surgery. Probing depths at the failing tooth and adjacent teeth were normal, in the range of 2–3 mm. The full-mouth bleeding score was 0% and the full-mouth plaque score was below 30%. The risk assessment for immediate implant placement and loading is outlined in Table 1, with several risk factors identified.

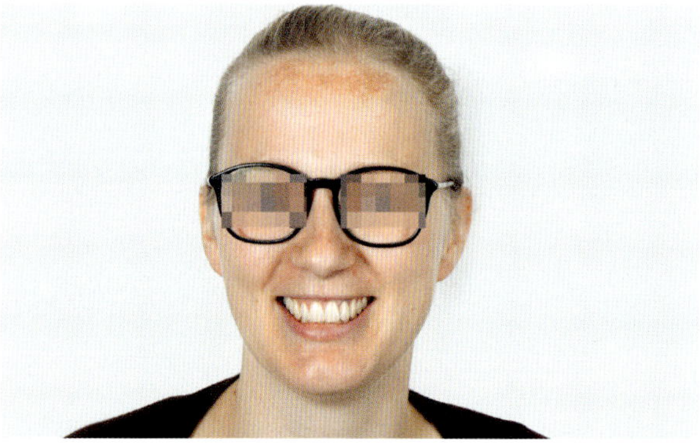

Fig 1 Portrait of the patient before treatment.

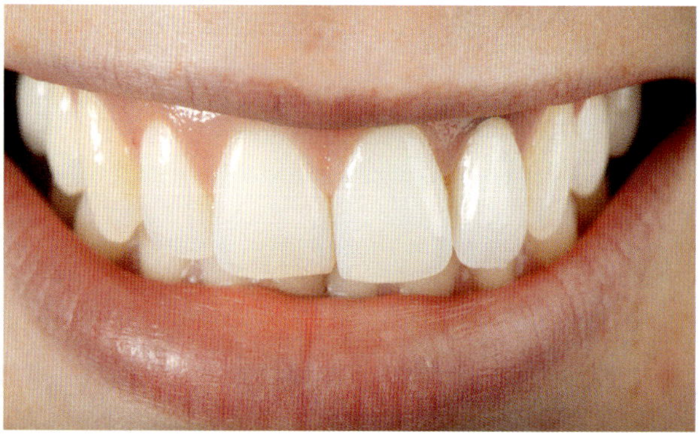

Fig 2 The patient's smile.

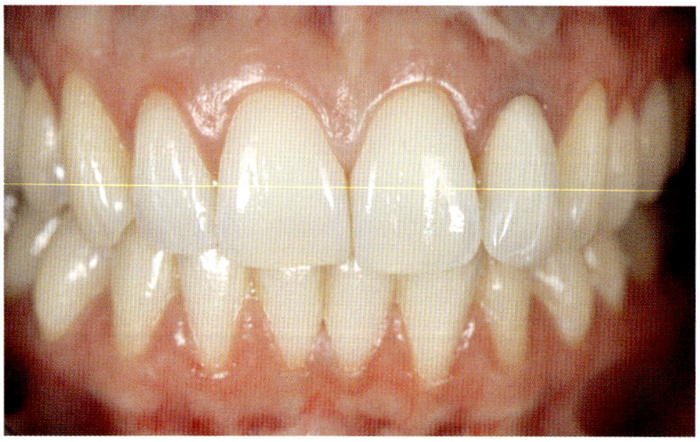

Fig 3 Failing maxillary left lateral incisor. The mesial papilla is shorter than the contralateral one.

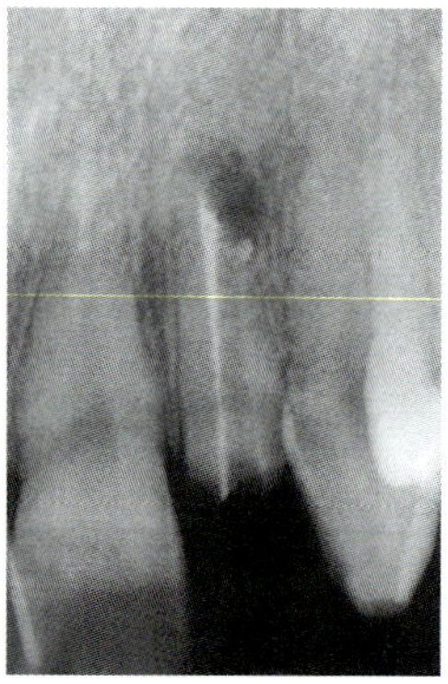

Fig 4 Periapical radiograph of the failing tooth.

Table 1 Risk assessment for immediate implant placement in single-tooth sites

	Low risk	**Medium risk**	**High risk**
Preoperative assessment			
Patient-related			
Medical status	Healthy, uneventful healing		Compromised healing
Esthetic risk	Low/medium esthetic risk	High esthetic risk	Significant esthetic compromise expected
Site-related			
Gingival-margin position	No recession	Minor gingival recession	Gingival recession ≥ 2 mm
Soft tissue quality	Thick gingival phenotype	Thin gingival phenotype or limited keratinized gingiva	No keratinized gingiva
Bone anchorage	Sufficient bone anchorage to achieve primary stability		Lack of bone anchorage to achieve primary stability
Facial bone wall	≥ 1 mm facial bone thickness	Facial bone plate < 1 mm thickness, or small fenestration or dehiscence defect	Significant fenestration or dehiscence of facial bone
Need for a mucoperiosteal flap	Sufficient alveolar bone for a flapless approach		Need for flapped bone augmentation
Socket position within alveolar envelope	Socket within the alveolar bone envelope		Socket and facial bone wall protruding out of the bone envelope
Presence of endodontic infection	No infection	Chronic periapical infection	Acute infection
Presence of periodontal disease	Periodontally healthy	Controlled periodontal disease	Active periodontal disease
Planning implant position	Ideal three-dimensional position with axis exiting through the cingulum or incisal edge		Facially positioned or over-angulated implant or excessive implant depth
Gap between buccal bone and planned implant position	≥ 2 mm	1–2 mm	< 1 mm
Intraoperative assessment			
Extraction	Minimally invasive tooth extraction	Damage to surrounding soft tissue, including severed/detached papillae	Significant damage to soft tissue and surrounding bone
Primary implant stability	Primary stability achieved		Lack of primary stability
Final implant position	Ideal three-dimensional position achieved		Facially positioned or over-angulated implant or excessive implant depth

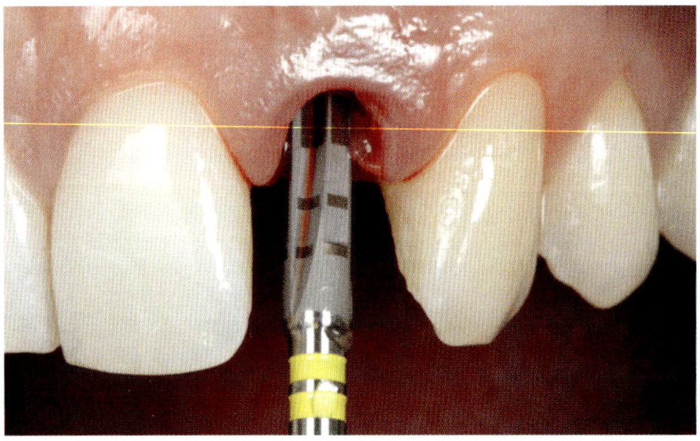

Fig 5 Preparing the implant bed with the 2.8 mm drill.

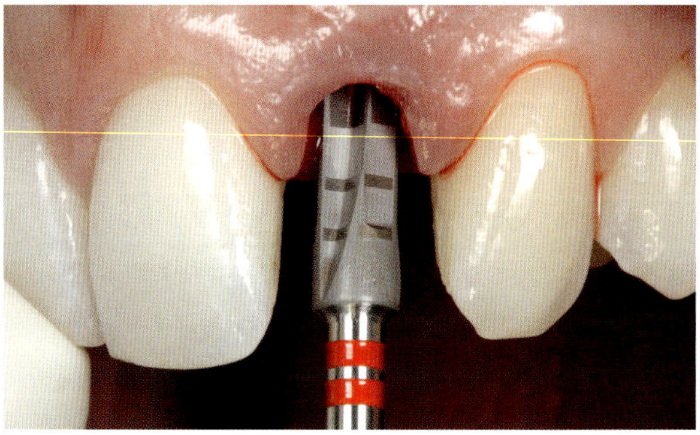

Fig 6 Preparing the implant bed with the 3.5 mm drill.

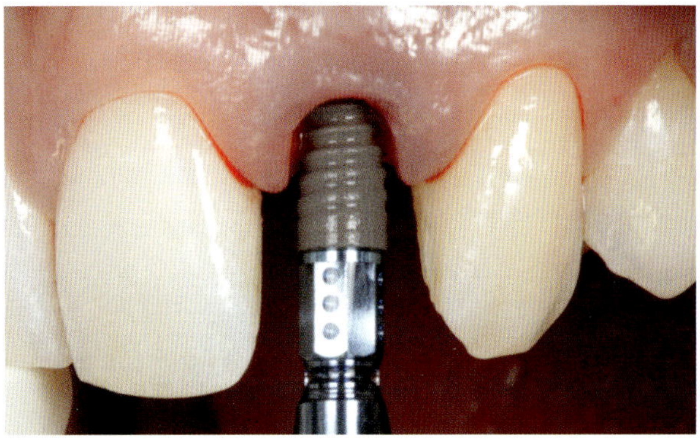

Fig 7 Inserting the implant in the palatal socket compartment.

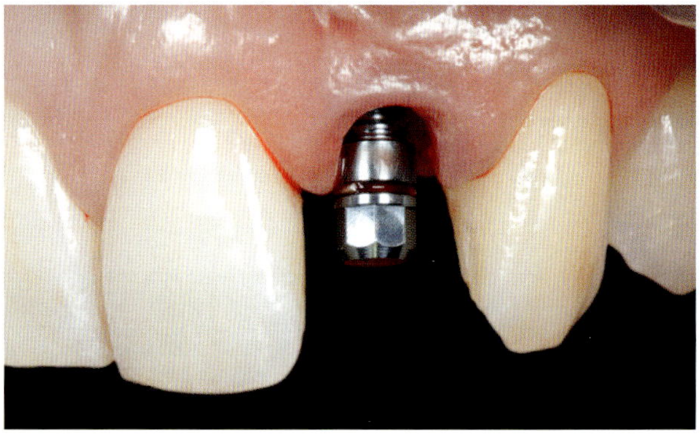

Fig 8 Final vertical position, 3.5 mm apical to the future soft tissue margin.

The periapical radiograph showed that an apicectomy had been performed in the past. There was sufficient bone height apical to the residual root for anchoring an implant, especially an implant with a tapered apical design that requires less bone width.

At the time of treatment, the quality of the available CBCTs was highly influenced by radiopaque root-canal filling material, which is why a CBCT was indicated to evaluate the buccal plate in this case. Today's CBCT devices use filters to reduce artifacts, and CBCTs in combination with planning software are now standard diagnostic tools for immediate implant treatments. The high smile line and the thin gingival phenotype were the only critical aspects identified preoperatively.

Based on the clinical examination, immediate implant placement and immediate provisionalization as per the type 1A placement and loading protocol (Gallucci and coworkers 2018) were planned. Immediate provisionalization was chosen to prevent collapse of the papillae in this high-scalloped soft tissue situation. Conventional impressions were taken for diagnostic casts and to facilitate a veneer for immediate provisionalization.

SURGICAL PHASE

After local anesthesia, the remaining root was carefully extracted. The buccal wall remained intact even though its thickness was less than 1 mm. A minimally invasive split-thickness flap was elevated on the facial aspect of the lateral incisor and extended beyond the mucogingival junction using a 15C blade and a tunneling knife in order to create pouch for a connective tissue graft (Tsuda 2011).

A Straumann BLT implant (diameter 4.1 mm, length 14 mm; Institut Straumann AG, Basel, Switzerland) was placed in the palatal socket compartment, leaving a gap of 2 mm between the implant and the buccal plate. The apical aspect of the implant was anchored in the apical third of the socket in the palatal bone. The implant diameter was chosen to reflect the size of the socket and the need for adequate primary stability, keeping a minimum distance of 1.5 mm from the adjacent teeth and 2 mm from the buccal plate.

The implant exhibited good primary stability at a torque of > 35 Ncm. The gap was filled with a combination of demineralized bovine bone mineral (90%) and collagen (10%) (BioOss Collagen, Geistlich, Wolhusen, Switzerland) (Figs 5 to 8).

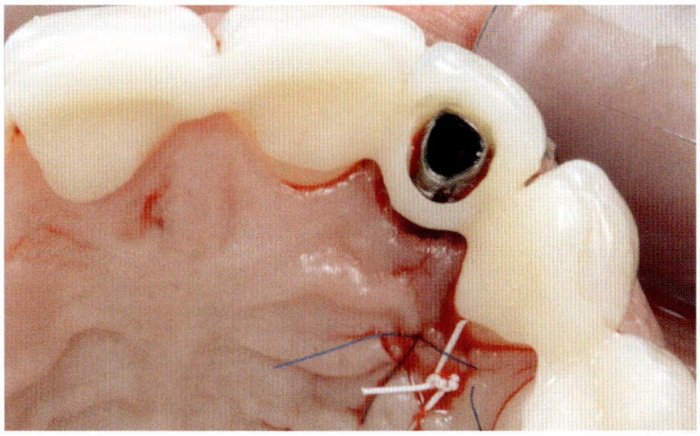

Fig 9 Prefabricated shell provisional with extensions for three-dimensional orientation.

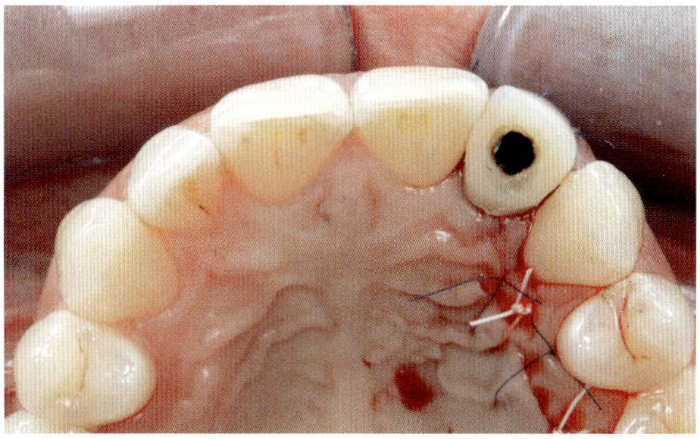

Fig 10 Final screw-retained provisional crown in place. Incision of the CTG donor site on the palatal aspect.

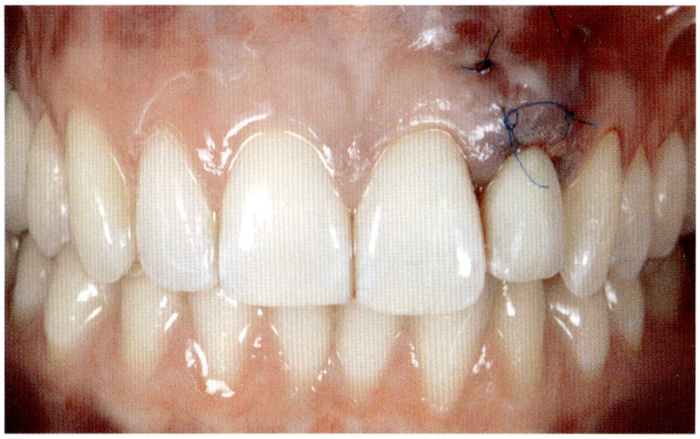

Fig 11 Postoperative view. The buccal tissue covers the CTG, secured with microsurgical sutures.

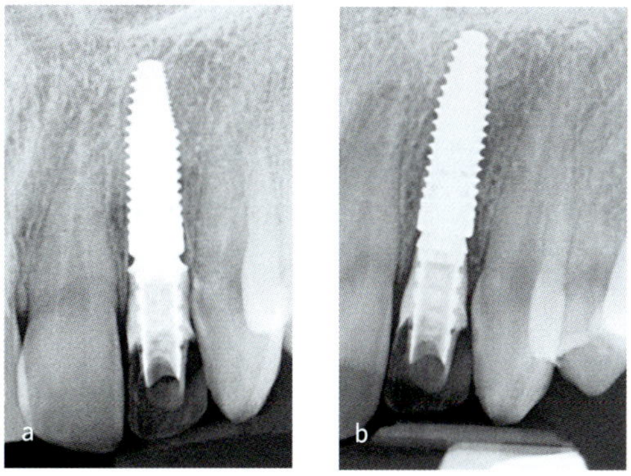

Figs 12a-b Periapical radiograph with the provisional in place. Due to the scalloping, the abutment was in contact with the adjacent bone (a). Situation after narrowing the apical aspect of the transmucosal part of the temporary restoration (b).

A subepithelial connective tissue graft was harvested from the premolar area of the palate on the same side of the maxilla, inserted in the buccal pouch, and secured with 6-0 monofilament sutures (Figs 9 to 11).

A temporary abutment made of titanium was used as the basis for the provisional restoration. Provisional resin veneers extended onto the adjacent teeth as supporting wings to provide guidance for three-dimensional orientation and an accurate fit (Fig 9). It was cemented with flowable temporary resin and polished, resulting in a screw-retained provisional crown. The additional wings were then removed, and the restoration was polished and cleaned (Fig 10).

In the submucosal area, the volume of the provisional crown was reduced to the diameter of the implant to avoid interference with the supporting tissues of the adjacent teeth. The coronal aspect of the transmucosal area of the provisional flared progressively to support the marginal mucosa (Figs 12a-b). Current research has shown that the shape to the transmucosal component may directly influence crestal bone remodeling (Souza and coworkers 2018; Finelle and coworkers 2015). The screw-retained temporary restoration was placed and the occlusion adjusted to maintain shimstock clearance in maximum intercuspation with no excursive contacts (Fig 11).

The site was left to heal for twelve weeks (Figs 13 and 14).

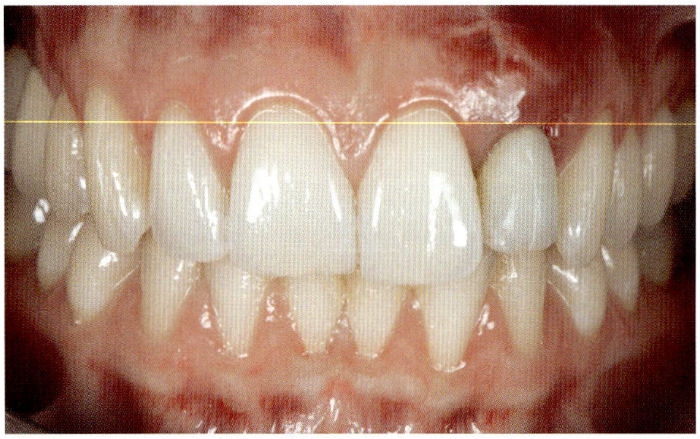

Fig 13 After two weeks of healing.

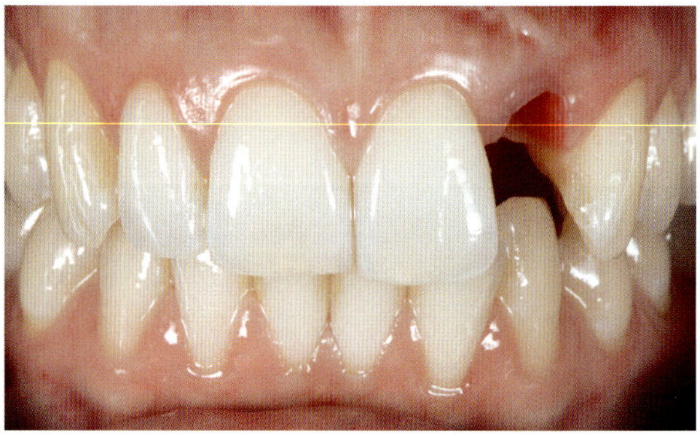

Fig 14 After twelve weeks of healing. The emergence profile was preserved.

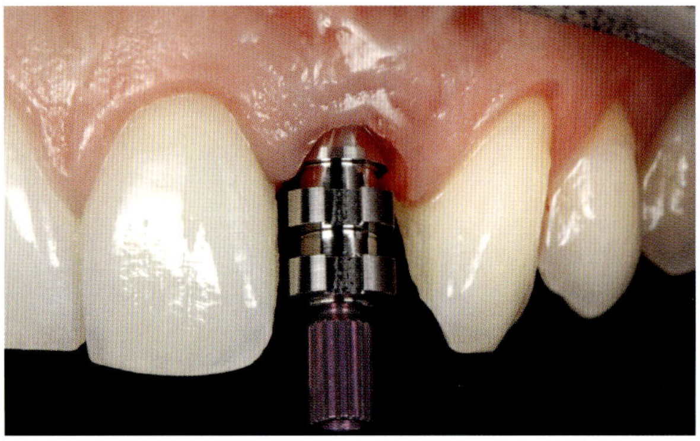

Fig 15 Impression coping in place.

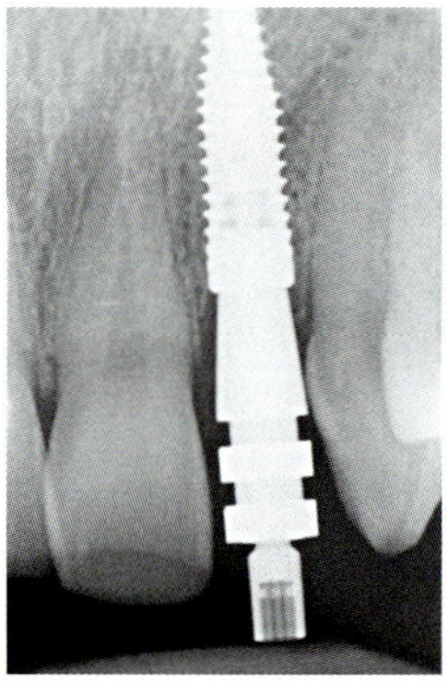

Fig 16 Radiographic control of the seating of the impression coping.

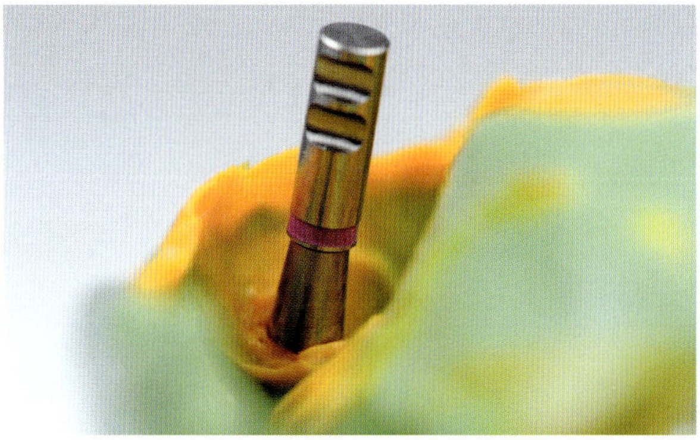

Fig 17 Conventional impression with silicone. Analog for fabrication of the cast in place.

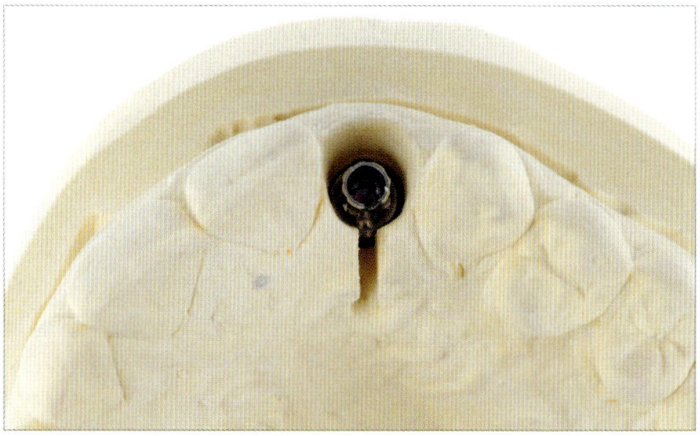

Fig 18 Variobase on the master cast.

PROSTHETIC PHASE

Following uneventful healing, the temporary restoration was removed and osseointegration was verified clinically. A conventional impression was taken for the final reconstruction (Figs 15 to 17). Digital dental photography was employed for shade taking and to communicate the anatomy of the contralateral reference tooth.

A zirconia framework was individually designed to fit on a prefabricated titanium base (Variobase; Institut Straumann AG) (Fig 18) using a CAD/CAM workflow. To ensure an adequate thickness of the ceramic veneer, the zirconia framework was designed based on a wax-up with the help of a silicone index (Figs 19 and 20).

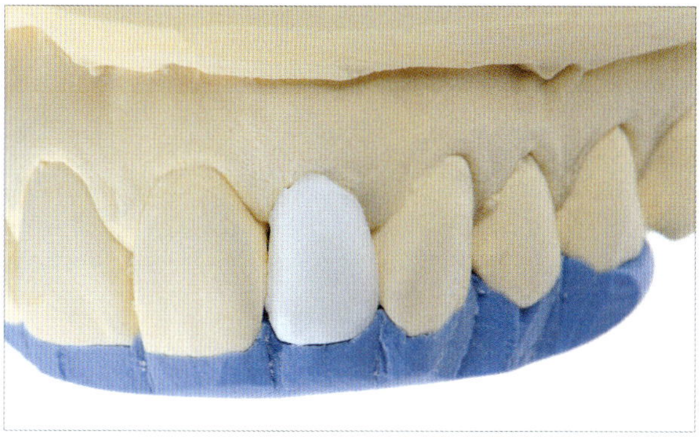

Fig 19 Wax-up and silicone index.

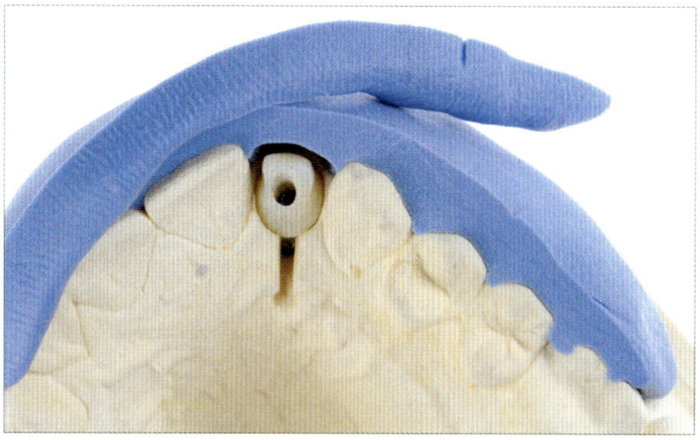

Fig 20 Silicone index and zirconia framework on the cast.

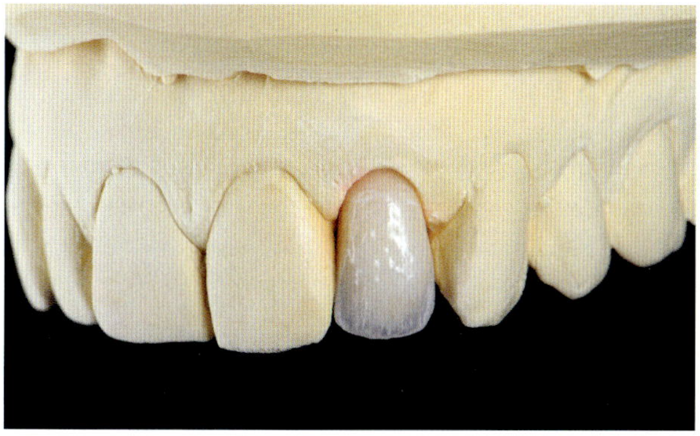

Fig 21 Ceramic build-up.

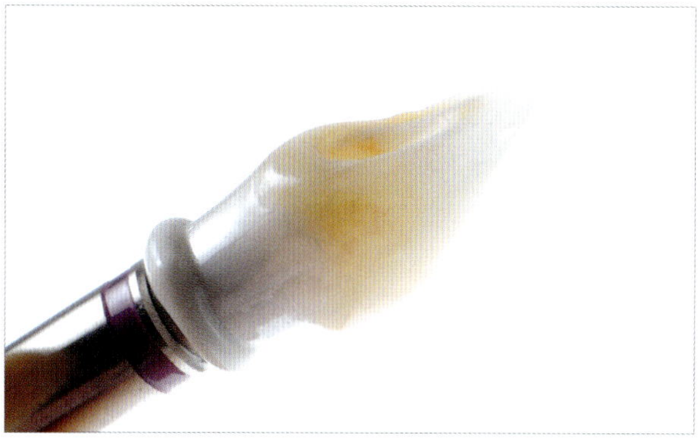

Fig 22 After the try-in, the crown was cemented to the titanium base.

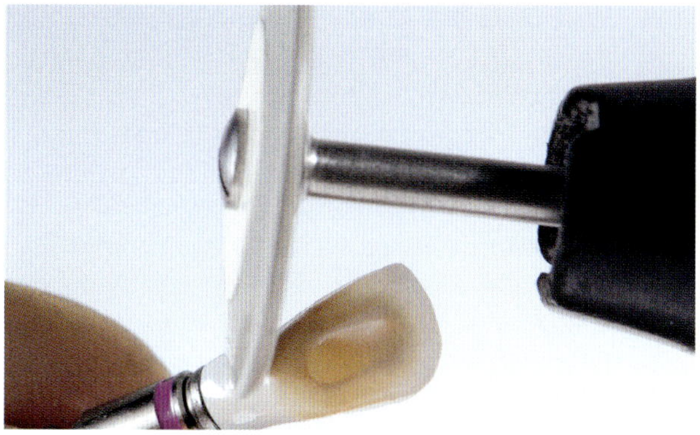

Fig 23 Finishing the submucosal area with rubber abrasive.

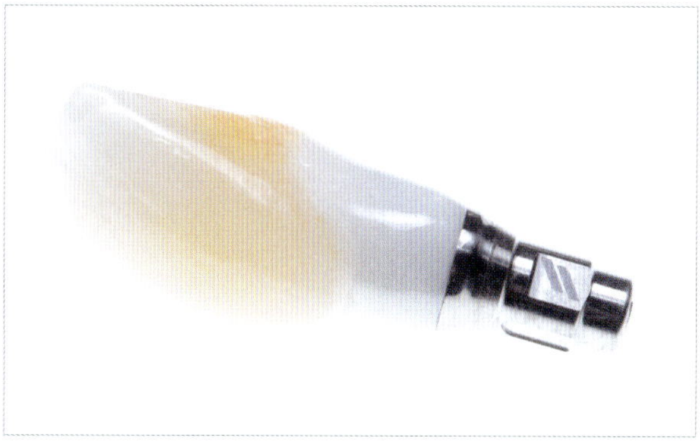

Fig 24 Final restoration ready for placement.

The framework was designed to provide sufficient support for the ceramic veneering to ensure adequate mechanical resistance. The crown was built up and fired, and the restoration was tried in, adjusted, and secured to the titanium base with resin cement, following the manufacturer's recommendations (Figs 21 and 22). The submucosal parts of the reconstruction, made of unveneered pure zirconia, were not polished to a high gloss, but smoothed with rubber abrasives and cleaned using a method proposed by Happe and coworkers (2015) (Figs 23 to 25).

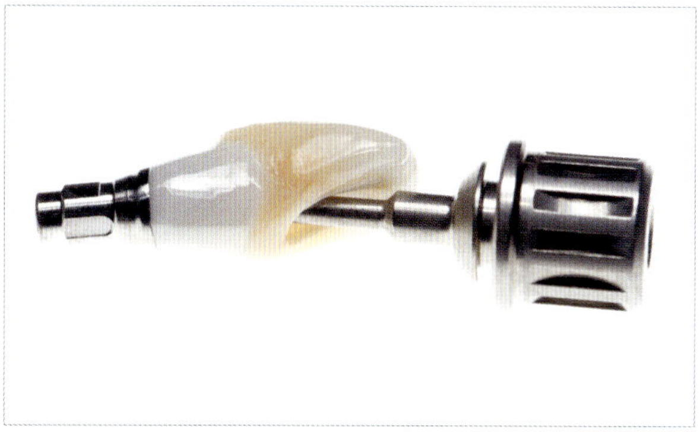

Fig 25 The screw access is visible on the palatal aspect of the restoration.

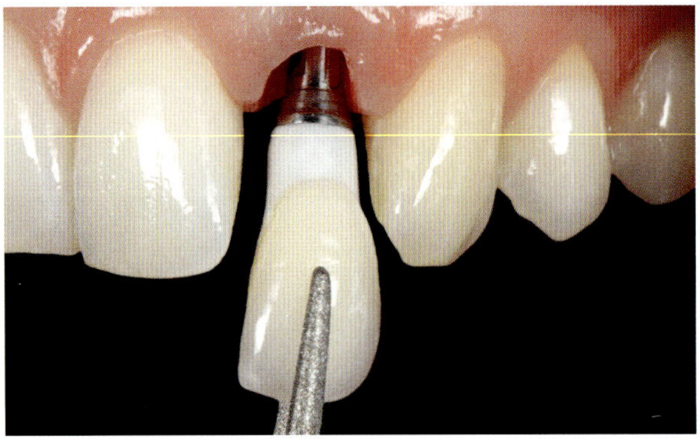

Fig 26 Placement of the screw-retained restoration.

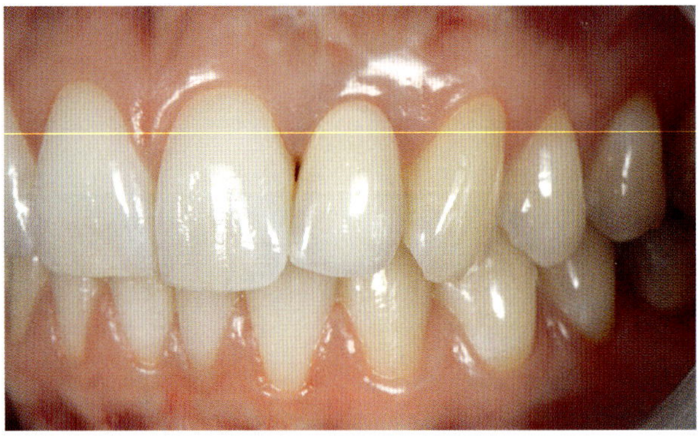

Fig 27 Lateral view several weeks after placement.

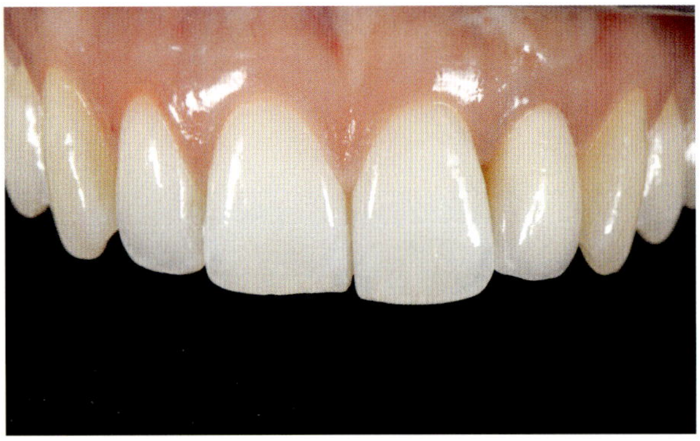

Fig 28 Frontal view of the treatment result.

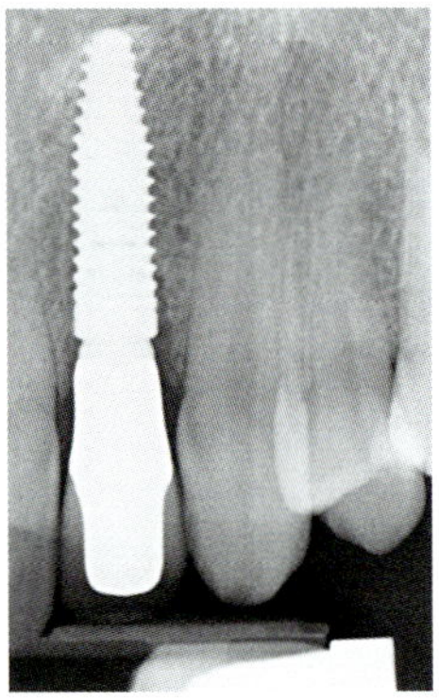

Fig 29 Periapical radiograph on delivery of the restoration.

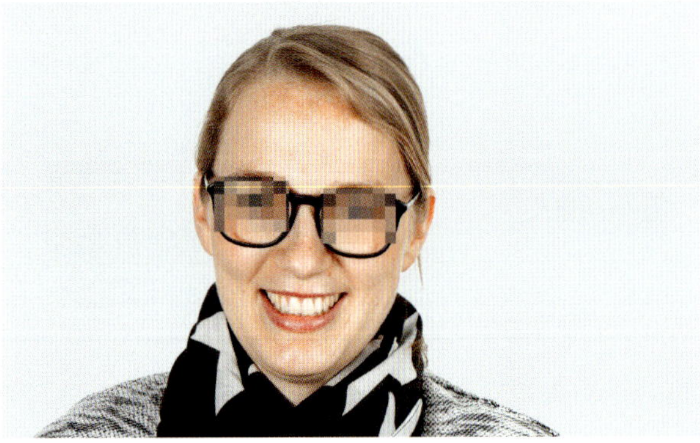

Fig 30 Portrait of the patient after the treatment.

The screw-retained restoration was placed and the abutment screw tightened to 35 Ncm as per the manufacturer's specifications. The screw was protected with PTFE, and the screw access hole was closed with composite resin. The occlusion was adjusted and the palatal surface polished to a high gloss. A periapical radiograph was taken to document the baseline situation for comparison with future radiographic follow-up (Figs 26 to 29).

The patient received oral hygiene instructions and was scheduled for oral hygiene and maintenance at twelve-month intervals. She was very happy with the result and the esthetic appearance of her implant-supported restoration (Fig 30).

At the five year follow-up, the periapical radiographs confirmed the presence of stable crestal bone (Fig 33). The clinical examination showed healthy mucosa with no signs of bleeding on probing or inflammation (Figs 31 to 34).

DISCUSSION

This case demonstrates the successful application of the concept of immediate implant placement with immediate provisionalization. While an implant diameter of 4.1 mm may seem rather wide for a lateral incisor, the anatomy of the socket permitted successful placement at a high torque while respecting the minimum distances to the adjacent teeth and the buccal plate.

Moreover, the nature of the implant/abutment connection provided a horizontal offset (platform switching), making it possible to install an implant of the selected size.

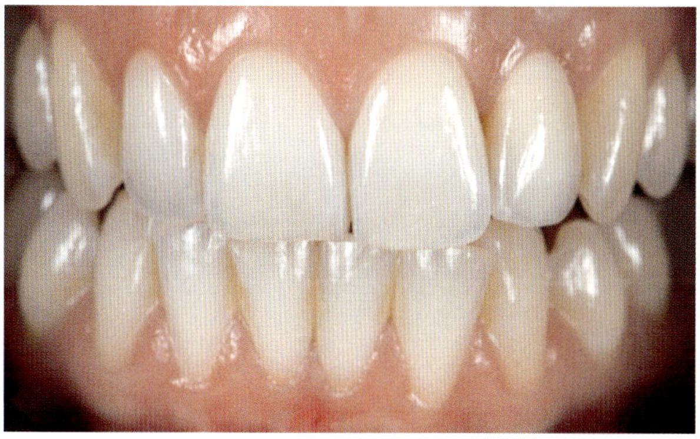

Fig 31 Frontal view in occlusion at the five year follow-up.

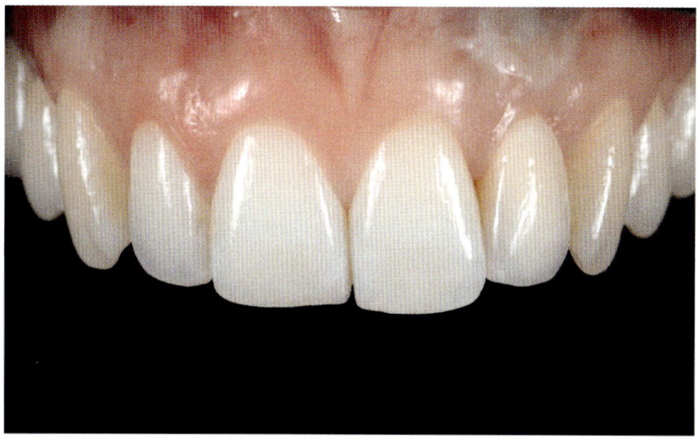

Fig 32 Intraoral view five years after the treatment.

The present approach was facilitated by the buccal plate being present and intact. Had the buccal plate not been preserved after the extraction, we would have had to choose a different treatment approach:

- *Option 1* would have been to raise a flap and augment the site with a GBR technique plus CGT and opt for immediate provisionalization in order to support the surrounding soft tissue, which is surgically very demanding and carries a high risk for complications.
- *Option 2* would have been to let the site heal and select a staged approach; the so-called "delayed implant placement." In that case, the reconstruction of the high-scalloped papillae would not have been very predictable.

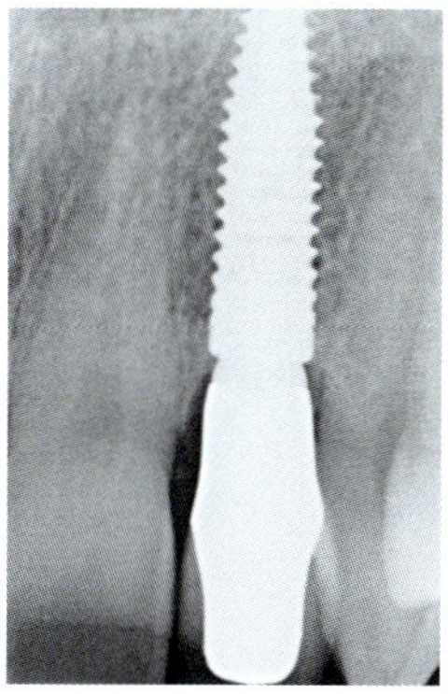

Fig 33 Periapical radiograph five years after the treatment. Stable interproximal bone conditions.

The high smile line and thin gingival phenotype were the only critical aspects identified preoperatively as risk factors. Intraoperatively, a thin but intact buccal bone plate became evident.

Key aspects of this successful treatment include:

- An intact buccal wall and the presence of sufficient bone apically and palatally to install an implant with high primary stability.
- Augmentation of the hard and soft tissues, and the resulting amount of tissue support—especially of the high-scalloped tissues associated with the temporary restoration.
- The carefully designed slim emergence profile of both the temporary and final restorations in the apical part of the transmucosal aspect of the suprastructure.

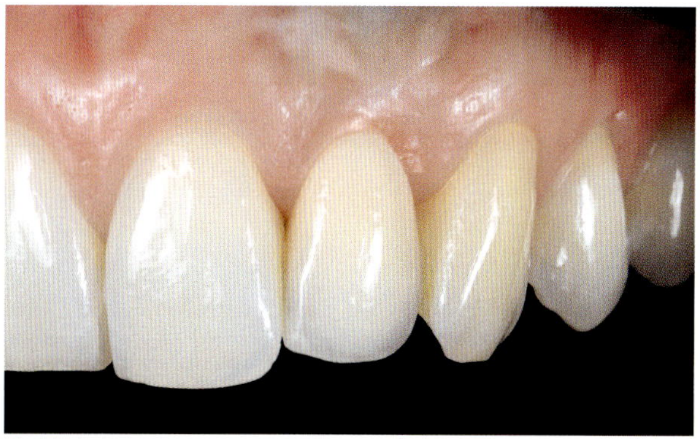

Fig 34 Close up of the peri-implant soft tissue.

ACKNOWLEDGMENT

Laboratory procedures

Pascal Holthaus – Münster, Germany

5.2 Immediate Implant Placement to Replace a Fractured Central Incisor in a Young Patient and Management of Long Term Implant Infraposition

A. Mainjot, F. Lambert

A healthy 20-year-old woman, a non-smoker, presented at the emergency department of the University Hospital of Liège in February 2011 with multiple vertical fractures of tooth 21, incisal fractures of tooth 31, and an enamel and dentin fracture of tooth 32 (Figs 1a-d). No tooth luxation was observed. Radiographs confirmed multiple root fractures on tooth 21, including a vertical infrabony fracture, indicating that the tooth was not restorable (Fig 2). A pulpectomy of tooth 21 and an indirect pulp cap on tooth 32 using resin-modified glass-ionomer cement (RMGIC) (Vitrebond; 3M, St. Paul, MN, USA) were performed. RMGC (Fuji IILC; GC, Tokyo, Japan) provisional restorations were placed on the injured teeth (Fig 3). The patient was sent for 3D imaging (multislice CT) the next day to determine the replacement strategy for tooth 21. Because of the vertical fractures, it was important to extract tooth 21 within a few days after the trauma to limit the risk of bacterial infection and consequent tissue loss.

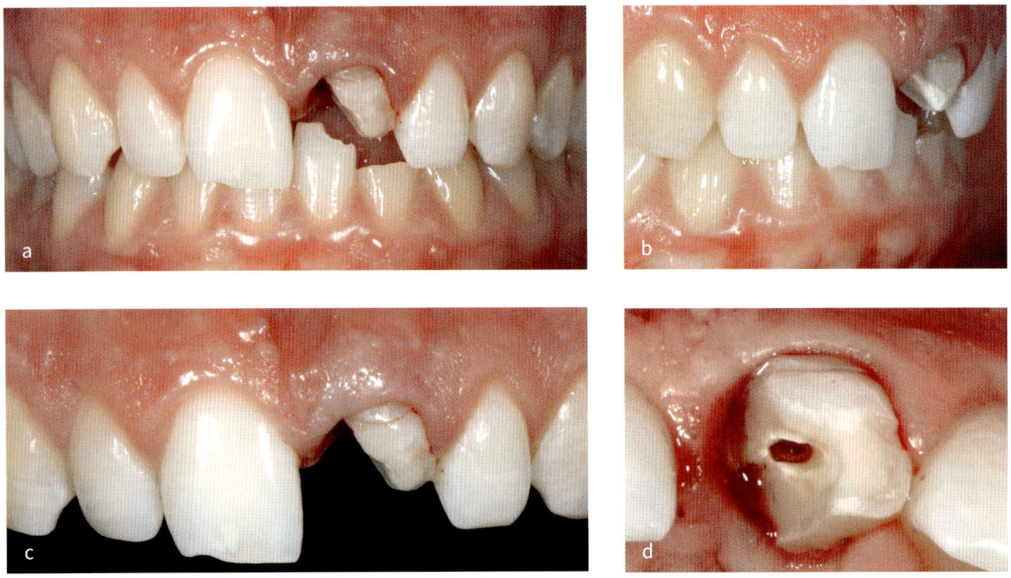

Figs 1a-d Preoperative situation showing the vertical fractures on tooth 21 and the coronal fractures on teeth 31 and 32.

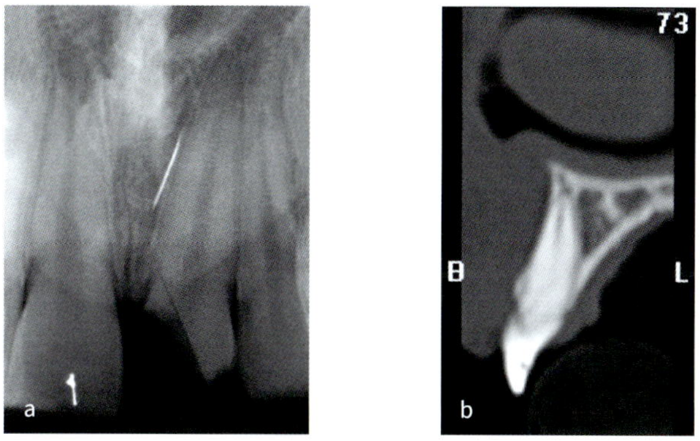

Figs 2a-b Preoperative radiograph and CT scan prior to extraction

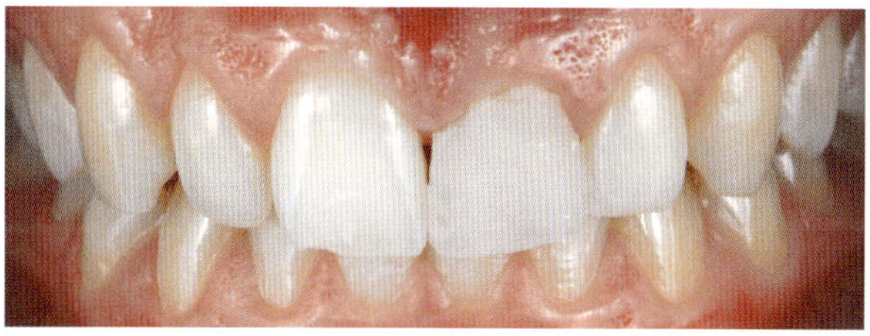

Fig 3 A provisional reconstruction in resin-modified glass-ionomer cement was placed on tooth 21.

DIAGNOSIS AND TREATMENT PLAN

The patient presented with mild localized gingivitis, and no occlusal pathology was detected. However, toothbrushing-related trauma with Stillman's clefts as well as a deep bite (4 mm) were found.

3D imaging revealed an intact buccal bone plate on tooth 21 and proximity of the nasal cavity at 3 mm from the apex on the buccal aspect; 6-7 mm apical bone anchorage was available on the palatal aspect. The bony environment combined with a thick periodontal phenotype and the ideal positioning of the gingival margin suggested that an immediate implant strategy could be possible. According to the risk assessment for immediate implant placement and immediate loading, an immediate implant placement procedure was selected. However, given the limited apical bone anchorage and the deep bite, a delayed loading procedure was preferred (Tables 1 and 2).

The treatment plan included (in chronological order):

- Oral hygiene instruction and professional tooth cleaning
- Minimally invasive extraction of tooth 21, immediate implant placement, and socket management using bone and soft tissue grafting
- Placement of a removable acrylic resin temporary
- Review of toothbrushing habits
- Slight bleaching on the canines and premolars
- Direct composites on teeth 11, 31, and 32
- Delayed implant loading with a screw-retained provisional crown
- Delivery of a definitive veneered zirconia screw-retained crown on implant 21

SURGICAL PHASE

The hard and soft tissue conditions allowed for extraction and immediate implantation. Three days after the initial trauma, a flapless and minimally invasive tooth extraction was performed to preserve the hard and soft tissues. Granulation tissue was debrided with a curette, and the transgingival epithelia (sulcular and junctional epithelia) were removed with a diamond bur in order to expose the underlying connective tissue. The integrity of the buccal bone was verified with a probe, and a bone-level implant was placed (Straumann Bone Level RN SLActive, diameter 4.1 mm, length 12 mm; Institut Straumann AG, Basel, Switzerland). The implant was inserted free-hand into the palatal wall of the socket to allow for a screw-retained final restoration and also to ensure a sufficient buccal distance for socket management. The vertical positioning of the implant was placed 4 mm below the future cervical margin of the restoration. Due to the limited apical bone, primary stability was restricted to 20 Ncm, and so immediate provisional restoration of the implant was not considered.

The remaining socket was filled with a slowly absorbed deproteinized bovine bone mineral (DBBM) (Bio-Oss; Geistlich, Wolhusen, Switzerland), and a connective tissue graft harvested from the palate was inserted transgingivally between the buccal soft tissue and the healing abutment and stabilized with 6-0 polypropylene sutures (HuFriedy, Chicago, IL, USA) (Figs 4a-d).

Table 1 Risk assessment for immediate implant placement in single-tooth sites

	Low risk	Medium risk	High risk
Preoperative assessment			
Patient-related			
Medical status	Healthy, uneventful healing		Compromised healing
Esthetic risk	Low/medium esthetic risk	High esthetic risk	Significant esthetic compromise expected
Site-related			
Gingival-margin position	No recession	Minor gingival recession	Gingival recession ≥ 2 mm
Soft tissue quality	Thick gingival phenotype	Thin gingival phenotype or limited keratinized gingiva	No keratinized gingiva
Bone anchorage	Sufficient bone anchorage to achieve primary stability		Lack of bone anchorage to achieve primary stability
Facial bone wall	≥ 1 mm facial bone thickness	Facial bone plate < 1 mm thickness, or small fenestration or dehiscence defect	Significant fenestration or dehiscence of facial bone
Need for a mucoperiosteal flap	Sufficient alveolar bone for a flapless approach		Need for flapped bone augmentation
Socket position within alveolar envelope	Socket within the alveolar bone envelope		Socket and facial bone wall protruding out of the bone envelope
Presence of endodontic infection	No infection	Chronic periapical infection	Acute infection
Presence of periodontal disease	Periodontally healthy	Controlled periodontal disease	Active periodontal disease
Planning implant position	Ideal three-dimensional position with axis exiting through the cingulum or incisal edge		Facially positioned or over-angulated implant or excessive implant depth
Gap between buccal bone and planned implant position	≥ 2 mm	1–2 mm	< 1 mm
Intraoperative assessment			
Extraction	Minimally invasive tooth extraction	Damage to surrounding soft tissue, including severed/detached papillae	Significant damage to soft tissue and surrounding bone
Primary implant stability	Primary stability achieved		Lack of primary stability
Final implant position	Ideal three-dimensional position achieved		Facially positioned or over-angulated implant or excessive implant depth

Table 2 Risk assessment for immediate loading of an immediately placed single implant

	Low risk	Medium risk	High risk
Preoperative assessment			
Patient-related			
Occlusal scheme	No direct occlusal contacts	Minimal occlusal contact and/or shared guidance	Main determinant of anterior guidance
Occlusal parafunction	Absent		Present
Site-related			
Bone anchorage	Sufficient bone anchorage to resist loading forces		Insufficient bone anchorage to resist loading forces
Tooth position	Incisor, premolars	Canine	Molars
Intraoperative assessment			
Primary implant stability	30–45 Ncm insertion torque	20–30 Ncm insertion torque	< 20 Ncm insertion torque

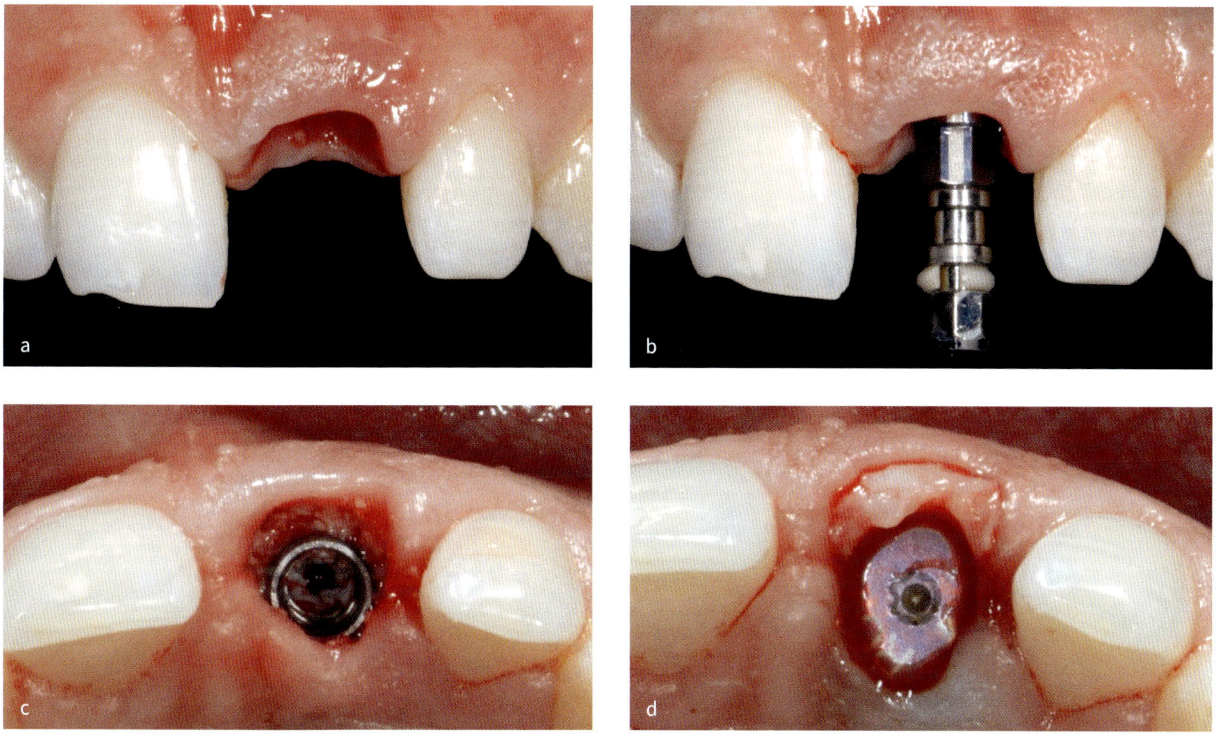

Figs 4a-d A minimally invasive extraction allowed the preservation of the hard and soft tissue architecture. The implant was placed in its ideal 3D position, and the remaining socket was grafted with a biomaterial to limit post-extraction bone remodeling. A connective tissue graft was performed to optimize the thickness of the soft tissue.

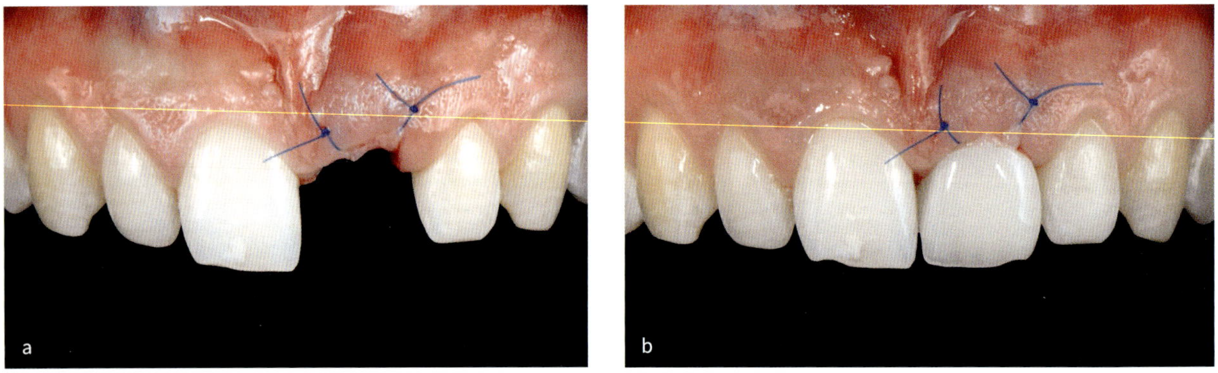

Figs 5a-b Placement of a removable acrylic resin temporary.

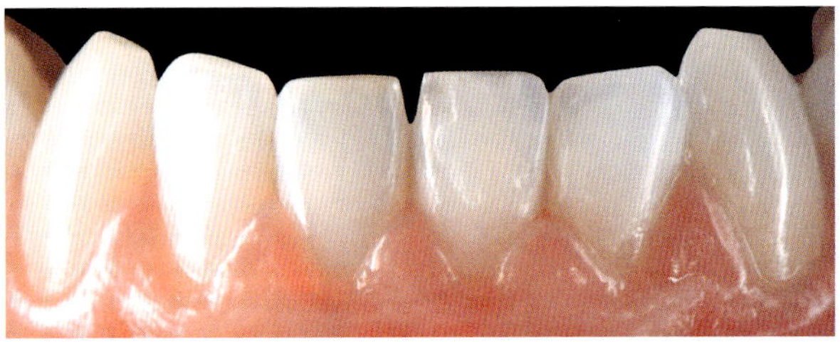

Fig 6 Direct composite restorations on teeth 31 and 32. Gingivitis was present despite the oral hygiene instructions given to the patient.

PROSTHETIC PHASE

A removable temporary acrylic resin prosthesis was placed directly after the extraction of tooth 21 (Figs 5a-b). It was designed to avoid contact with the implant and reduce compression of the soft tissue.

During the osseointegration phase, direct composite restorations were performed on teeth 11, 31, and 32 (Optibond FL adhesive; Kerr, Brea, CA, USA; or Miris 2 direct composite; Coltene-Whaledent, Altstätten, Switzerland) (Fig 6). A home bleaching procedure was carried out on the canines and the premolars using 10% carbamide peroxide gel in custom nightguards for one to two weeks.

Five weeks after implant placement, an open-tray impression was taken using a silicone-based material (double-mix technique: Aquasil; Dentsply, York, PA, USA), and the implant was loaded with a provisional screw-retained acrylic resin crown in slight infraocclusion nine weeks after the implant placement. The concave transmucosal contour of the provisional restoration was designed to promote the stability of the peri-implant soft tissues. Ideally, this part should be made in a highly biocompatible material, preferably titanium, but in the present case a temporary cylinder covered with acrylic resin was used (Fig 7a). The emergence contour of the provisional crown was designed to mimic the contralateral natural tooth. The soft tissues were compressed at the time of delivery, allowing immediate conditioning of the soft tissues in the ideal position (Fig 7b).

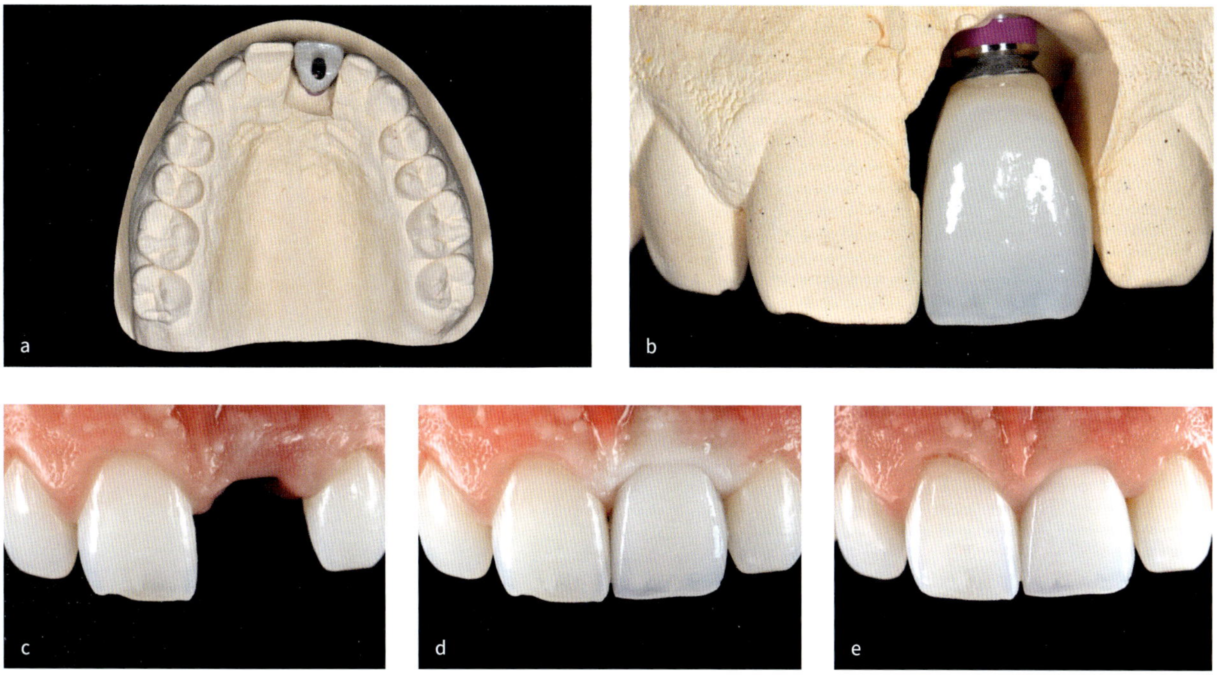

Figs 7a-e Provisional screw-retained acrylic resin crown on tooth 21 (a); soft tissue level prior to provisional crown placement, right after placement and three weeks later (b).

The final screw-retained restoration was placed thirteen weeks after implant placement. A 3 mol-% yttria-doped tetragonal zirconia polycrystal material (3Y-TZP, a first-generation zirconia material) CAD/CAM framework was designed (Cares abutment; Institut Straumann AG) (Figs 8a-f). The gingival contour was idealized on the model, and the buccal margin of the ceramic veneer was placed just below the ideal mucosal margin, as compared to the contralateral tooth. The infrastructure was designed to match the shape of the final crown, with the thickness of the veneering material being limited to promote mechanical resistance. The framework also mimicked the dentine anatomy, showing mamelons to create the final esthetic result (Fig 8a). The lack of palatal space did not allow veneering of the palatal aspect of the framework, which was merely glazed supramucosally (Fig 8b), while the transmucosal aspect was left untreated to preserve the biocompatibility of the zirconia and to allow proper integration the peri-implant soft tissues.

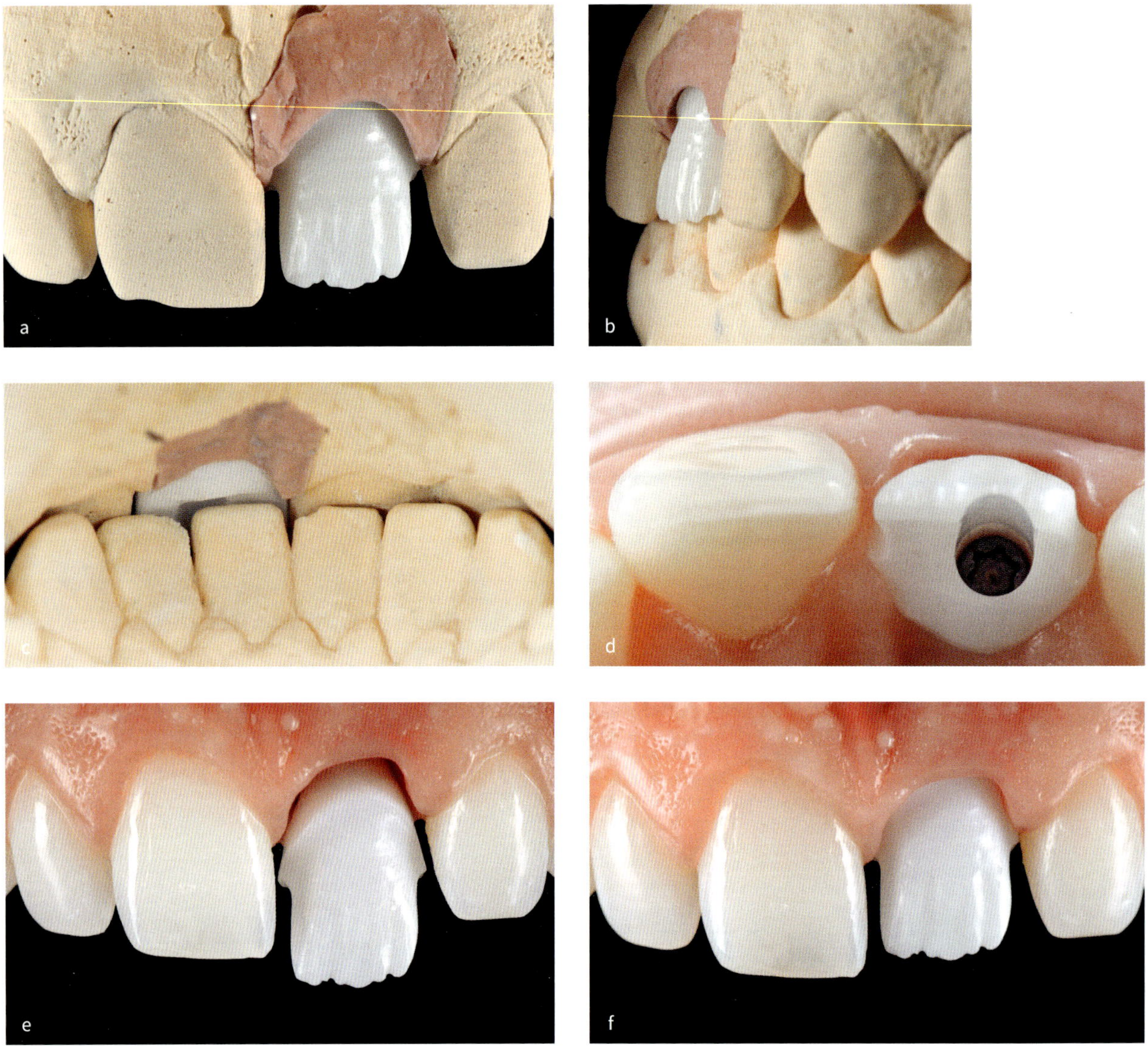

Figs 8a-f 3-YTZP zirconia framework for a screw-retained restoration.

Figure 9 shows the zirconia framework prior to and after veneering. Advantages of this one-piece zirconia framework include its optical properties and the biocompatibility of the transmucosal aspect, which must remain unglazed because veneering ceramics are not as biocompatible as zirconia. A disadvantage of this type of infrastructure is the risk of fracture of the internal connection, which occurs usually at the time of connecting the screw, particularly when the restoration is not inserted following the correct axis. Therefore, manufacturers have developed secondary metallic components for the connection. The transmucosal profile of the restoration is concave to thicken the peri-implant soft tissue and to allow the organization of a soft tissue ring around the transgingival aspect of the restoration, which is supposed to provide vertical tissue stability. The emergence contour of the prosthesis is usually located around 0.5–1.0 mm below the ideal mucosal level. Fig 9c shows how much soft tissue was required to enhance the cervical convexity in comparison with the provisional restoration to push back the mucosa and to replicate the mucosal level of tooth 11 (Fig 10).

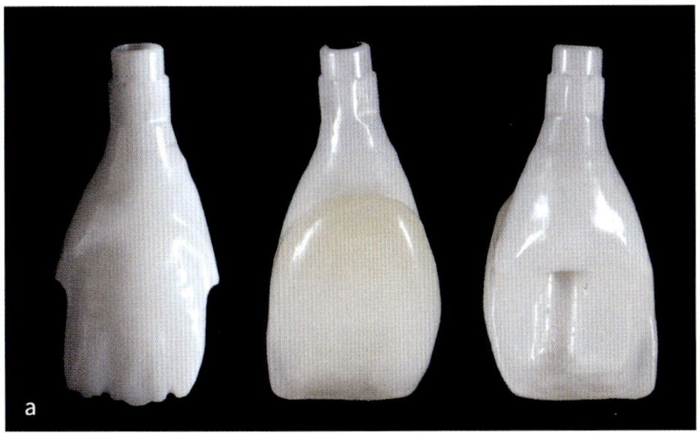

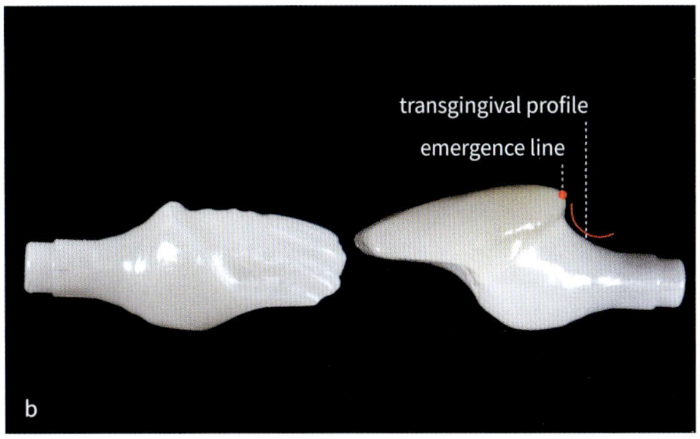

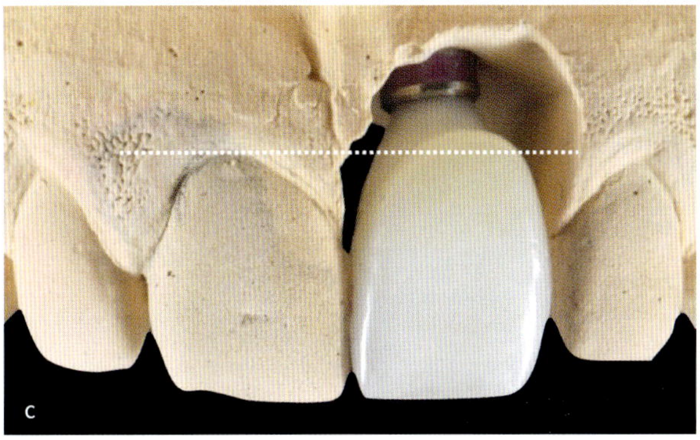

Figs 9a-c Zirconia framework before and after veneering.

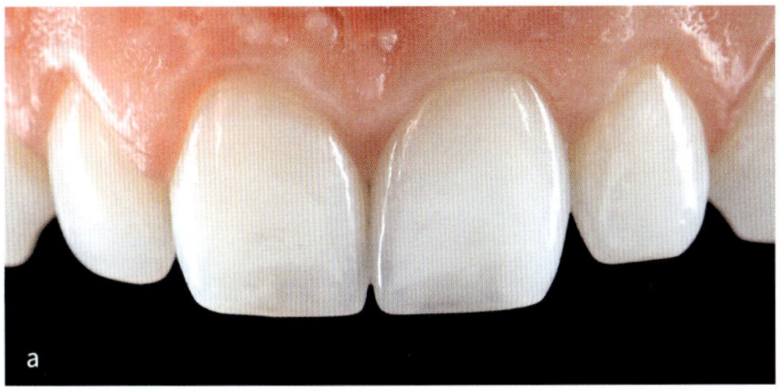

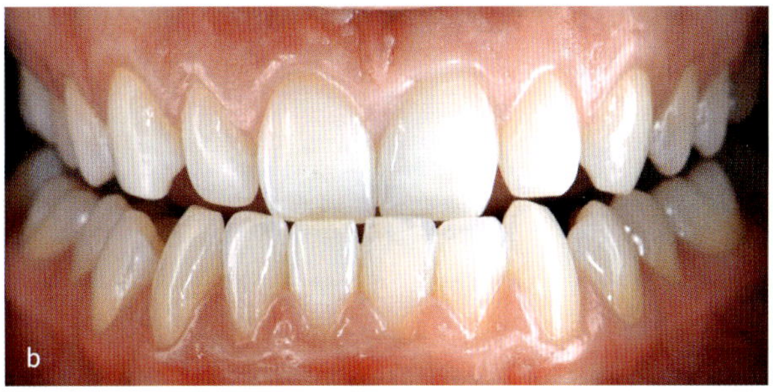

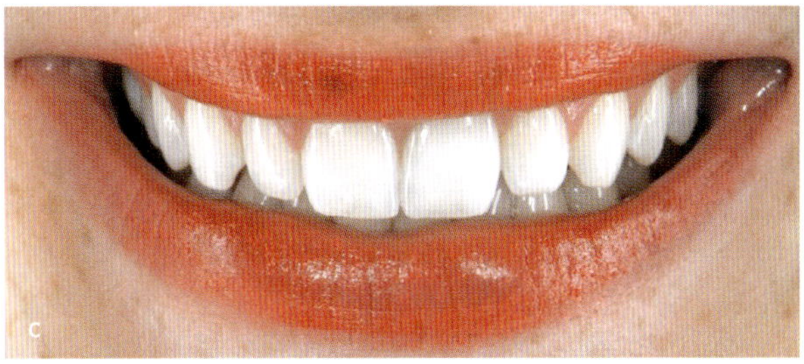

Figs 10a-c Final restoration three months after implant placement.

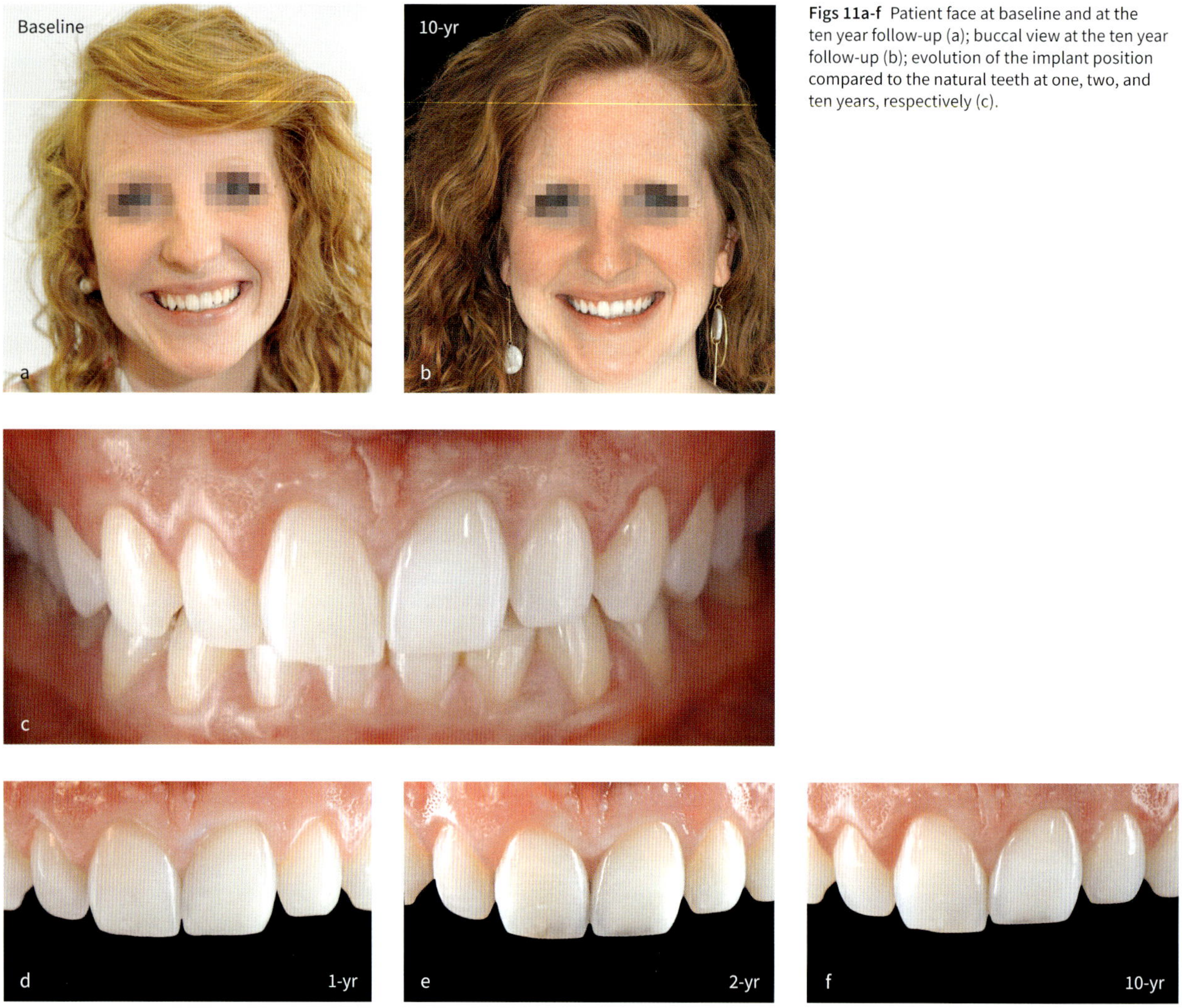

Figs 11a-f Patient face at baseline and at the ten year follow-up (a); buccal view at the ten year follow-up (b); evolution of the implant position compared to the natural teeth at one, two, and ten years, respectively (c).

The patient was seen at one- and two year intervals after treatment but was then lost to follow-up for several years. After ten years, she returned because she was concerned about a discrepancy between the incisal edges of teeth 21 and 11. The implant was infrapositioned due to facial growth, resulting in an esthetic problem (Figs 11a-e). While the peri-implant tissue remained thick, the mucosal margin was no longer symmetrical to that of tooth 11. Looking back at the details of the follow-up images, the result of facial growth had already been somewhat noticeable at two years (Fig 11e).

IMPLANT INFRAPOSITION MANAGEMENT

After discussing the options with the patient, who for financial reasons did not wish to have the crown remade, and the dental technician, who did not recommend adding veneering ceramics to the original crown because of the high risk of deterioration during firing, it was proposed to adhesively connect a chip of feldspathic ceramic to lengthen the restoration. Moreover, to compensate for the soft tissue mismatch, it was decided to recontour the crown, and particularly the transmucosal profile, in order to relocate the soft tissue margin (Figs 12a-i).

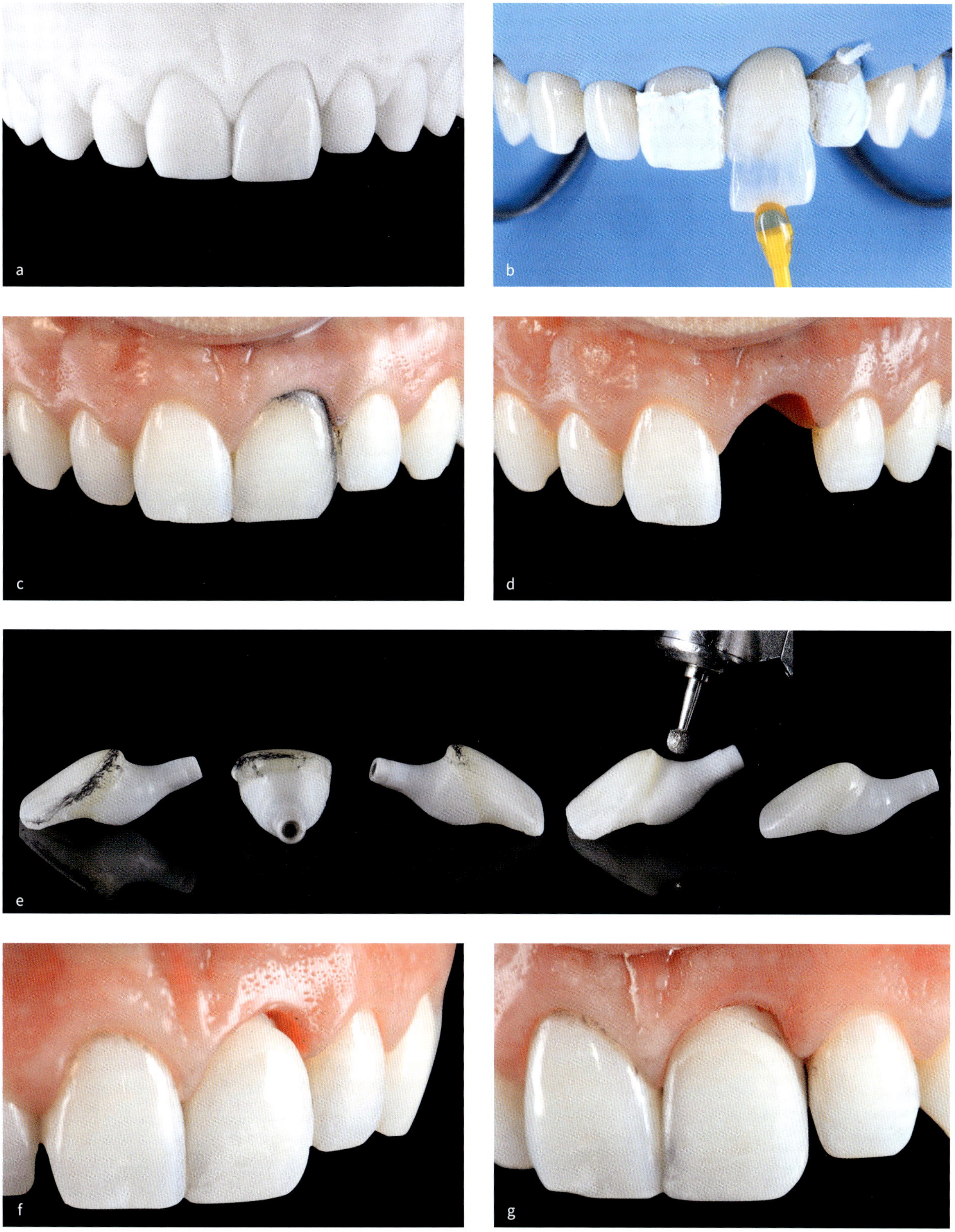

Figs 12a-i Feldspathic ceramic chip before bonding (a and b); analysis of the cervical and distal areas for recontouring, highlighting the gingival level mismatch between teeth 11 and 21 (c and d); recontouring of the transmucosal profile (e); gap between the soft tissue and the restoration and a diastema between teeth 21 and 22 that arose after the restoration was recontoured (f and g).

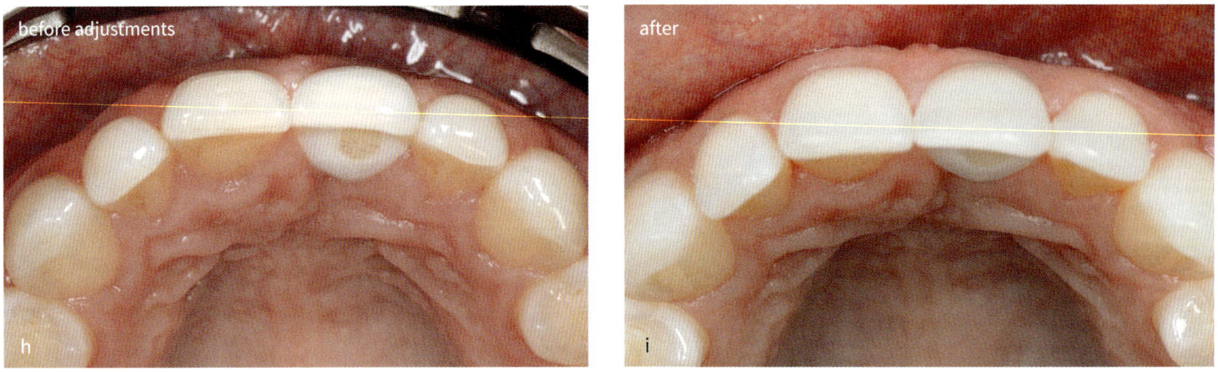

Figs 12a-i (continued)

An intraoral scan was made and a chip of feldspathic ceramic (Vita VM9; Vita Zahnfabrik, Bad Säckingen, Germany) was manufactured (Figs 12a-b). After isolation with rubber dam, the intaglio surface of the chip and the surface of the veneer were etched with 10% hydrofluoric acid for one minute, and a silane layer was applied according the to manufacturer's recommendations (Monobond Plus; Ivoclar Vivadent, Schaan, Liechtenstein). The chip was then bonded with a composite resin cement (Variolink Esthetic DC; Ivoclar Vivadent).

The restoration was subsequently unscrewed, and the transgingival profile, incisal edge, and distal and buccal surfaces were adjusted using diamond followed by Arkansas stone burs, and ceramic diamond polishing instruments for the final finish (Optrafine; Ivoclar Vivadent) (Figs 12c-e). As a result of facial growth, the buccal and distal profiles of teeth 11 and 21 were no longer symmetrical (Figs 12h-i). The transmucosal profile of the restoration was revised by moving down the transmucosal concavity and the emergence line, creating a gap between the restoration and the soft tissue (Figs 12f-g). Since the convexity corresponding to the emergence line had been reduced slightly too far, a small amount of direct composite (Inspiro; Edelweiss, Wolfurt, Austria) was added on the surface after proper ceramic pretreatment. Finally, a combination of facial growth and the recontouring of the distal surface to achieve identical widths for teeth 11 and 21 had created a diastema (Figs 12f-g). This diastema was closed by adding direct composite (Inspiro; Edelweiss, Wolfurt, Austria) on the mesial surface of tooth 22.

The adjusted restoration was cleaned and disinfected using successive ultrasonic baths (soapy solution, water, and 90% alcohol). Once properly dried, it was screwed in at 35 Ncm, and the screw channel was closed with direct composite.

The gingival gap was already closed after one week (Figs 13a-g), which clearly illustrates the effect of the transmucosal and emergence profiles of the prosthesis on the soft tissues. Figure 14 shows radiographs after implant placement, after restoration placement, and at the two and ten year follow-ups. It demonstrates the excellent peri-implant bone level stability over time. Figure 15 shows the situation one year after the restoration had been recontoured.

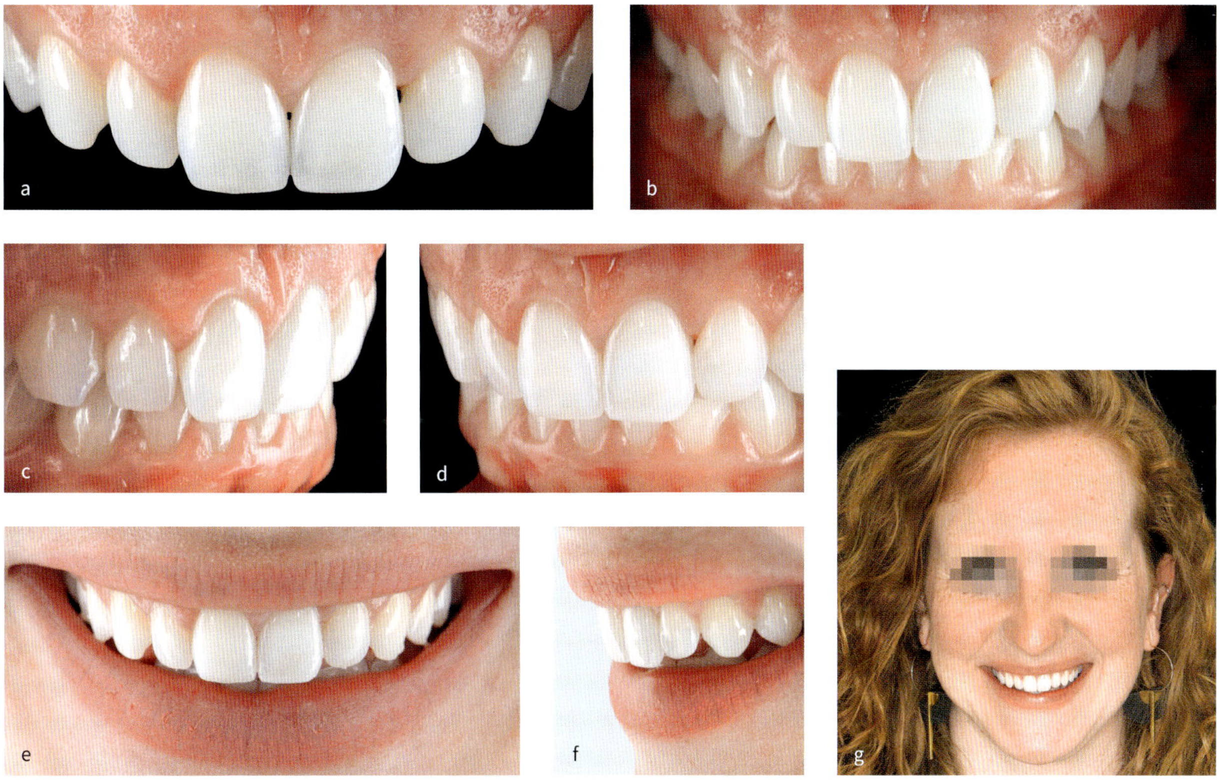

Figs 13a-g Final restoration one week after recontouring (eleven year follow-up).

Fig 14 Radiographs after implant placement, after restoration placement, and at the two and ten year follow-ups.

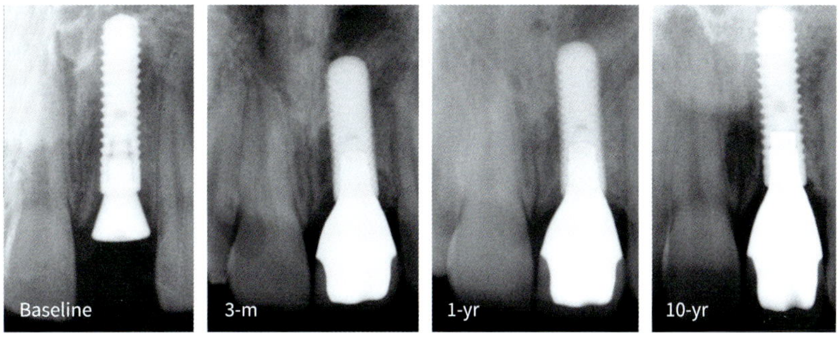

Fig 15 Restoration one year after recontouring.

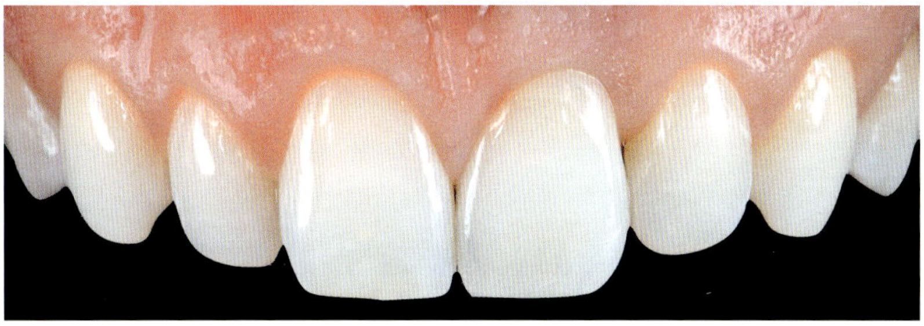

DISCUSSION

The management of trauma cases is always a challenge, especially since the practitioner has to deal with an emergency situation and psychological stress. From the very first emergency visit, decision-making and treatment strategy are of the utmost importance to minimize hard and soft tissue loss, which is critical for the success of the future implant-supported rehabilitation. These tissues play a crucial role in the final esthetic result. In case of multiple and infrabony fractures, well-considered decisions have to be made quickly to avoid secondary infection. Furthermore, each surgical and prosthetic step, from the extraction to the choice of material and the prosthetic design, must be considered as part of an overall treatment strategy.

Surgical strategy. Despite the emergency, the patient was healthy and exhibited adequate hard and soft tissue conditions to facilitate an extraction and immediate implant placement. Indeed, the patient had a rather thick gingival phenotype, the cervical level was favorable, and no recession was observed (Tonetti and coworkers 2019). On the 3D images, an intact buccal plate was observed, and the sagittal root position relative to the anterior maxillary osseous housing was class I according to Kan and coworkers, designating a favorable anatomy for immediate implant placement (Kan and coworkers 2011a). However, apical bone availability was not extensive; because of the unfavorable occlusion type (deep bite), delayed implant loading was considered.

To limit post-extraction bone remodeling, and as recommended in recent consensus reports (Avila-Ortiz and coworkers 2014; Tonetti and coworkers 2019), the socket defect that had remained after implant placement was filled with a bone graft biomaterial. Although there is no consensus in this respect, a slowly resorbable biomaterial was preferred to enhance long-term three-dimensional stability (Botilde and coworkers 2020). However, this type of socket management in combination with immediate implant placement requires proper implant positioning in the buccolingual direction, limiting the distance between the facial aspect of the implant and the inner aspect of the remaining buccal plate to at least 2 mm (Caneva and coworkers 2010). Filled with the biomaterial, this gap may act as a shield and could provide sufficient buccal bone volume after the expected buccal plate remodeling (Lambert and coworkers 2012; Avila-Ortiz and coworkers 2014).

Soft tissue grafting was also considered to compensate for the expected post-extraction bone loss (Vanhoutte and coworkers 2014), which is especially evident in esthetic cases such as this. The connective tissue grafting technique employed in this case does not involve a pouch and relies on the transgingival vascular bed. It entails thickening of the soft tissue in the most critical area (Avila-Ortiz and coworkers 2014); however, adequate removal of the junctional and sulcular epithelium and proper graft stabilization are key aspects for graft integration.

Prosthetic rehabilitation. The peri-implant soft tissue can also be optimized by the prosthodontic procedures, but this requires good communication between the surgeon, the prosthodontist, and the dental laboratory. Despite limited scientific evidence regarding the effect of transgingival and emergence profile designs on soft tissue behavior, the present case shows that when combined with surgical thickening, a concave transgingival profile and convex emergence line located just below the ideal gingival level provided soft tissue stability over time.

In this particular case, a provisional restoration might not even have been necessary. Indeed, by relying on prosthetically guided soft tissue management, comparable results might have been observed, delivering the final crown with the ideal design once osseointegration was achieved.

Implant position is crucial to screw-retained restorations and to optimized transmucosal profiles and emergence contours. The buccolingual implant position must be 1.5 to 2.0 mm palatal to the incisal margin; vertically, the implant needs to be at least 4 mm deep to accommodate the biologic width and to provide enough height for the transmucosal profile (Testori and coworkers 2018). Therefore, proper planning is mandatory; nowadays this is usually a systematic digital process in order to visualize the final outcome and improve communication within the team.

Despite the absence of scientific evidence favoring screw-retained restorations over cemented restorations (Alqutaibi 2017; Lemos and coworkers 2016), the former have several advantages, such as:

- Easier management of emergence profiles
- Avoidance of excess submucosal cement and related complications (Staubli and coworkers 2017)
- Reintervention option in case of complications such as chipping or implant infraposition

In addition, screw-retained restorations reduce the risk of chipping because of the favorable ratio between the thickness of the infrastructure and the ceramic veneer (Mainjot and coworkers 2012a; Mainjot and coworkers 2012b).

Finally, screw-retained implant restorations probably constitute the best indication for zirconia (3-YTZP) in prosthodontics for the following reasons:

- Zirconia exhibits biocompatibility properties at least equivalent to titanium in terms of promoting the adhesion of fibroblasts and keratinocytes on the transmucosal components and, thus, peri-implant soft tissue integration (Grenade and coworkers 2016; Grenade and coworkers 2017)
- Zirconia has better optical properties than titanium, which improves the color match between the peri-implant mucosa and the natural tooth (Cai and coworkers 2017).
- The long-term survival rate of zirconia abutments is very high and similar to titanium (Fabbri and coworkers 2017; Sailer and coworkers 2009; Koenig and coworkers 2018)

Implant infraposition management. According to a systematic review, the prevalence of implant infraposition reaches around 50% of cases after five to fifteen years following implant placement (Papageorgiou and coworkers 2018). The discrepancy is greater than 1 mm in 20% of cases; loss of proximal contact points is observed in 43% of cases. It correlates significantly with age, with younger patients being more vulnerable. Implant infraposition also seems to be more frequent in the maxilla, in female patients, and in patients with an elongated face type. Partially edentulous patients must be informed about this potential long-term adverse effect; alternatives such as ceramic Maryland bridges should be considered in young patients, particularly when replacing lateral incisors. However, the present case shows that solutions exist to manage this type of complication in a simple and minimally invasive way, and that the lifespan of the restoration can be extended.

CONCLUSIONS

The present clinical case shows the long-term success of immediate implant placement in the esthetic zone in a young patient. Key concepts of this treatment strategy include hard and soft tissue preservation, implant positioning, biomaterial selection (both for socket management and for the implant crown), transmucosal and emergence profiles (to shape and optimize the soft tissues), and the choice of a screw-retained restoration to allow the adjustment of this profile design over time, to be able to manage complications successfully, as demonstrated by the present case. Effective communication between the surgeon, the dental technician, and the prosthodontist is mandatory for treatment success. Digital tools greatly facilitate adequate planning and the sharing of information.

Finally, while implant infraposition was successfully managed in this case, the treatment selection must consider the age factor, especially in the case of young patients, and weigh the advantages of providing an implant-supported restoration in the esthetic zone against the not inconsiderable risk of implant infraposition, something that should always be explained to the patient. In the present case, the choice of a screw-retained restoration clearly facilitated the management of this complication.

ACKNOWLEDGMENTS

Laboratory procedures

Mirko Picone – Liège, Belgium (zirconia screw-retained restoration)

Luc and Patrick Rutten – Dental Team, Tessenderlo, Belgium (feldspathic ceramic chips)

5.3 Immediate Implant Placement and Restoration of a Maxillary Left Central Incisor with a Provisional Crown

L. Pariente, K. Dada

A 34-year-old female patient with high esthetic expectations, a non-smoker with no relevant medical history (ASA class 1), was referred to our practice (62LTM, Paris, France) for replacement of her failing maxillary left central incisor (tooth 21), which exhibited a vertical root fracture as diagnosed by the referring endodontist under the microscope (Fig 1).

This case illustrates a type 1A treatment protocol (Gallucci and coworkers 2018) complete with diagnosis, treatment decisions, and clinical and laboratory steps.

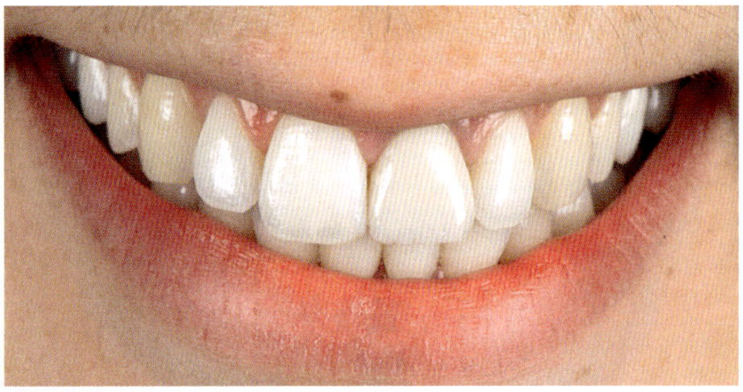

Fig 1 Extraoral view of the patient's smile. The failing tooth and its periodontal environment are exposed during smiling: the medium lip line reveals the papillae.

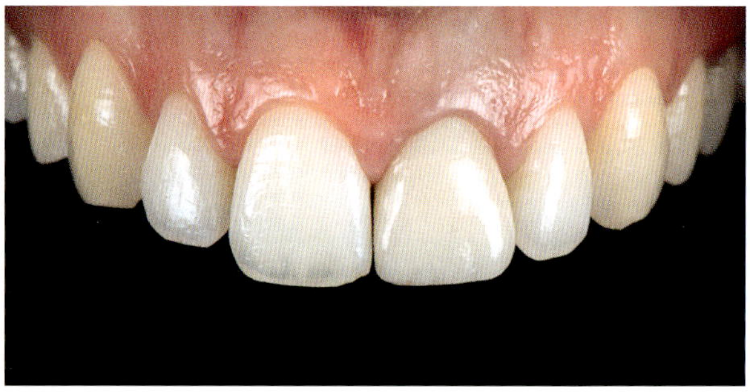

Fig 2 Intraoral view revealing a medium-scalloped, medium-thick gingival phenotype. The crown shapes are slightly triangular. There were no soft tissue defects.

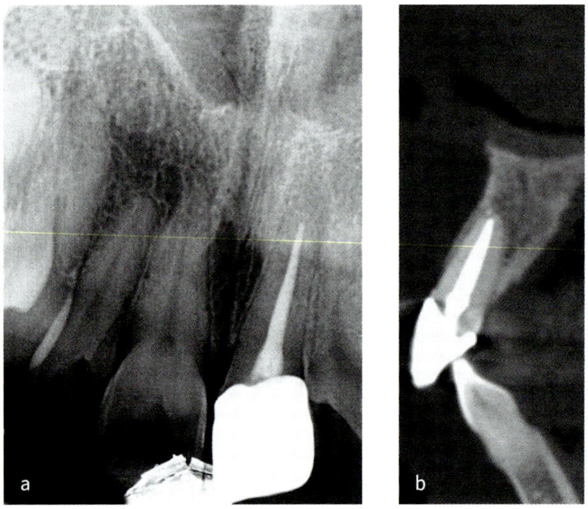

Figs 3a-b Preoperative periapical radiograph and CBCT.

INITIAL EXAMINATION

The clinical examination revealed a healthy periodontal status, good oral hygiene and compliance, and intact gingival contours and interproximal papillae (Fig 2). The failing tooth and the surrounding periodontal tissues were exposed during smiling; the medium lip line revealed the adjacent papillae.

The initial radiological examination (Fig 3a) revealed no infection at the future implant site. The interdental proximal papillae were sufficiently supported, as the height of the bone crest to the contact point of the adjacent teeth ranged from 5.5 to 6.5 mm. The neighboring teeth were unrestored.

The CBCT (Fig 3b) revealed no palatal or buccal bone defects (class I, Elian and Cho 2007) and an adequate bone volume for implant placement beyond the root apex of the hopeless tooth (class I, Kan and coworkers 2011a).

Several treatment choices were presented to the patient, including all relevant options in terms of the timing of the implant placement and possible modes of provisionalization.

The clinical and radiographical parameters detailed in the risk-assessment table (Table 1) favored immediate implant placement and immediate provisionalization.

Table 1 Risk assessment for immediate implant placement in single-tooth sites

	Low risk	Medium risk	High risk
Preoperative assessment			
Patient-related			
Medical status	Healthy, uneventful healing		Compromised healing
Esthetic risk	Low/medium esthetic risk	High esthetic risk	Significant esthetic compromise expected
Site-related			
Gingival-margin position	No recession	Minor gingival recession	Gingival recession ≥ 2 mm
Soft tissue quality	Thick gingival phenotype	Thin gingival phenotype or limited keratinized gingiva	No keratinized gingiva
Bone anchorage	Sufficient bone anchorage to achieve primary stability		Lack of bone anchorage to achieve primary stability
Facial bone wall	≥ 1 mm facial bone thickness	Facial bone plate < 1 mm thickness, or small fenestration or dehiscence defect	Significant fenestration or dehiscence of facial bone
Need for a mucoperiosteal flap	Sufficient alveolar bone for a flapless approach		Need for flapped bone augmentation
Socket position within alveolar envelope	Socket within the alveolar bone envelope		Socket and facial bone wall protruding out of the bone envelope
Presence of endodontic infection	No infection	Chronic periapical infection	Acute infection
Presence of periodontal disease	Periodontally healthy	Controlled periodontal disease	Active periodontal disease
Planning implant position	Ideal three-dimensional position with axis exiting through the cingulum or incisal edge		Facially positioned or over-angulated implant or excessive implant depth
Gap between buccal bone and planned implant position	≥ 2 mm	1–2 mm	< 1 mm

SURGICAL PROCEDURE

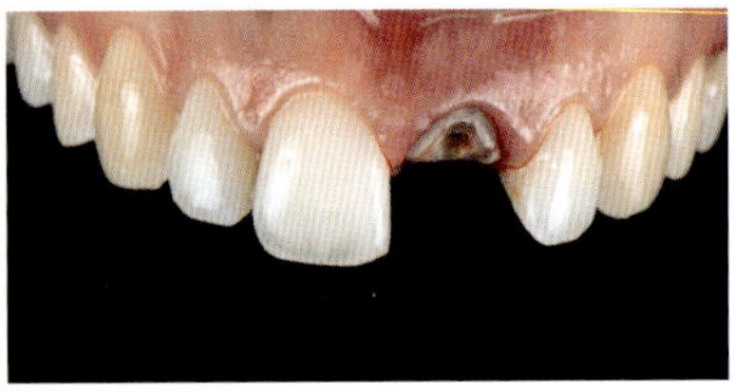

Fig 4 The first surgical step was to remove the crown of the failing tooth.

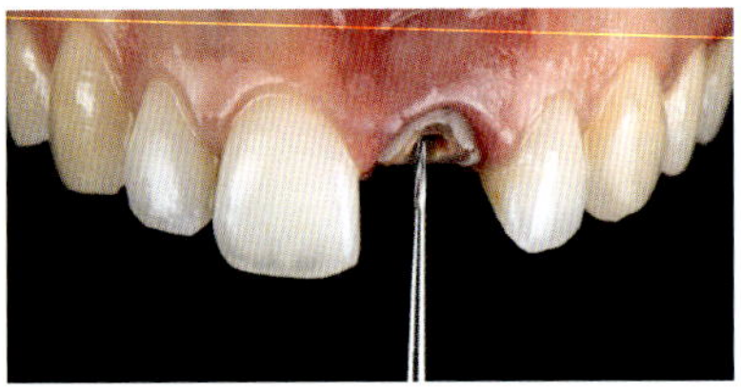

Fig 5 The failing tooth was then sectioned horizontally to protect the buccal bone from damage by the surgical bur and to perform a minimally invasive extraction.

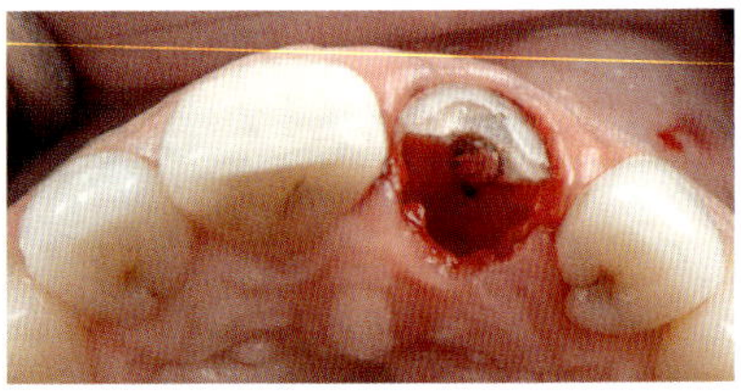

Fig 6 The palatal aspect of the root was removed to facilitate the luxation of the remaining fragment without exerting pressure on the buccal bone.

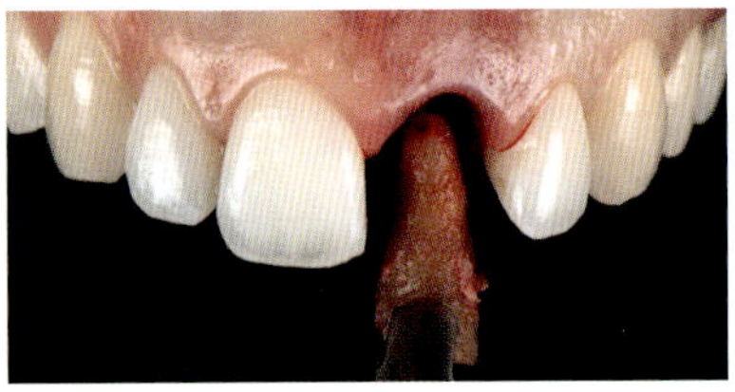

Fig 7 The remaining root fragment was carefully extracted with minimal trauma, without damaging the soft tissue and the surrounding bone.

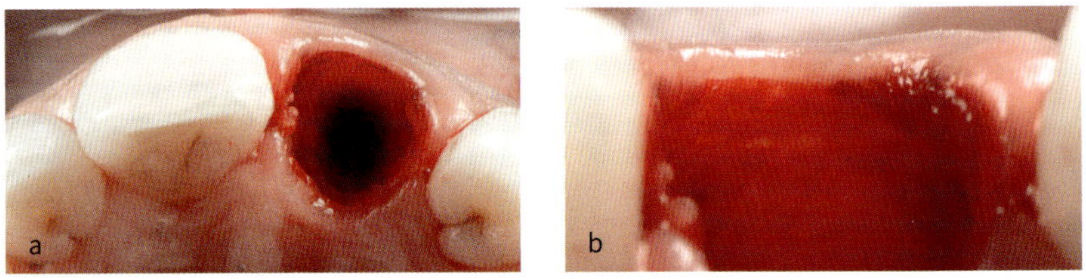

a

b

Figs 8a-b The assessed integrity of the buccal bone plate supported immediate implant placement.

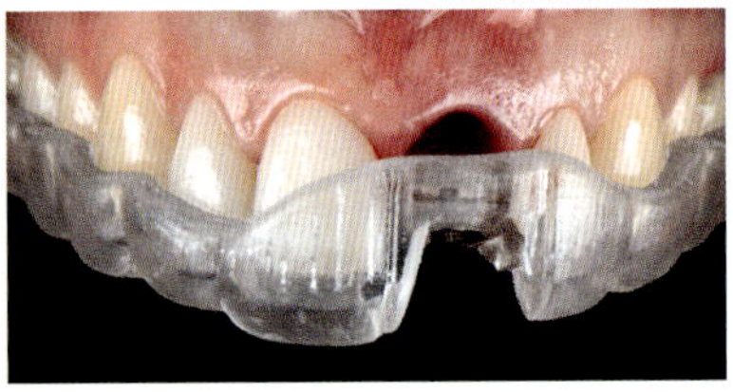

Fig 9 A surgical template (NobelProcera; Nobel Biocare, Kloten, Switzerland) assisted in preparing the osteotomy.

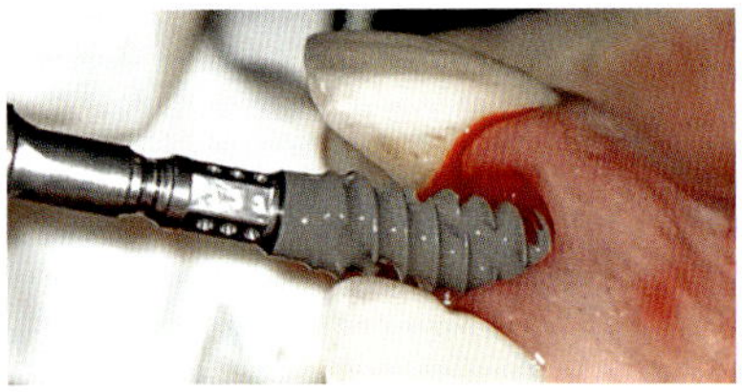

Fig 10 A BLX implant (diameter 4 mm, length 12 mm; Institut Straumann AG, Basel, Switzerland) was placed in the fresh socket at 45 Ncm insertion torque.

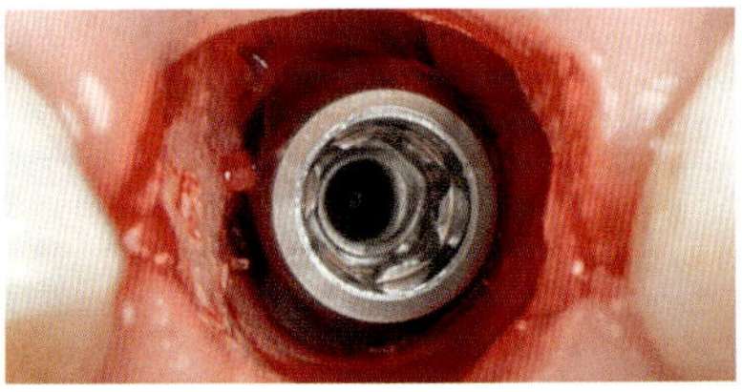

Fig 11 A sufficient gap around the implant faces the buccal bone plate, providing space for the bone regeneration material.

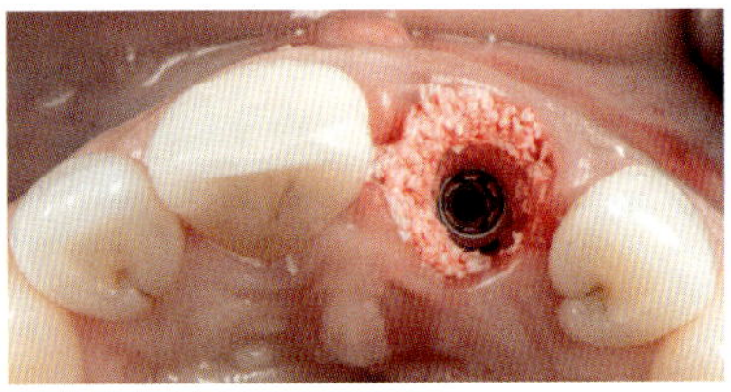

Fig 12 A particulate xenograft (Bio-Oss; Geistlich Pharma, Wolhusen, Switzerland) was used to fill the residual gap.

PROSTHETIC PROCEDURE

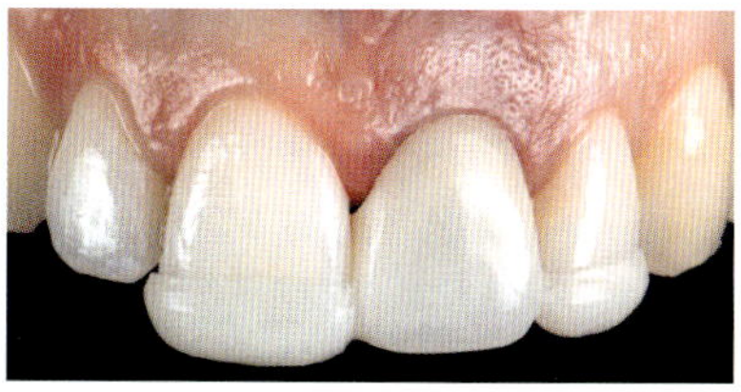

Fig 13 A provisional restoration was fabricated from a prefabricated polymethyl methacrylate (PMMA) shell attached to an engaging temporary abutment using composite resin.

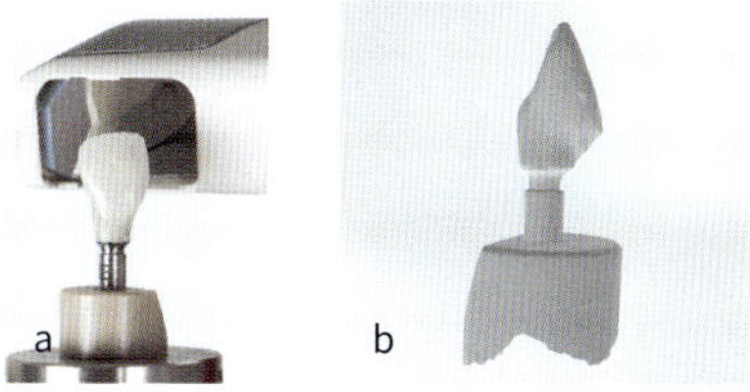

Figs 14a-b Following the E-merge protocol, the provisional restoration and its emergence profile were scanned with an IOS (a), shown here on a prototype of the holder, to obtain a STL file of the indexed provisional (b).

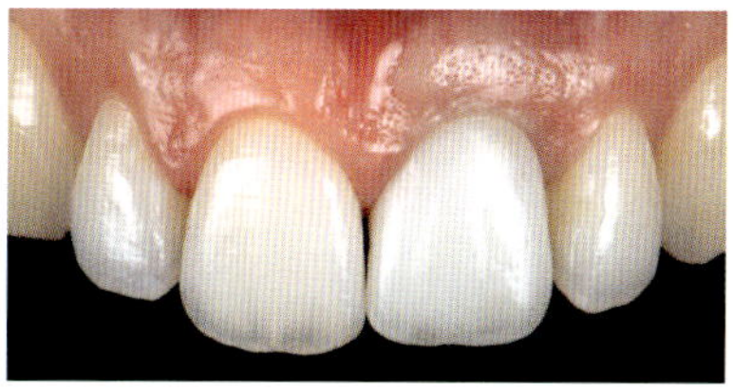

Fig 15 The provisional restoration was inserted and tightened to 35 Ncm.

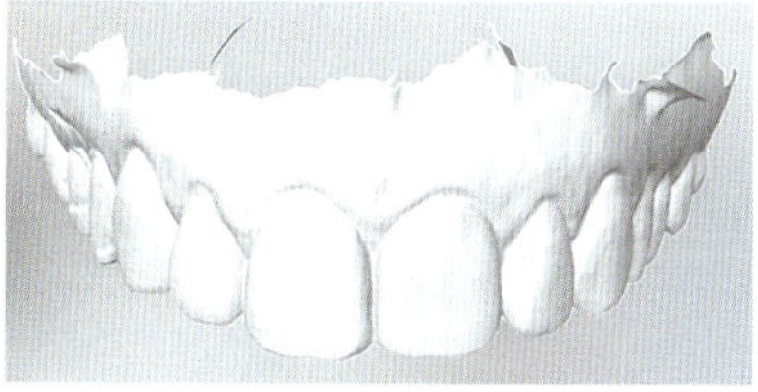

Fig 16 The patient was seen again at the three-month follow-up. A full arch intraoral scan was performed without removing the provisional restoration.

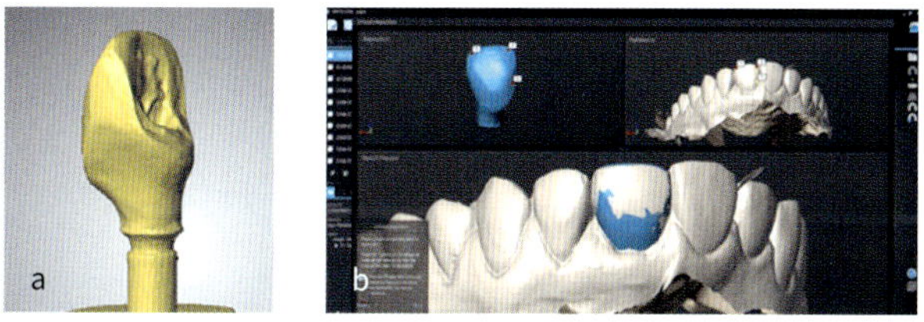

Figs 17a-b The STL files obtained from the scan of the provisional restoration (on the day of the surgery) (a) and the full-arch scan (taken after three months) (b) were merged using the E-merge feature in the CAD software (Dental Wings, Montreal, Canada) to obtain a virtual model and to design the final crown.

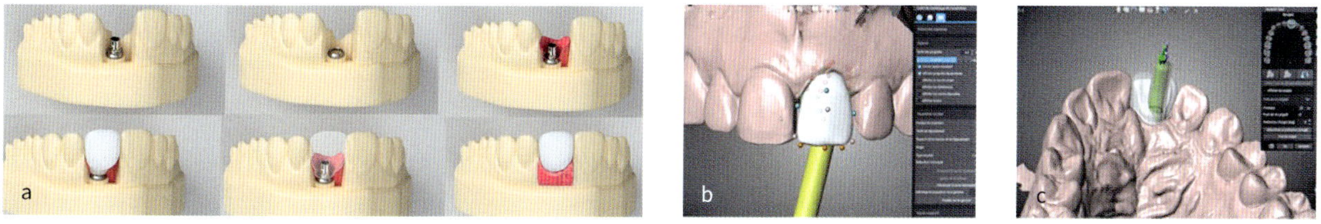

Figs 18a-c The framework of the final crown was designed according to the prosthetic envelope, maintaining the emergence profile previously established with the provisional crown. The STL file of the model was then exported for printing (b and c) (Cares; Institut Straumann AG).

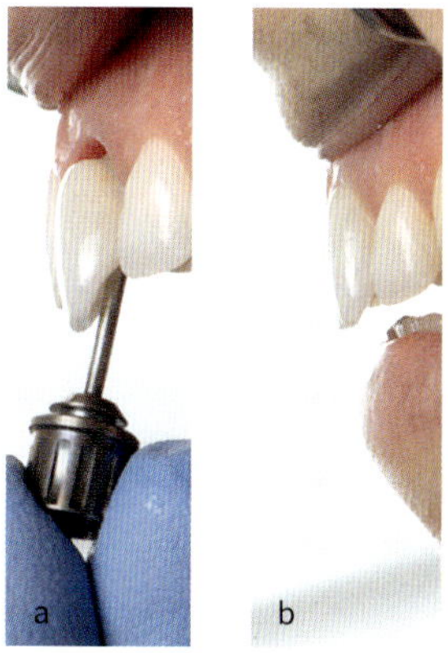

Figs 19a-b The final restoration was tried in and fitted, showing no soft tissue compression.

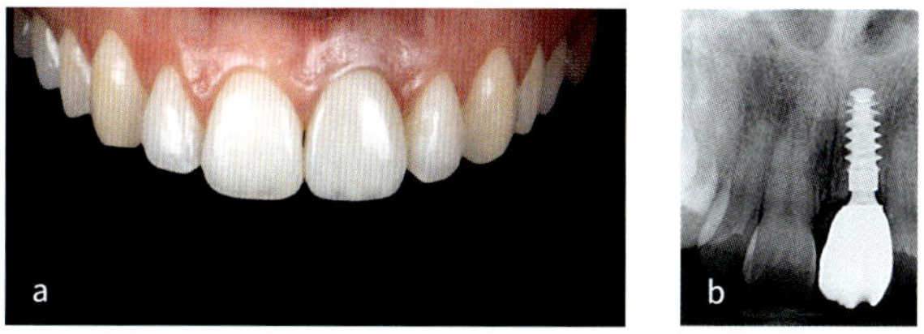

Figs 20a-b At the one year follow-up, the clinical and radiographic views show the implant integrated with stable bone levels.

DISCUSSION

Implant placement immediately after tooth extraction offers multiple advantages—especially shorter treatment times than with the delayed approach and fewer surgical procedures—but could present difficulties relating to primary stability or the fabrication of the provisional restoration. Immediate implant loading shortens the overall treatment and eliminates the need for a provisional removable prosthesis or a resin-bonded bridge during the healing process, improving patient comfort. Furthermore, the option of an implant-supported provisional restoration has shown to help preserve the gingival contour and papillae when combined with filling the gap between the implant and the buccal plate with a xenograft (Tarnow and coworkers 2014).

Achieving an ideal esthetic outcome using immediate implant placement requires careful patient selection and precise implant positioning. The risk-assessment tools presented in this Treatment Guide are a safe approach to determining the most appropriate treatment option.

As for the optimal buccolingual position, Buser and coworkers (2004) recommended the implant shoulder to be placed 1 to 2 mm lingual to the emergence line of the adjacent teeth, in order to ensure an adequate width of buccal bone and stable mucosa across the buccal implant surface. This recommendation is supported by the findings of another study, in which the buccolingual position of the implant shoulder was found to be a highly significant factor in determining the degree of buccal marginal tissue recession (Bittner and coworkers 2019). Ideally, the impression technique should replicate the emergence profile created by the provisional prosthesis while minimizing the number of steps and number of disconnections of the provisional restoration, so as not to disrupt the soft tissue architecture.

It has been demonstrated that abutment disconnection and reconnection adversely affect peri-implant marginal bone levels to a significant extent. The resulting bone loss appears to be mainly due to the reduction of the connective tissue aspect of the peri-implant mucosa resulting from abutment manipulations (Koutouzis and coworkers 2017; Bressan and coworkers 2017).

These findings pave the way for revisiting current restorative protocols to prevent incipient marginal bone loss). Even if the clinical significance of these studies is still controversial (de Carvalho Barbara and coworkers 2019), minimizing the number of abutment disconnections is still a topic of debate between clinicians.

The digital protocol for emergence profile capture meets all expectations in these delicate situations:

- It is easy to apply.
- It does not require any particular CAD skills.
- It reduces the number of disconnections to a strict minimum, minimizing patient discomfort and reducing chair time.

When a modification of the provisional restoration is necessary, or when an esthetic result requires additional trial sessions, the E-merge protocol will always require one fewer disconnection step than all other methods used today, and it can often reproduce the emergence profile developed by the provisional prosthesis.

In addition, in case of a fracture of the provisional restoration during the healing phase, the E-merge protocol allows a new identical provisional to be fabricated promptly without additional clinical steps.

CONCLUSION

The present case report indicates that immediate implant placement and restoration with a provisional crown is a suitable method to replace a failing single anterior tooth. It helps maintain the hard and soft tissue architecture with a fixed provisional, providing an esthetic and comfortable immediate solution. Combining immediate implant placement with emergence profile management—with STL superimposition of digital impressions of the retained provisional before and after healing—appears to be a practical way to create and transfer the emergence profile which is a key factor in obtaining a pleasing esthetic result.

5.4 Immediate Implant Placement with Static Computer-Aided Implant Surgery and Immediate Loading in the Esthetic Zone with Prefabricated CAD/CAM Provisional Implant Restorations

A. Lanis, L. Gonzaga, A. Hamilton

The type 1A protocol for immediate implant placement and immediate loading is defined as a surgical and prosthodontic procedure where dental implants are placed in the extraction socket on the same day the tooth is extracted and a restoration is delivered immediately (Morton and coworkers 2018; Gallucci and coworkers 2018). In the esthetic zone, the success of this approach depends on several factors, such as an adequate diagnosis, appropriate patient selection, favorable alveolar anatomy, suitable conditions at and characteristics of the surgical site, and proper training and sufficient experience on the part of the clinician (Levine and coworkers 2017; Chappuis and coworkers 2013; Belser and coworkers 2009; Chen and Buser 2014). Although long-term treatment predictability is intimately related to the described variables in these cases, and only a limited patient cohort meets all the criteria for this type of treatment, "immediacy" has been gaining popularity with clinicians and patients worldwide (Sans-Sánchez and coworkers 2015; Buser and coworkers 2017a).

Different approaches have been described for immediate implant placement in the esthetic zone (Gallucci and coworkers 2018). Most techniques contemplate procedures complementary to implant placement, such as the use of bone substitutes and soft tissue management to stabilize the surgical region and to counteract bone resorption following tooth extraction (Evans and Chen 2008; Fürhauser and coworkers 2015; Araújo and coworkers 2005; Chappuis and coworkers 2017; Li and coworkers 2018; Kuchler and coworkers 2016; van Nimwegen and coworkers 2018; Frizzera and coworkers 2019; Noelken and coworkers 2018).

From a surgical aspect, primary stability is considered a crucial parameter for immediate loading (Papaspyridakos and coworkers 2014). Primary implant stability is influenced by many factors, including local bone quality and quantity, implant macrodesign, and surgical technique (Javed and coworkers 2013). Manufacturers have developed different implant designs to achieve greater implant stability during insertion.

A novel implant concept was launched recently. Its shape and threads were especially designed to both compress soft bone and to cut into hard bone (Arcuri and coworkers 2019). This fully tapered implant was designed with a view to obtaining high insertion torques in different anatomic situations, and it was specifically created to promote "immediacy."

From a restorative perspective, a crucial factor to consider in single-tooth replacement is the correct three-dimensional implant position. This has been amply documented and plays a significant role in achieving esthetic restorative results (Buser and coworkers 2000; Tarnow and coworkers 2000). Thus, virtual Implant planning combines radiographic, prosthetic, surgical, and laboratory aspects in a common virtual scenario, permitting a detailed surgical simulation based on a prosthetic proposal (Lanis and coworkers 2015). The CAD/CAM template used in static computer-aided implant surgery (s-CAIS) links the virtual treatment plan and the actual surgery by accurately transferring the resulting simulation to the surgical site (Matta and coworkers 2017). Therefore, when an indication requires an immediate implant, s-CAIS may be considered the gold standard to obtain a precise and adequate three-dimensional implant position (Lanis and coworkers 2017).

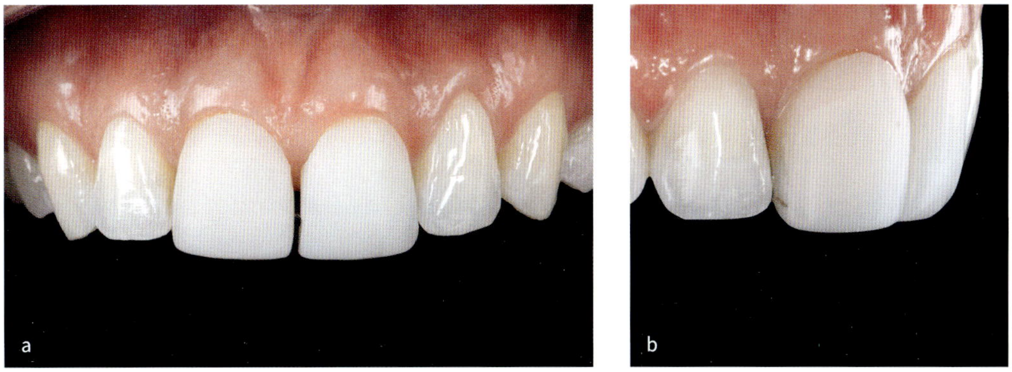

Figs 1a-b Initial situation. Intraoral frontal view and lateral close-up.

DWOS Synergy was developed to interact with two different software environments simultaneously and in real time. One environment is the surgical planning for s-CAIS; the other is the design and fabrication of restorative structures. When the two are linked, it is possible to design and fabricate CAD/CAM restorations prior to implant placement, taking into consideration the planned implant position and its abutment—as if they were already present intraorally. The implant and restoration function as a single unit, and modifying one of them will affect the other.

This concept allows for a precise refinement of the three-dimensional implant position, with real-time communication between the surgical, restorative, and laboratory team members during implant planning. If, when planning the restoration, the resulting contours appear to be incorrectly designed, the implant position can be virtually modified to provide an ideal balance between biological, mechanical, and esthetic success. This also permits the visualization of the prospective emergence profiles relative to the bone crest in situations where the implant is placed subcrestally and can aid in designing more biologically favorable emergence profiles.

This case report describes the planning phase and treatment sequence of an esthetic reconstruction based on this innovative technology. It addresses the replacement of two central incisors with immediate implants and immediate restorations using s-CAIS and the Synergy concept. The provision of the final CAD/CAM restorations for the implants is also described.

CASE DESCRIPTION

A 32-year-old female patient was referred to Prime Clinic in Santiago, Chile for a specific evaluation of teeth 11 and 21. Her chief complaint was the esthetic discrepancy between her two central incisors and the discomfort produced by moderate mobility of these two teeth. She had suffered a dentoalveolar trauma in 2016, leading to non-complex crown fractures of both 11 and 21. Two direct composite veneers were delivered at that time. These restorations showed a poor marginal seal and were overcontoured and opaque, resulting in an unpleasant esthetic relationship with the rest of the maxillary anterior teeth. Both teeth exhibited grade 1 to 2 mobility. The patient reported permanent discomfort in the anterior region. A palatal bonded wire was present that splinted the two incisors (Figs 1a-b).

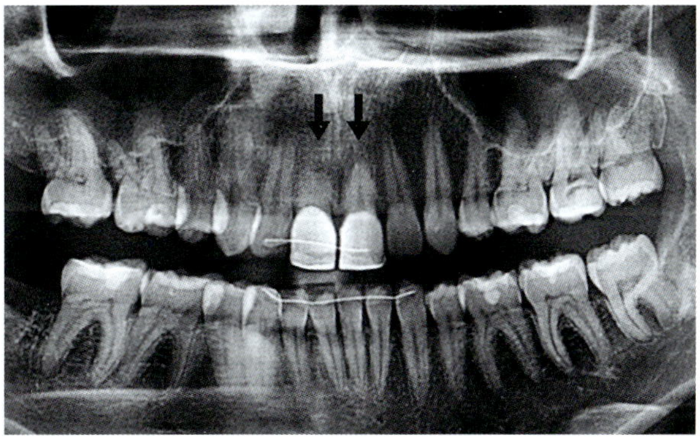

Fig 2 Orthopantomogram (OPG) of the Initial situation. External root resorption on teeth 11 and 21.

The patient practiced good oral hygiene and visited her dentist regularly for checkups and supportive periodontal care. No contributory systemic or dental findings were registered. Clinical and radiological examination showed that teeth 11 and 21 were affected by advanced root resorption (Fig 2).

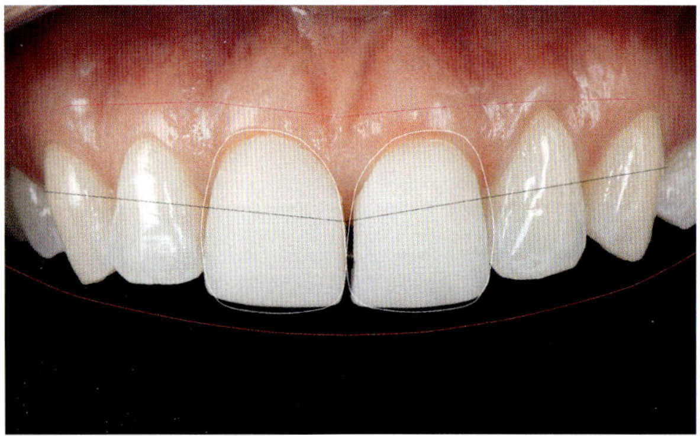

Fig 3 DSD analysis.

TREATMENT PLANNING

A complete photographic and Digital Smile Design (DSD) analysis was performed to provide diagnostic and planning information for the patient and the lab technician (Coachman and coworkers 2016). Both central incisors were digitally modified in shape to obtain a more feminine and harmonious relationship between the six anterior maxillary teeth (Magne and coworkers 1995) (Fig 3).

Digital Imaging and Communication in Medicine (DICOM) files obtained from the CBCT and a Standard Tessellation Language (STL) file from a digital impression of the maxilla were imported to the virtual planning software (coDiagnostiX 9; Dental Wings, Montreal, Canada). To analyze in detail the integrity and thickness of the buccal bone wall in relation with the central incisors, the CBCT was taken with lip retraction (Januário and coworkers 2008). The clinical situation and proposed treatment was considered to be "high risk" by the Esthetic Risk Assessment (ERA) tool (Dawson and coworkers 2021), mainly based on the region of the teeth to be extracted, tissue exposure, extraction of multiple adjacent teeth, and the selected clinical protocol. Comprehensive diagnosis and treatment risk assessment were also performed (Dawson and coworkers 2021) (Tables 1 and 2).

A comprehensive prosthetically driven digital implant placement simulation was carried out. BLX implants (diameter 3,75 mm, length 12 mm; Institut Straumann AG, Basel, Switzerland) were selected for the intervention in both sites (Figs 4a-c).

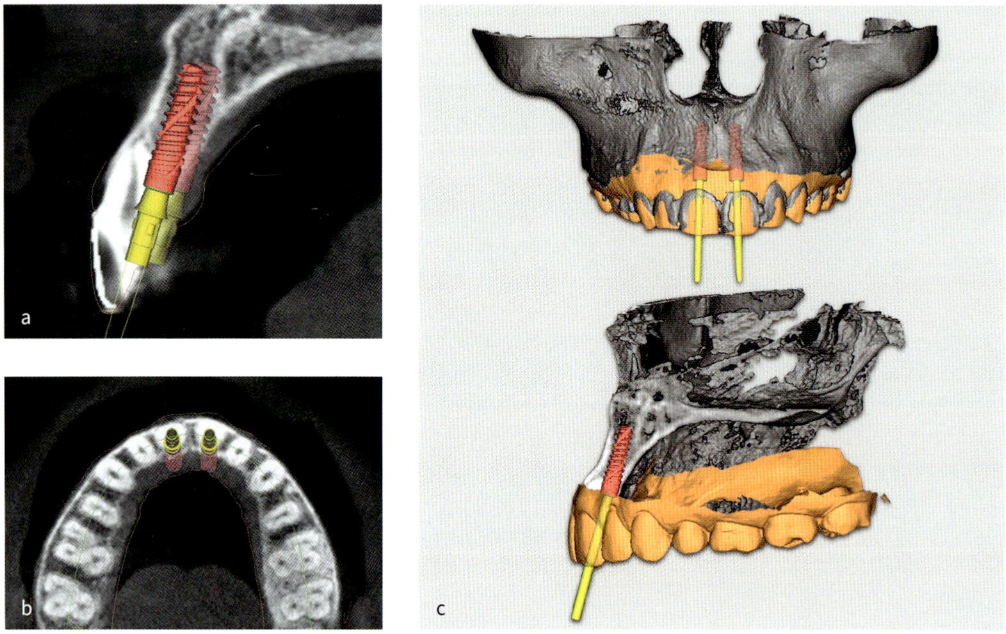

Figs 4a-c Digital surgical simulation. Sagittal (a) and axial (b) radiographic views. Frontal and lateral 3D views (c).

Table 1 Risk assessment for immediate implant placement in single-tooth sites

	Low risk	Medium risk	High risk
Preoperative assessment			
Patient-related			
Medical status	Healthy, uneventful healing		Compromised healing
Esthetic risk	Low/medium esthetic risk	High esthetic risk	Significant esthetic compromise expected
Site-related			
Gingival-margin position	No recession	Minor gingival recession	Gingival recession ≥ 2 mm
Soft tissue quality	Thick gingival phenotype	Thin gingival phenotype or limited keratinized gingiva	No keratinized gingiva
Bone anchorage	Sufficient bone anchorage to achieve primary stability		Lack of bone anchorage to achieve primary stability
Facial bone wall	≥ 1 mm facial bone thickness	Facial bone plate < 1 mm thickness, or small fenestration or dehiscence defect	Significant fenestration or dehiscence of facial bone
Need for a mucoperiosteal flap	Sufficient alveolar bone for a flapless approach		Need for flapped bone augmentation
Socket position within alveolar envelope	Socket within the alveolar bone envelope		Socket and facial bone wall protruding out of the bone envelope
Presence of endodontic infection	No infection	Chronic periapical infection	Acute infection
Presence of periodontal disease	Periodontally healthy	Controlled periodontal disease	Active periodontal disease
Planning implant position	Ideal three-dimensional position with axis exiting through the cingulum or incisal edge		Facially positioned or over-angulated implant or excessive implant depth
Gap between buccal bone and planned implant position	≥ 2 mm	1–2 mm	< 1 mm
Intraoperative assessment			
Extraction	Minimally invasive tooth extraction	Damage to surrounding soft tissue, including severed/detached papillae	Significant damage to soft tissue and surrounding bone
Primary implant stability	Primary stability achieved		Lack of primary stability
Final implant position	Ideal three-dimensional position achieved		Facially positioned or over-angulated implant or excessive implant depth

Table 2 Risk assessment for immediate loading of an immediately placed single implant

	Low risk	Medium risk	High risk
Preoperative assessment			
Patient-related			
Occlusal scheme	No direct occlusal contacts	Minimal occlusal contact and/or shared guidance	Main determinant of anterior guidance
Occlusal parafunction	Absent		Present
Site-related			
Bone anchorage	Sufficient bone anchorage to resist loading forces		Insufficient bone anchorage to resist loading forces
Tooth position	Incisor, premolars	Canine	Molars
Intraoperative assessment			
Primary implant stability	30–45 Ncm insertion torque	20–30 Ncm insertion torque	< 20 Ncm insertion torque

The virtual implant planning software was then linked to CAD/CAM software with the synergy feature (Straumann CARES, Institut Straumann AG). Titanium base abutments 2,5 mm in height (Variobase abutment, Institut Straumann AG) were selected. Two provisional restorations were digitally designed, improving the anatomy of the incisors, and connected to each abutment separately. Minor modifications to implant positions were performed to refine the restorative contours and biological positions of the implants within the alveolar process (Figs 5a-d).

Once the implant position and restorative design were finalized, the provisional implant restorations were exported and milled in polymethylmethacrylate (PMMA) (Straumann PMMA/CARES M Series; Institut Straumann AG). Both provisional crowns were cemented on the selected abutments (Multilink; Ivoclar Vivadent, Schaan, Liechtenstein). A surgical guide was designed in the virtual implant planning software, exported, and 3D-printed (P30, Institut Straumann AG) (Fig 6).

Marks designed and printed in the surgical guide (as a reference for the correct rotational position of the implant connection during implant placement) were outlined in black ink (Fig 7).

TREATMENT SEQUENCE

A local anesthetic (Scandicaine 2%; Septodont, Lancaster, PA, USA) was delivered on the buccal and palatal aspects of the maxillary anterior region. Using periotomes (PT5-PT6, Hu-Friedy, Chicago, IL, USA) and anterior forceps (Hu-Friedy), teeth 11 and 21 were carefully extracted with minimal trauma (Figs 8a-b).

The alveolar sockets were debrided and irrigated with saline solution. The fit of the 3D-printed surgical guide was verified by visualization in the inspection windows, and guided osteotomies were performed.

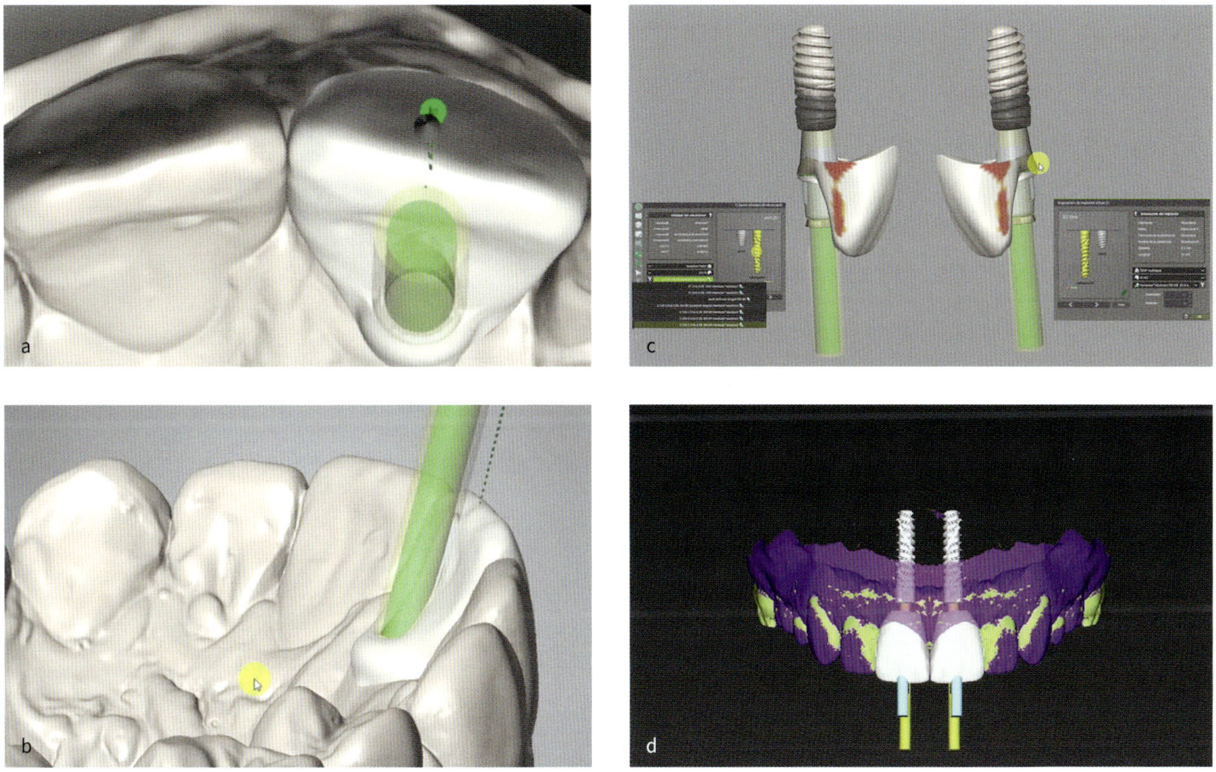

Figs 5a-d Digital restorative simulation. Occlusal (a) and lateral 3D (b) view on the Straumann CARES screen. Provisional restoration design process). Straumann Cares screen (c). Restorations and implants 3D, frontal view, coDiagnostiX screen (d).

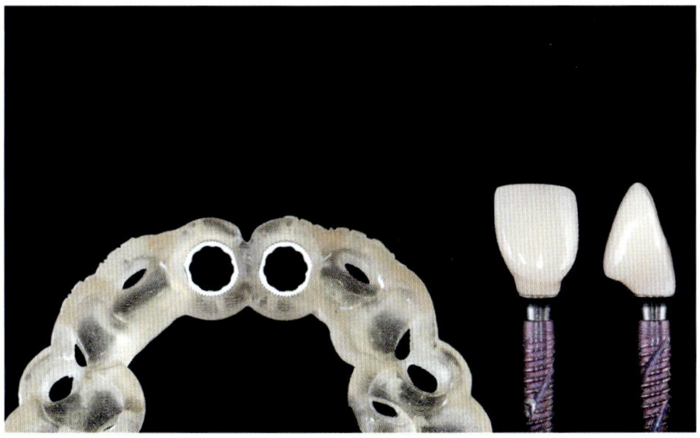

Fig 6 3D-printed surgical guide with surgical sleeves in position. Internal surface. The provisional restorations were milled and polished. Both crowns were adhesively cemented to the Variobase abutments.

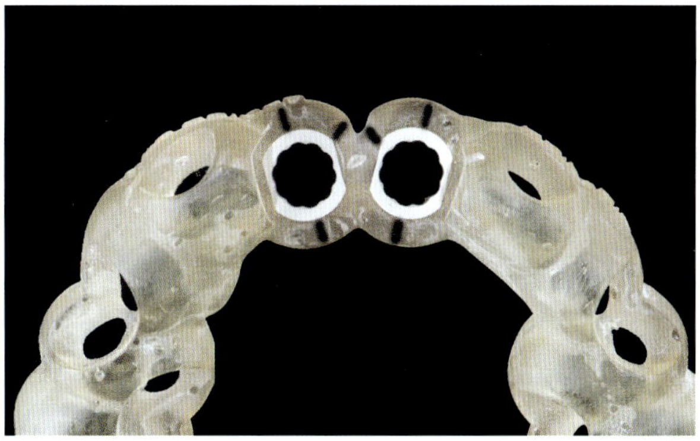

Fig 7 External surface of the 3D-printed surgical guide. The surgical sleeves are already in position. Black marks at the 3D printed reference channels.

Use this QR code to view a highlight video of the guided osteotomy following s-CAIS protocol using a 2.8 mm diameter by 20 mm length drill in region 21.

Use this QR code to view a highlight video of the guided osteotomy following s-CAIS protocol using a 2.8 mm diameter by 20 mm length drill in region 11.

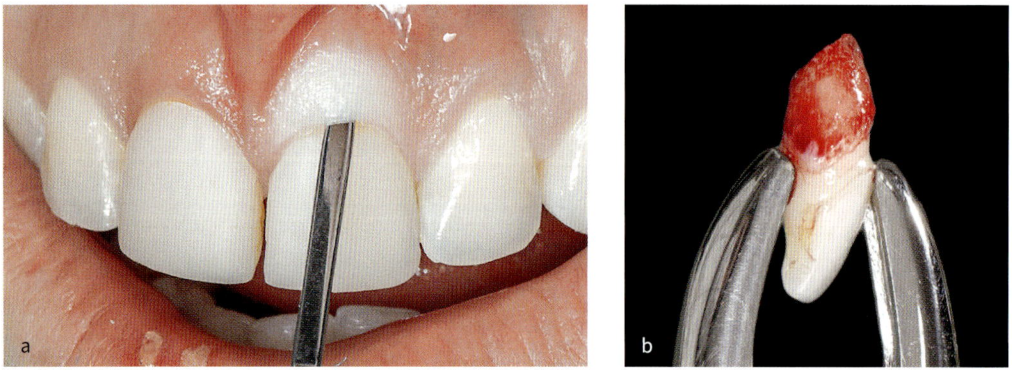

Figs 8a-b The central incisors were luxated with periotomes and carefully extracted with anterior forceps using rotational movements.

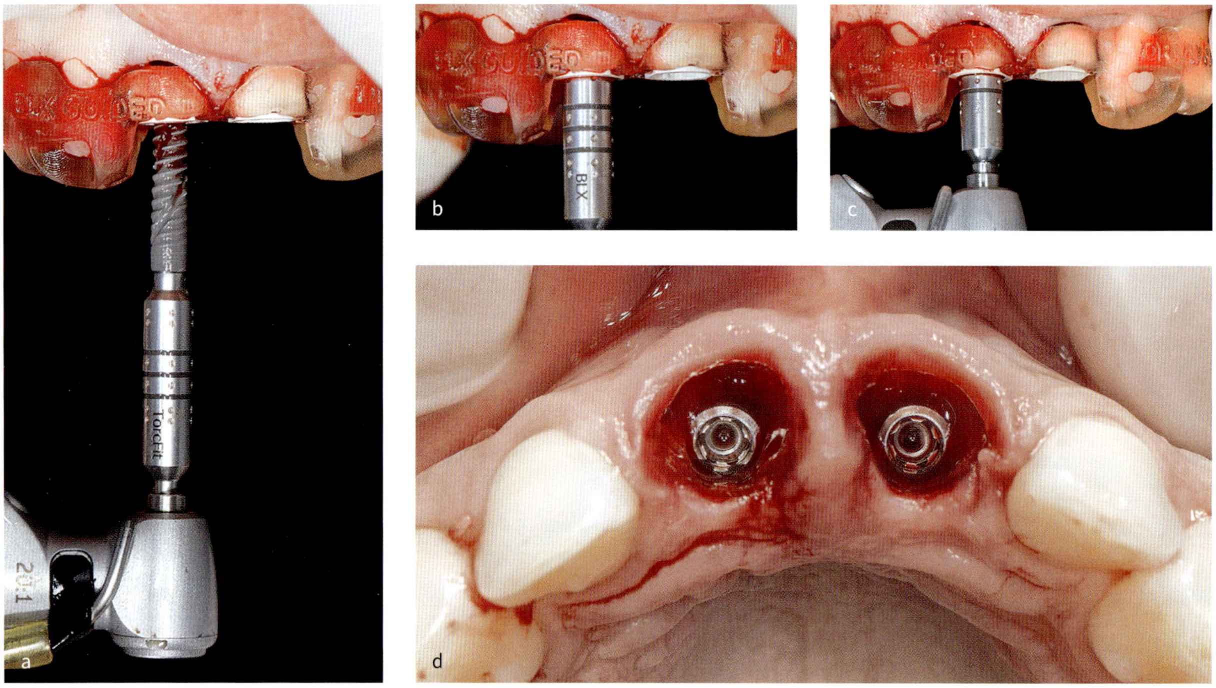

Figs 9a-d Guided osteotomies were performed based on the surgical protocol obtained from the software (a-c), and the implants were place following a fully guided protocol (d).

Implants (STML BLX RB SLActive, diameter 3.75 mm, length 12 mm; Institut Straumann AG) were placed in a fully guided protocol. An insertion torque of 60 Ncm was achieved at both sites (Figs 9a-d).

Healing abutments (RB; Institut Straumann AG) were placed on the implants. To fill the gap between the implants and the buccal bone walls of the two sockets, a deproteinized bovine bone mineral substitute (DBBM) was gently introduced and packed (Cerabone; Botiss, Zossen, Germany) (Figs 10 and 11).

The healing abutments were removed to allow for the delivery of the prefabricated CAD/CAM provisional restorations and the abutment screws tightened to 15 Ncm.

Use this QR code to view a highlight video of the removal of the healing abutment for the insertion of the CAD/CAM prefabricated provisional restoration.

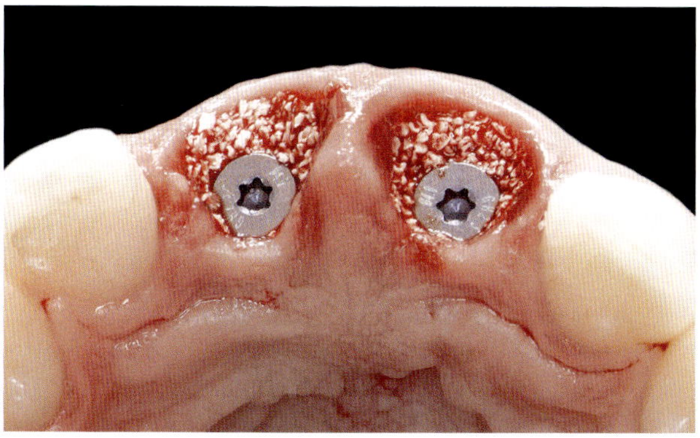

Fig 10 DBBM bone substitute filling the gap between the implants and surrounding bone.

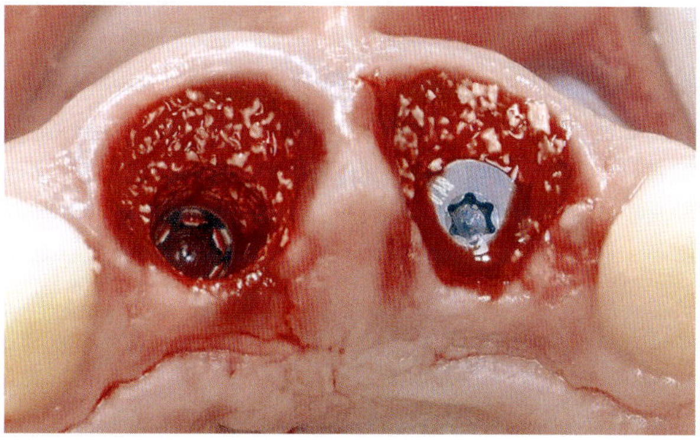

Fig 11 Same situation as in Figure 10, with healing abutments were removed to install the provisional restorations.

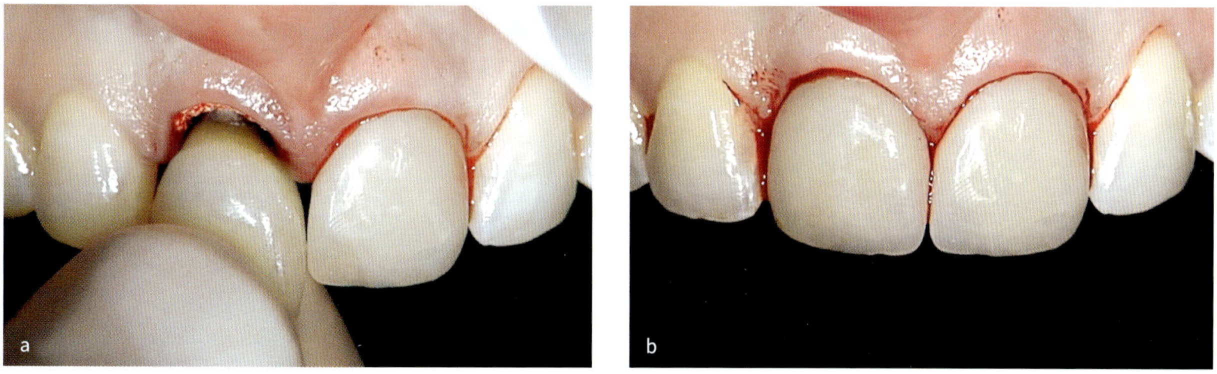

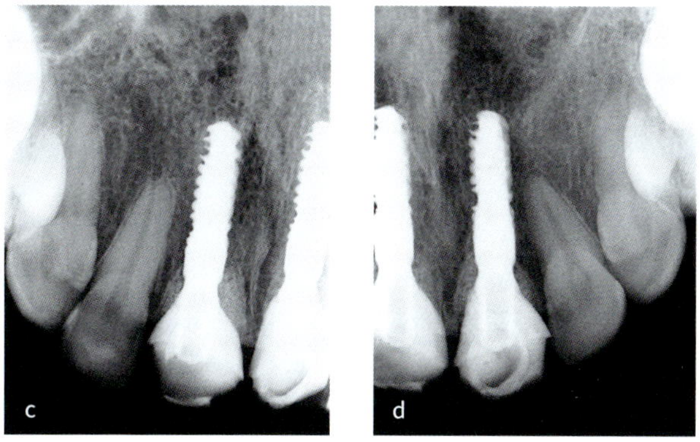

Figs 12a-d Provisional restorations installed and torqued at 15 Ncm (a-b). Periapical radiographs were requested (c-d).

The screw holes were covered with polytetrafluoroethylene (PTFE) tape and composite resin (Tetric N-Ceram Flow; Ivoclar Vivadent). The occlusion was checked to ensure the provisional restorations had no contacts in maximum intercuspation and eccentric mandible movements. A small layer of direct composite resin was added buccally to both crowns to improve the color match and mask the grayish color of the metallic abutments (Tetric N-Ceram, Ivoclar Vivadent). Periapical radiographs were evaluated after the surgery to confirm the restorations were fully seated (Figs 12a-d). Ketoprofen 100 mg twice a day (Profenid; Sanofi-Aventis, Bridgewater, NJ, USA) was prescribed for three days, as well as Amoxicillin 875 mg twice a day (Optamox; Pharma-Investi, Santiago, Chile) for seven days. The patient was dismissed and followed up at 3, 15, 21, 30 days and at four months. No complications were reported.

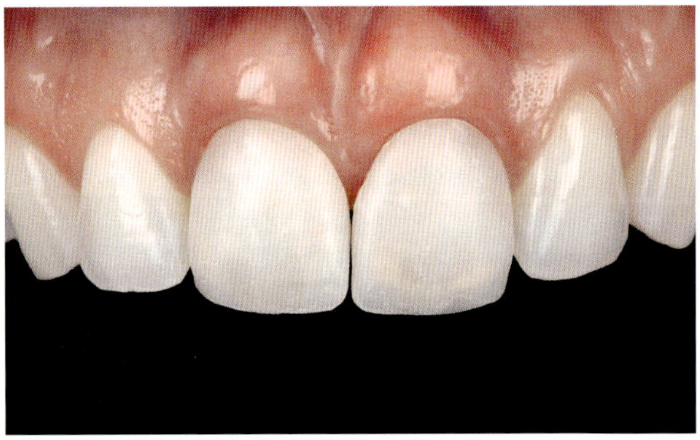

Fig 13 Provisional restorations in place for four months. The desired emergence profile was obtained based on the design of the provisionals.

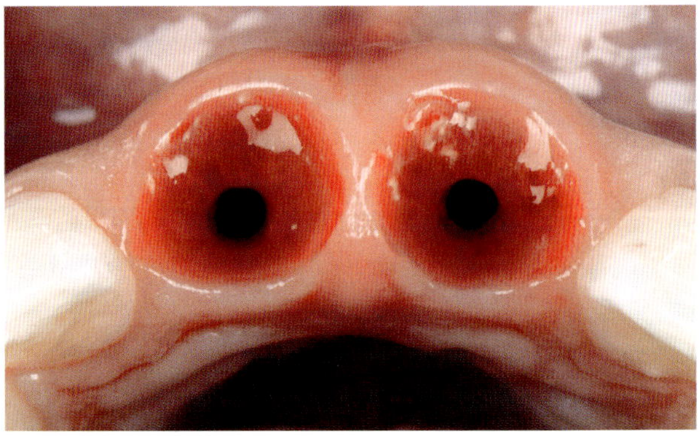

Fig 14 The provisional crowns were removed four months after implant placement.

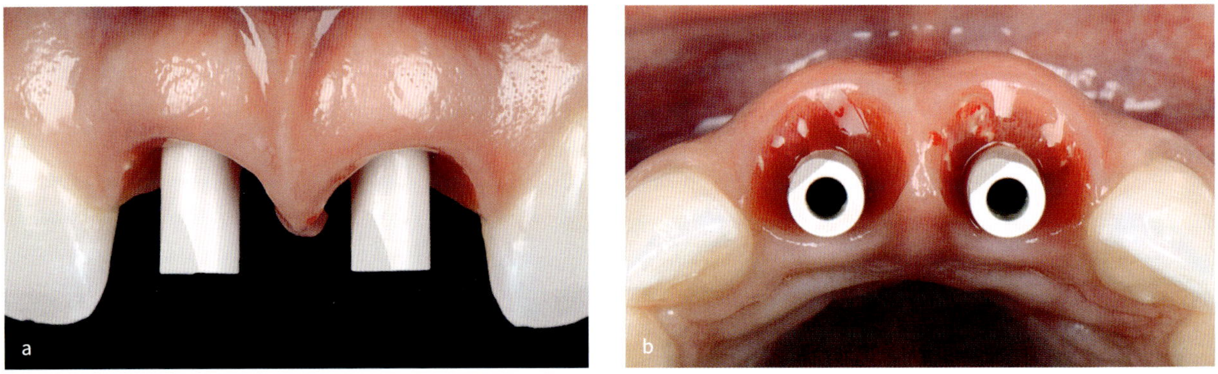

Figs 15a-b Scanbodies in position for the digital impression.

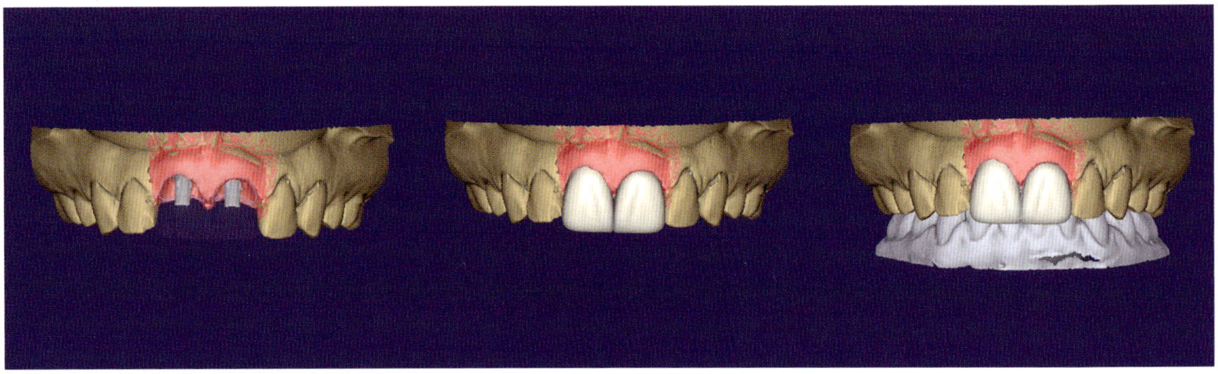

Fig 16 Digital design of the ceramic restorations in the Exocad software.

At four months, the desired emergence profile of both central incisors had been achieved. The provisional crowns were removed (Figs 13 and 14) and digital implant impressions were performed (Trios 2; 3Shape, Copenhagen, Denmark, and RB Scan Body; Institut Straumann AG) (Figs 15a-b).

Digital information was imported into CAD software (Exocad; Align Technology, Darmstadt, Germany). Two ceramic crowns were designed to be cemented over titanium-base abutments with a direct palatal screw access (Fig 16).

The files were exported and the restorations milled (Emax CAD MO; Ivoclar Vivadent). A 3D-printed model was also generated to be used for a minimal esthetic ceramic build-up of the crowns and for final adjustments (Emax Ceram; Ivoclar Vivadent) (Figs 17a-c).

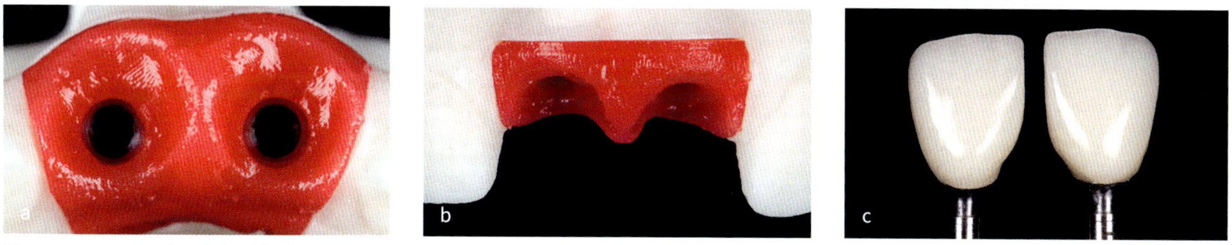

Figs 17a-c 3D-printed model and final restorations.

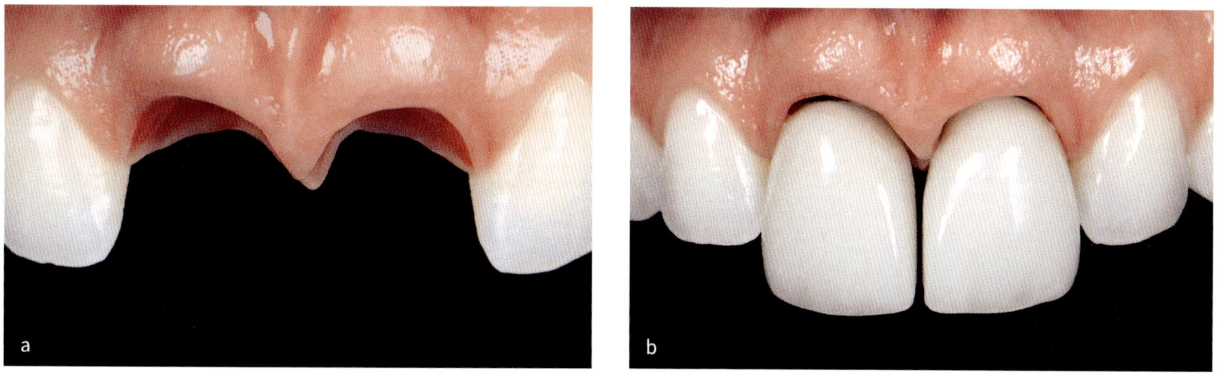

Figs 18a-b Trying in the final restorations for final checking. Small adjustments were requested.

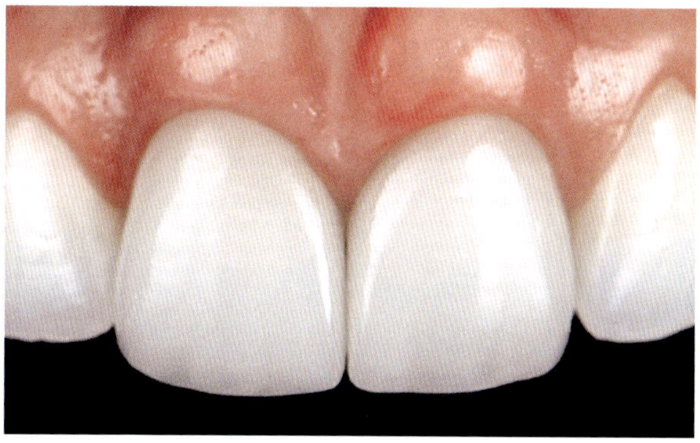

Fig 19 Definitive crowns delivered and abutment screws tightened.

The ceramic structures were fitted and tried in on the implants (Figs 18a-b). Minor modifications were requested from the laboratory.

At the next appointment, the final restorations were tried in. After approval, the ceramic crowns were cemented onto the definitive implant abutments (VarioBase RB; Institut Straumann AG, and Multilink Hybrid; Ivoclar Vivadent) The hybrid crowns for the implants were delivered and the abutment screws tightened to 35 Ncm. The screw access holes were sealed with PTFE and composite resin (Fig 19 and Figs 20a-b)

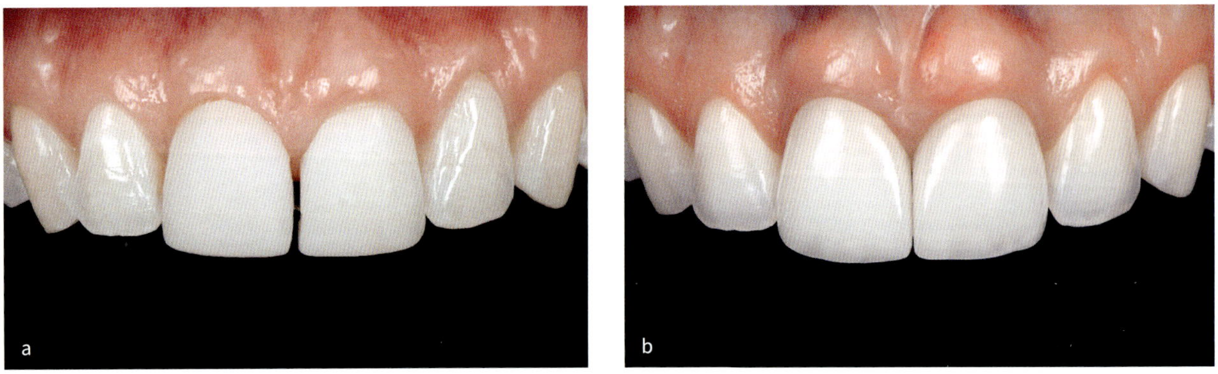

Figs 20a-b Comparison between the initial situation and the situation with the final restorations delivered.

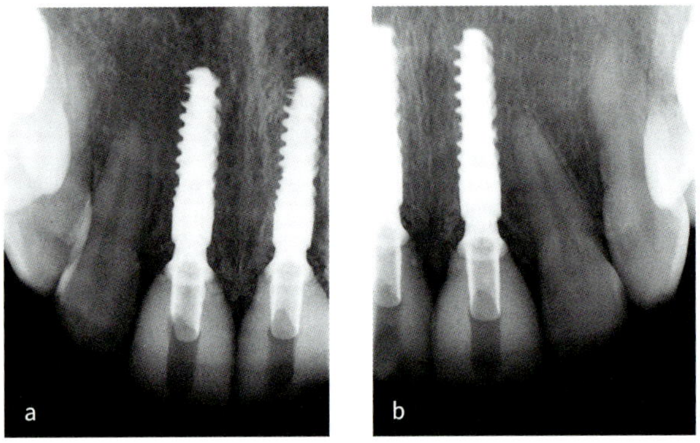

Figs 21a-b Periapical radiographs after delivery of the restorations.

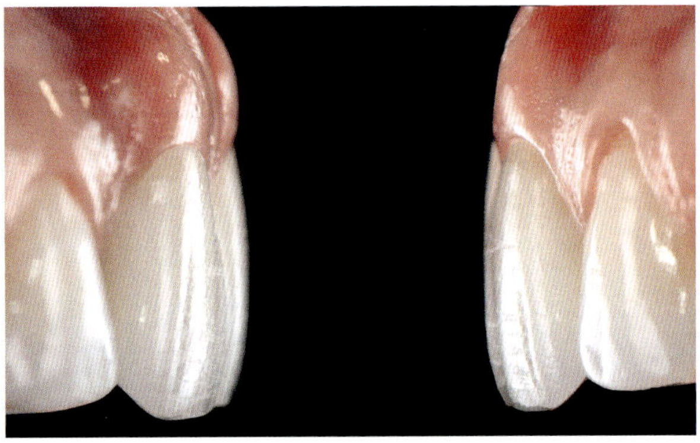

Fig 22 Six-month follow-up. Lateral close-up of the final restorations.

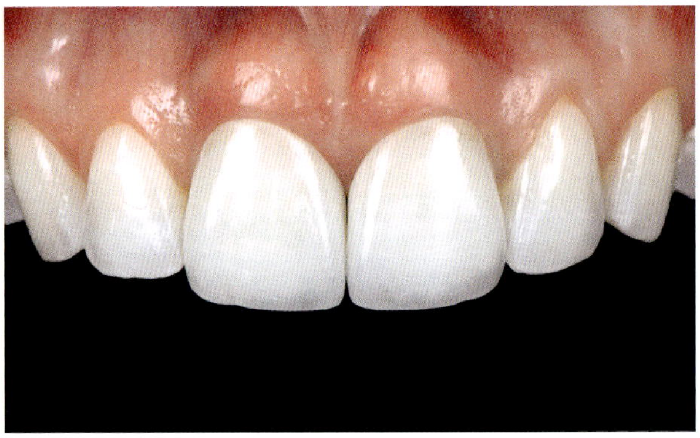

Fig 23 Two year follow-up. Intraoral frontal view.

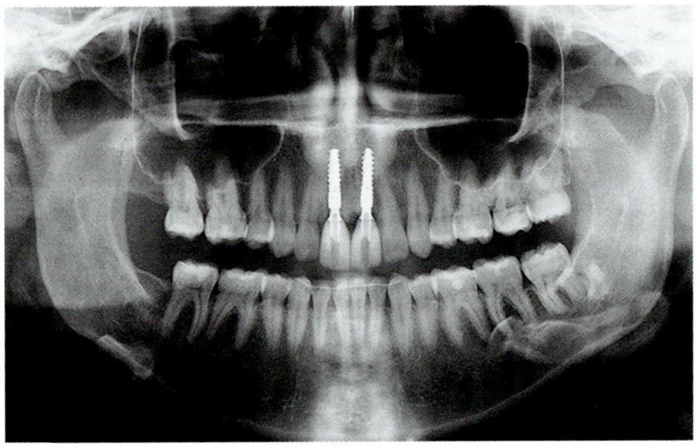

Fig 24 Two year radiographic follow-up. Orthopantomogram.

Periapical radiographs were requested (Figs 21a-b). The patient has been periodically followed for two years; no complications have been reported (Figs 22 to 24).

DISCUSSION

It is well documented that the long-term success of immediate implants in the esthetic zone depends on multiple factors (Morton and coworkers 2018; Gallucci and coworkers 2018; Levine and coworkers 2017). Proper patient selection and adequate treatment are fundamental in achieving ideal esthetic outcomes with implant-supported restorations. Anatomical conditions at the surgical site are considered a key factor for treatment predictability (Chappuis and coworkers 2013; Belser and coworkers 2009). In the clinical situation described, the two upper central incisors presented with grade 1 to 2 mobility due to advanced external root resorption, and the patient was highly uncomfortable with the situation. At sites 11 and 21, the patient presented with an intact buccal bone wall, a thick gingival phenotype, no signs of acute infection, and a bone quantity adequate for supporting an immediate implant. It was therefore decided to proceed with a 1A clinical protocol, as presented in the Proceedings of the 6th ITI Consensus Conference (Gallucci and coworkers 2018).

The use of a specific reduced-diameter implant helped keep the shoulder far enough from the buccal bone wall while allowing more space for socket management and helping to reduce buccal bone resorption (Evans and Chen 2008; Fürhauser and coworkers 2005; Araújo and coworkers 2005; Chappuis and coworkers 2017; Li and coworkers 2018).

In the same way, the utilization of a low-rate resorption bone substitute to fill the gap was considered to counteract a potential shrinkage of the tissues after extraction (Kuchler and coworkers 2016; van Nimwegen and coworkers 2018; Frizzera and coworkers 2019; Noelken and coworkers 2018). In this particular case, due to the presence of thick a gingival phenotype in the extractions sites, a connective tissue graft was not indicated.

The novel design of the implants permitted an insertion torque of more than 60 Ncm, providing more than adequate primary stability for immediate loading (Papaspyridakos and coworkers 2014; Javed and coworkers 2013).

One obstacle to the precise placement of an implant in an extraction socket is that drills tend to follow the path of least resistance, resulting in implant positions that are more buccal than desired as a consequence of the dense cortex of the palatal socket (Arcuri and coworkers 2019; Buser and coworkers 2000; Tarnow and coworkers 2000). Therefore, the use of a rigid surgical guide may reduce placement errors resulting from any resistance that the more dense palatal bone can offer to the implant as the osteotomy is being prepared and the implant is inserted (Lanis and coworkers 2017; Matta and coworkers 2017).

The synergy concept was developed to unite the prosthetic and surgical worlds in a single virtual scenario to design and fabricate implant restorations prior to implant placement. This provides benefits, including detailed prosthetically driven implant planning, shorter surgical procedures, and lower patient morbidity (Lanis and coworkers 2017).

Often the negative impact of compromised implant positions on the esthetic outcomes will not be recognized until the final restoration is fabricated. The present approach allows for the detailed visualization of the final implant-prosthodontic outcome ahead of the treatment, which will help minimize esthetic complications.

For technical reasons, the fabrication of restorations prior to implant placement is highly dependent on precise implant positions based on digital planning. In the clinical situation described, implants were placed following a fully guided protocol for precise replication of the virtual implant planning. For the technique to be successful, the mesiodistal and buccolingual positions, angulation, rotation, and placement depth of the implant all have to be extremely well controlled since the position of the prosthetic connection will determine the crown position. To master this challenge, a guided implant mount is recommended, with specific rotational markings designed and integrated into the surgical guide. This ensures that, as the implant is installed, the reference marks from the implant mount and the surgical guide will coincide. Moreover, the surgical procedure has to be performed under extreme precautions and taking into consideration the guided surgery protocol obtained from the planning software.

CONCLUSION

Comprehensive virtual implant planning in combination with s-CAIS and the synergy protocol can aid in obtaining an ideal implant positioning and therefore, may be considered as a valuable tool when immediate implant placement is performed. This case report shows proof of concept that a restoration can be fabricated and delivered based on a virtually planned implant position.

ACKNOWLEDGMENTS

Intrasurgical photography

Dr. Orlando Álvarez – Santiago, Chile

5.5 Replacement of a Maxillary Left Canine with a Cemented Crown on an Immediately Placed Bone-Level Tapered Implant Using a One-Abutment, One-Time Approach

K. Chmielewski, B. Roland

A 42-year-old woman was a regular maintenance patient at our office. During a recall and hygiene appointment, signs of external resorption were noticed on the vestibular root surface of tooth 23 (Figs 1 and 2).

A detailed examination was performed including a CBCT and Esthetic Risk Assessment. The patient, a non-smoker, was in good general health.

The intraoral examination showed slight soft tissue recession of tooth 23. A resorption chamber in the root of the upper left canine was filled with granulation tissue below the soft tissue zenith, without a visible dentin barrier. According to the Heithersay clinical classification of hyperplastic invasive dental resorptions (Heithersay 2007), the case qualified for the initial phase of class 3 invasive cervical resorption due to the lack of a visible dentin barrier.

The recommended treatment for Heithersay class 3 situations includes the topical application of 90% trichloroacetic acid to the resorptive tissue, curettage, elective pulpectomy, and root canal preparation; intracanal dressing with Ledermix paste (Esteve; Torre Esteve, Barcelona, Spain), followed by root-canal filling and a final glass-ionomer cement restoration. In some cases, a periodontal flap must be reflected for better access (Heithersay 2007).

Following a discussion with the patient about the expected outcomes of this treatment, including the potential recurrence of resorption and esthetic complications, it was decided to extract and replace the tooth with a dental implant.

The vestibular external root resorption was clearly visible in cross-section in the cone-beam computed tomography (CBCT) image (Fig 3).

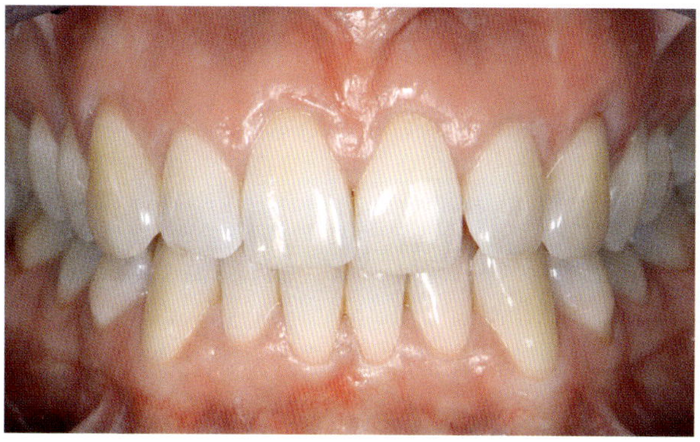

Fig 1 Initial situation.

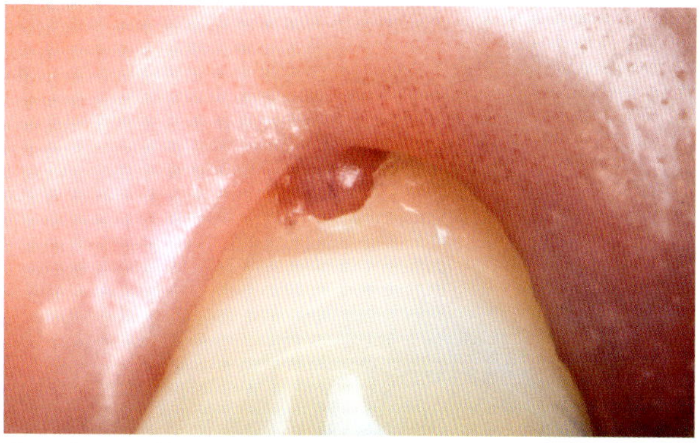

Fig 2 Close-up of the cervical aspect of tooth 23. Visible external resorption.

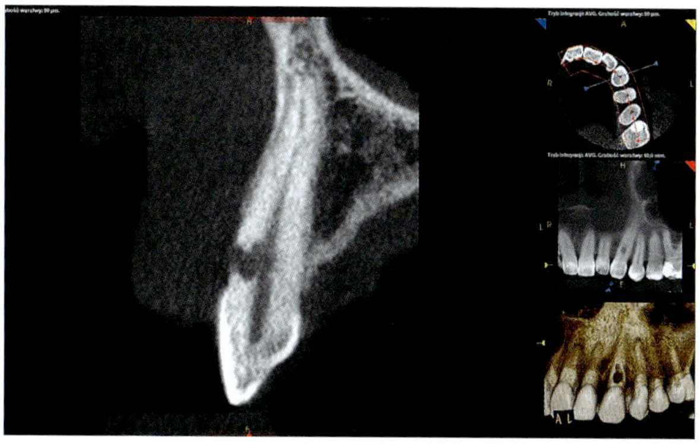

Fig 3 Cross-sectional view of tooth 23 showing external root resorption.

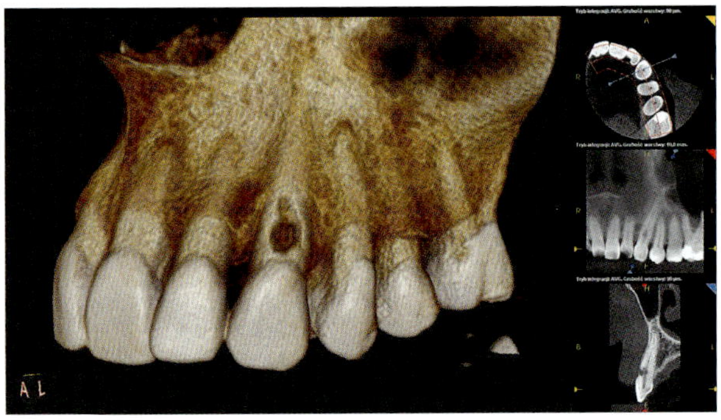

Fig 4 CBCT 3D reconstruction. External root resorption of root 23.

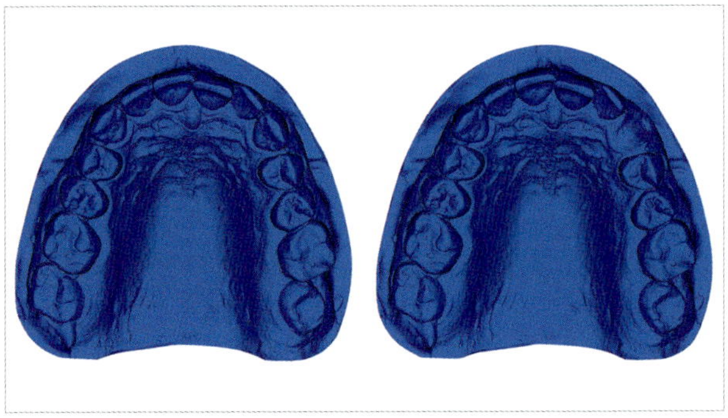

Fig 5 STL files (right: without tooth 23).

An additional 3D reconstruction highlighted the size of the defect (Fig 4).

The tooth was located in the esthetic zone, and the patient exhibited a high smile line. The case was therefore assessed as "high risk" according to the ITI Esthetic Risk Assessment (ERA) (Martin and coworkers 2017).

Tables 1 and 2 highlight the risk factors associated with the case.

Assuming that the optimal 3D implant position can be achieved and primary stability of the implant allows immediate loading, the case can be classified as "medium difficulty." The main risk factors are of an esthetic and anatomical nature (tissue phenotype), including the position of the tooth in the dental arch.

TREATMENT PLAN

The situation and available treatment scenarios were discussed with the patient. The following treatment plan was agreed on:

- Planning of the implant position
- Fabrication of a surgical guide
- Planning and fabrication of the final abutment and temporary crown
- Extraction of tooth 23
- Immediate implantation with guided surgery
- Post-extraction socket augmentation with a xenograft
- Immediate non-functional loading of the implant with the final hybrid abutment and a cemented temporary crown
- Evaluation of implant integration and soft tissue maturation and shape after four months of loading
- Delivery of the final restoration with a cemented ceramic crown after a further five months

The surgical protocol called for immediate implant placement (type 1A; Gallucci and coworkers 2018) and immediate loading.

However, an alternative plan was also prepared in the event that insufficient primary stability was encountered (type 1C; Gallucci and coworkers 2018):

- Immediate implantation, filling the remaining socket gap with a biomaterial with a low substitution rate
- Temporary adhesive bridge
- Temporary restoration and progressive implant loading after four months and upon completion of shaping of the soft tissue
- Final restoration after six months

Alginate impressions were taken of both jaws and casts were poured in dental stone. The two casts were scanned and digitalized using the laboratory desktop scanner to obtain Standard Tesselation Language (STL) files. For planning purposes and to design the surgical guide for guided surgery, tooth 23 had to be removed from the maxillary cast. A second scan yielded a digital STL file (Fig 5).

Table 1 Risk assessment for immediate implant placement in single-tooth sites

	Low risk	Medium risk	High risk
Preoperative assessment			
Patient-related			
Medical status	Healthy, uneventful healing		Compromised healing
Esthetic risk	Low/medium esthetic risk	High esthetic risk	Significant esthetic compromise expected
Site-related			
Gingival-margin position	No recession	Minor gingival recession	Gingival recession ≥ 2 mm
Soft tissue quality	Thick gingival phenotype	Thin gingival phenotype or limited keratinized gingiva	No keratinized gingiva
Bone anchorage	Sufficient bone anchorage to achieve primary stability		Lack of bone anchorage to achieve primary stability
Facial bone wall	≥ 1 mm facial bone thickness	Facial bone plate < 1 mm thickness, or small fenestration or dehiscence defect	Significant fenestration or dehiscence of facial bone
Need for a mucoperiosteal flap	Sufficient alveolar bone for a flapless approach		Need for flapped bone augmentation
Socket position within alveolar envelope	Socket within the alveolar bone envelope		Socket and facial bone wall protruding out of the bone envelope
Presence of endodontic infection	No infection	Chronic periapical infection	Acute infection
Presence of periodontal disease	Periodontally healthy	Controlled periodontal disease	Active periodontal disease
Planning implant position	Ideal three-dimensional position with axis exiting through the cingulum or incisal edge		Facially positioned or over-angulated implant or excessive implant depth
Gap between buccal bone and planned implant position	≥ 2 mm	1–2 mm	< 1 mm
Intraoperative assessment			
Extraction	Minimally invasive tooth extraction	Damage to surrounding soft tissue, including severed/ detached papillae	Significant damage to soft tissue and surrounding bone
Primary implant stability	Primary stability achieved		Lack of primary stability
Final implant position	Ideal three-dimensional position achieved		Facially positioned or over-angulated implant or excessive implant depth

Table 2 Risk assessment for immediate loading of an immediately placed single implant

	Low risk	Medium risk	High risk
Preoperative assessment			
Patient-related			
Occlusal scheme	No direct occlusal contacts	Minimal occlusal contact and/or shared guidance	Main determinant of anterior guidance
Occlusal parafunction	Absent		Present
Site-related			
Bone anchorage	Sufficient bone anchorage to resist loading forces		Insufficient bone anchorage to resist loading forces
Tooth position	Incisor, premolars	Canine	Molars
Intraoperative assessment			
Primary implant stability	30–45 Ncm insertion torque	20–30 Ncm insertion torque	< 20 Ncm insertion torque

PLANNING THE IMPLANT POSITION AND DESIGNING THE GUIDE

The implant position was planned and the surgical guide designed using a virtual implant planning software package (coDiagnostiX; DentalWings, Montreal, Canada). After importing the uncompressed Digital Imaging and Communications in Medicine (DICOM) files from the CBCT examination, the process of planning followed these steps:

Step 1. Segmentation of the data to create the maxillary digital 3D model of the bone and teeth. The color green was chosen for better differentiation between the layers (Fig 6).

Step 2. Superimposition of the maxillary STL model with the teeth (blue) on the segmented DICOM model (green) (Fig 7).

Step 3. Superimposition of the teeth of the second maxillary STL model (without the removed tooth 23): the compound model (Fig 8).

Step 4. Planning of the optimal 3D position for an implant at site 23 (Fig 9) to obtain the best possible axis for the prosthetic restoration and to provide additional bone anchorage. The STL models also represent the soft tissue, which allows adjustment of the position of the implant prosthetic platform to the soft tissue level. A BLT SLA Roxolid RC implant (diameter 4.1 mm, length 14 mm; Institut Straumann AG, Basel, Switzerland) was selected.

Step 5. Planning of a drilling sleeve 5 mm in diameter to depth stop H4 to ensure the correct position and avoid collision with the soft tissue. H4 means a 4 mm distance of the sleeve from the implant platform and is the maximum distance for a 14 mm implant, given the length of the available drills (Fig 9).

Step 6. Designing the guide based on the STL file of the maxillary model. Following the onscreen instructions, the guide is designed with additional information regarding the implant index position to obtain the correct orientation (Fig 10). To facilitate the final fitting of the guide during the surgical procedure, windows were created in the guide before printing (Fig 11).

Step 7. Using a virtual implant planning software (coDiagnostiX; DentalWings), the planning was sent to the dental technician.

The dental technician (Björn Röland) also received the STL files of the models via a file-transfer service (WeTransfer, Amsterdam, Netherlands),

Depending on the settings, the guide may be either printed or milled. In this case the guide was printed on the SLA Printer (Form 2; Formlabs, MA, USA) with clear medical resin. The guide was rinsed in fresh isopropanol and fully post-cured to maximize its mechanical properties.

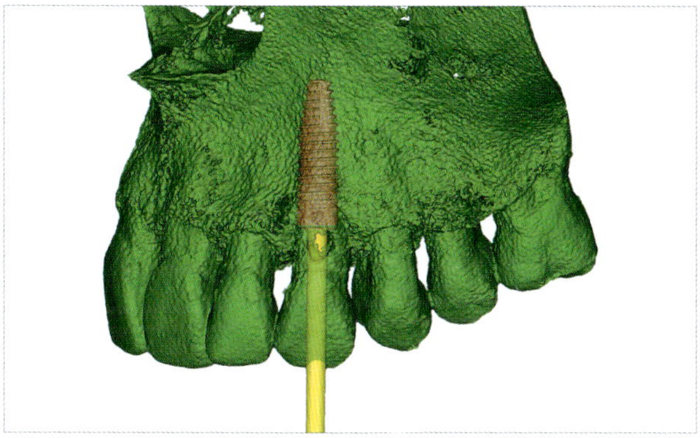

Fig 6 3D segmentation of the hard tissue and the implant position.

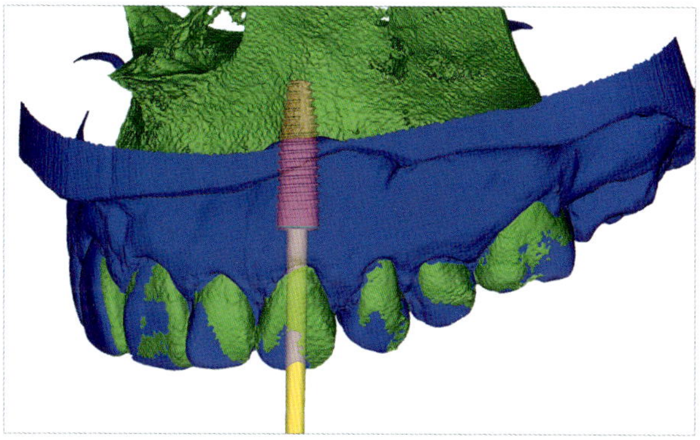

Fig 7 Superimposed DICOM and STL files showing the implant position.

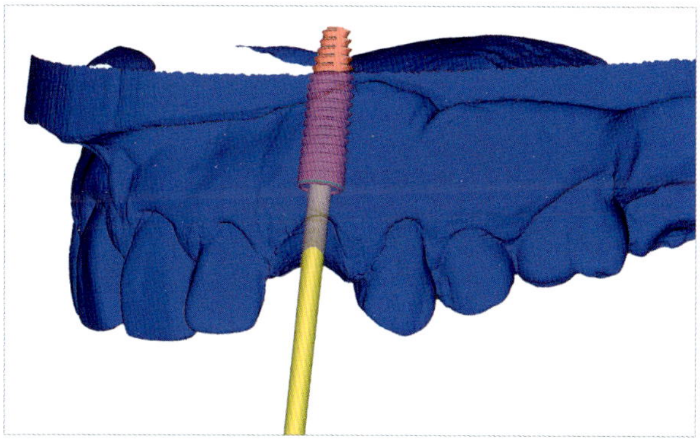

Fig 8 Maxillary 3D digital model without tooth 23.

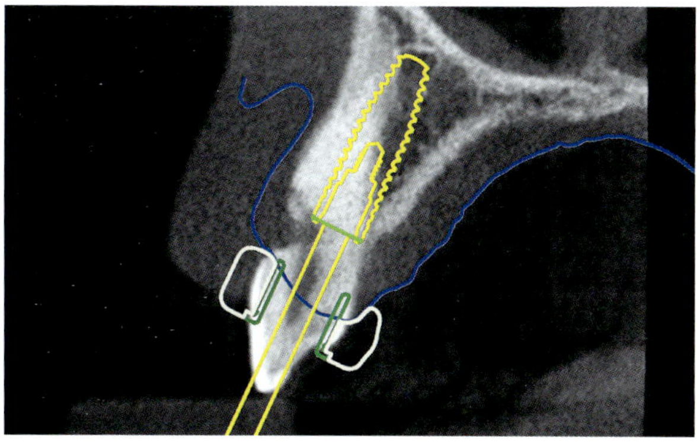

Fig 9 Cross-sectional view with implant 23. The green outline visualizes the drilling sleeve in the relation to the soft tissue (blue). The implant platform platform was planned 3.5 mm below the soft tissue zenith.

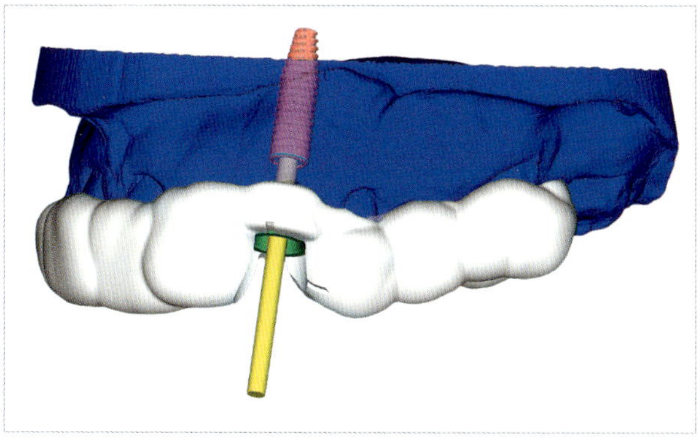

Fig 10 Surgical guide design (lateral view).

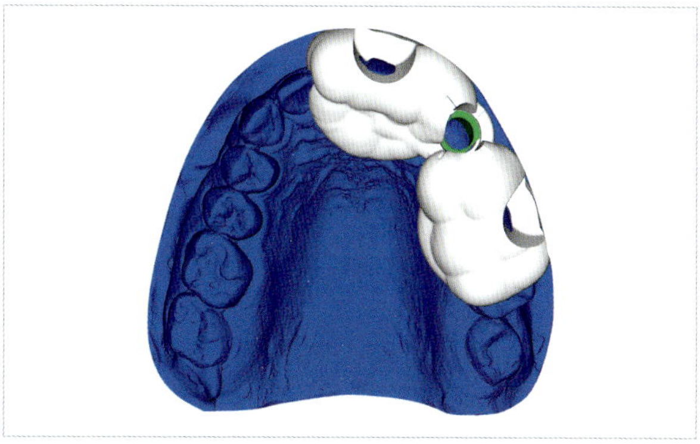

Fig 11 Surgical guide design with inspection windows.

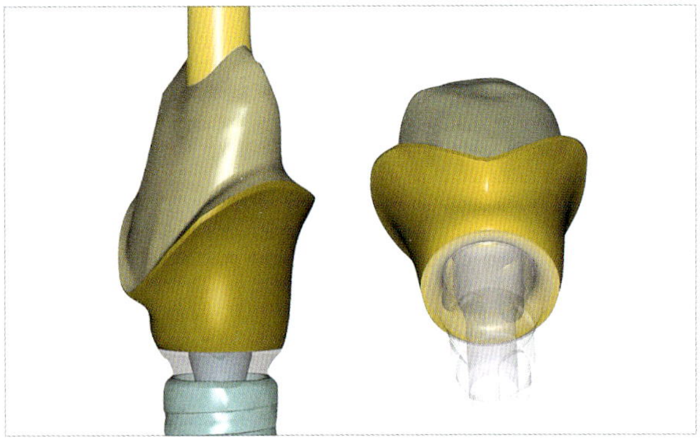

Fig 12 Design of the hybrid abutment based on the RC Variobase abutment.

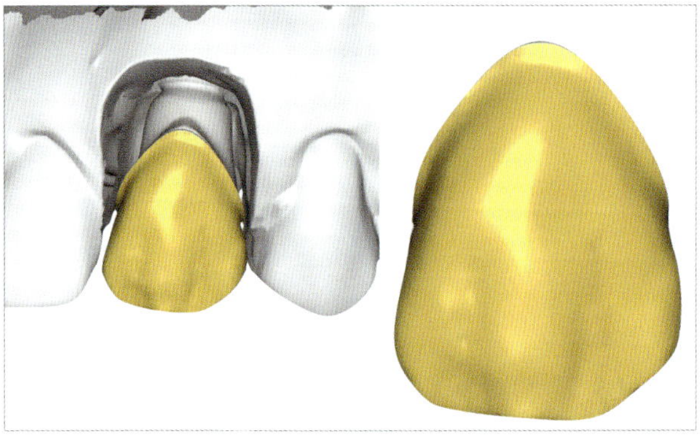

Fig 13 Design of the coping for the final crown.

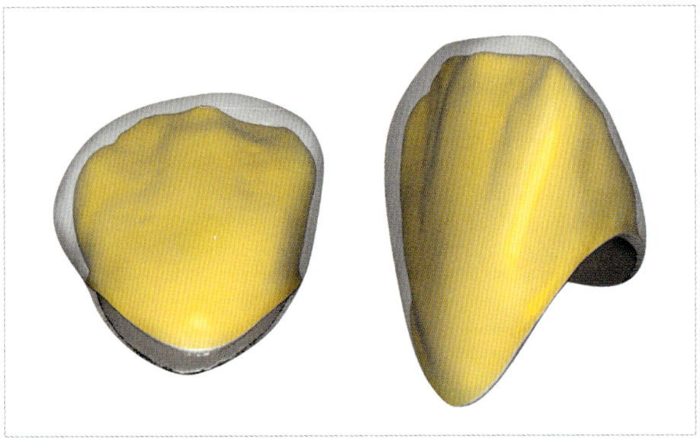

Fig 14 Design of the coping for the final crown with reduction for final layering with ceramic.

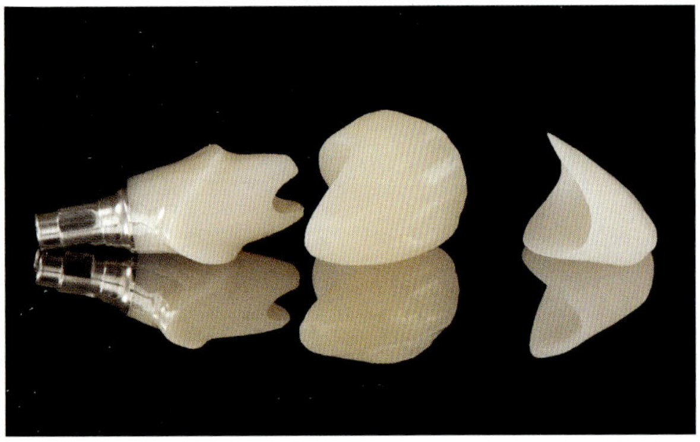

Fig 15 Custom hybrid abutment, temporary crown, and zirconia coping for the final crown.

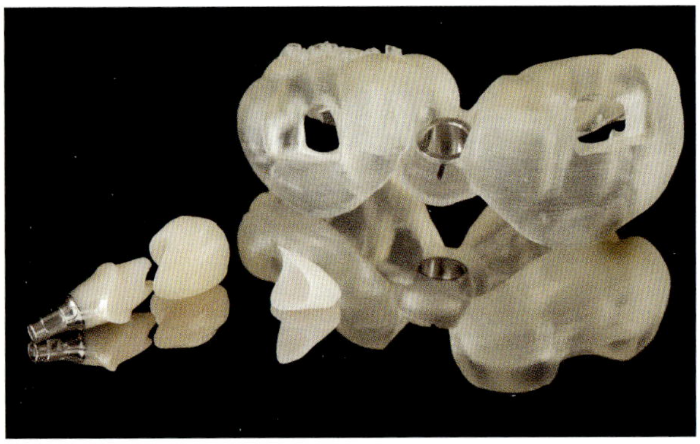

Fig 16 The surgical guide, individual hybrid abutment, temporary crown, and zirconia coping for the final crown.

PREPARATION OF THE ABUTMENT, TEMPORARY CROWN, AND COPING FOR THE FINAL CROWN.

The shape of the custom abutment with an optimized emergence profile was designed in CAD software (ExoCad, Darmstadt, Germany) (Fig 12).

The temporary and final crown were then designed, taking into consideration the final esthetic outcome (Figs 13 and 14).

The custom abutment was created using a zirconia material (Katana HT 12; Kuraray Noritake, Hattersheim, Germany) and bonded with an opaque cement (Panavia V5; Kuraray Noritake) to a titanium base abutment (RC Variobase; Institut Straumann AG).

The temporary crown was milled from a composite blank Bio (HIPC A2; Bredent, Poznań, Poland).

The dental laboratory delivered the surgical guide, individual hybrid abutment, temporary crown, and coping for the final crown (Fig 15).

Assembled with a metal guide, the sleeve was prepared for disinfection prior to intraoperative use. For a clearer view, index marks were created with a black marker on the printed guide (Fig 16).

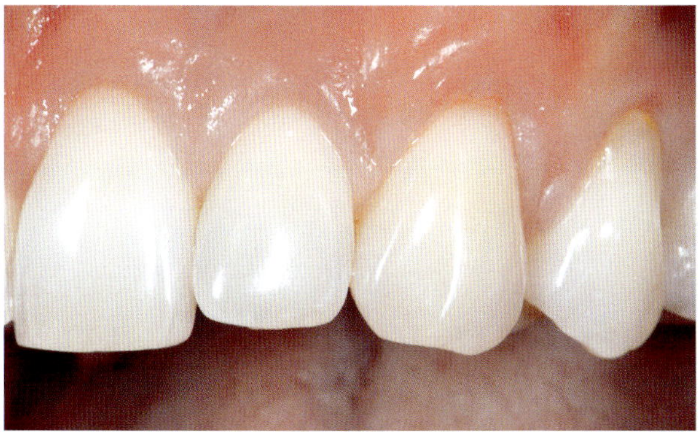
Fig 17 Initial situation on the day of the surgery.

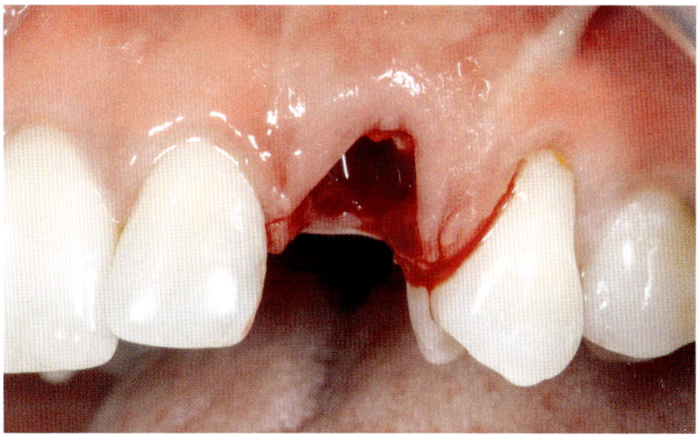
Fig 18 The crown of tooth 23 has been separated.

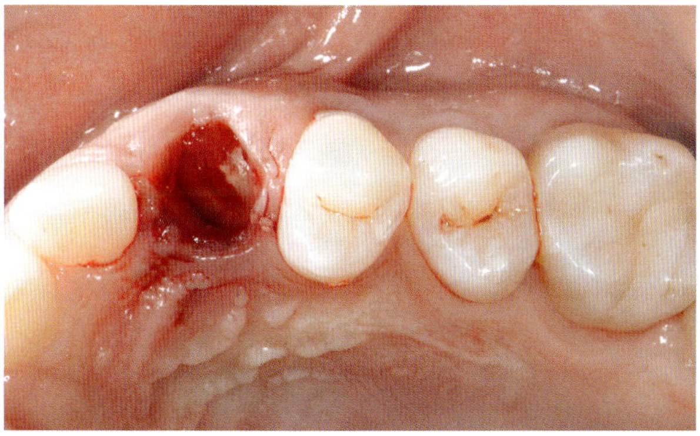
Fig 19 Residual root of tooth 23.

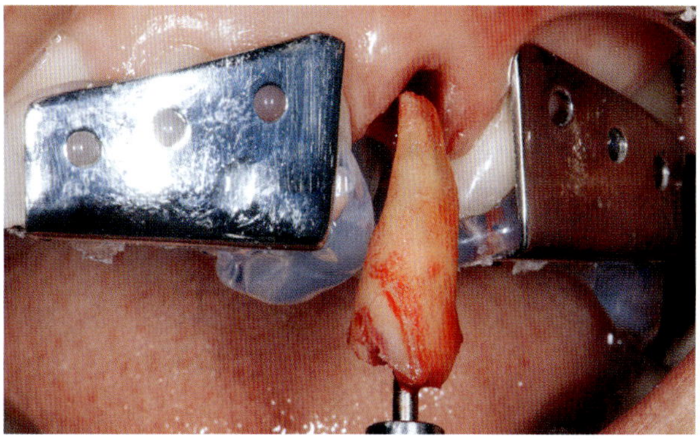
Fig 20 Removal of root 23 with a minimally invasive extraction system.

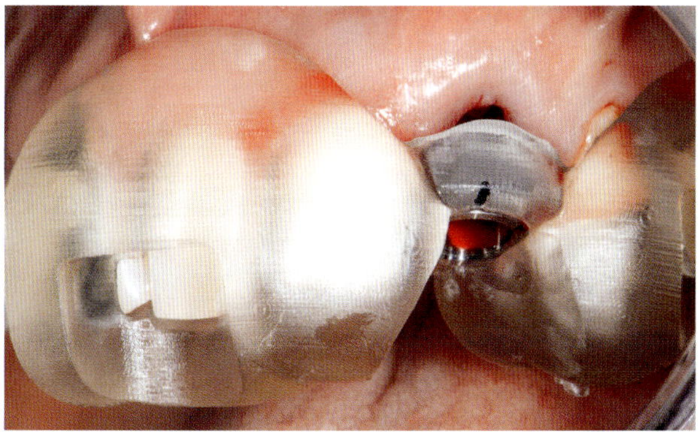
Fig 21 Checking the fit of the surgical guide.

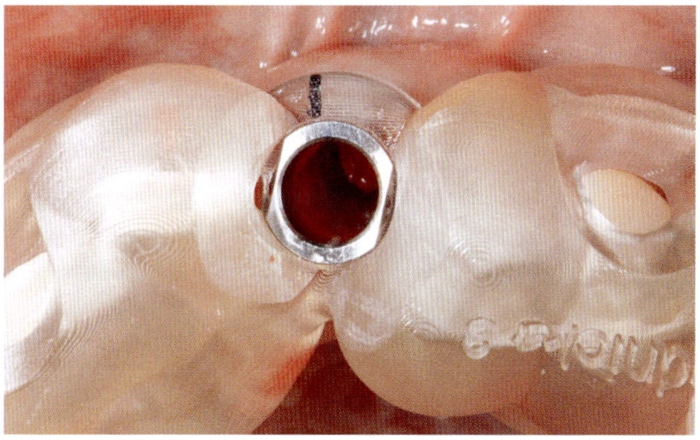
Fig 22 Checking the fit of the drilling sleeve.

SURGICAL PHASE

On the day of the surgery, no contraindications were observed. The soft tissue was healthy and stable (Fig 17).

After delivery of the local anesthesia (Ubistesin Forte, 4% articaine with adrenaline 1 : 100,000; 3M Espe, Seefeld, Germany), the crown of the tooth was removed (Fig 18).

The crown was easy to separate from the remaining root structure because of external root resorption in the cervical area (Fig 19).

The fractured root 23 was removed with a minimally invasive extraction system (Benex, Luzern, Switzerland) (Fig 20).

The fit of the printed surgical guide was checked immediately after the extraction (Figs 21 and 22).

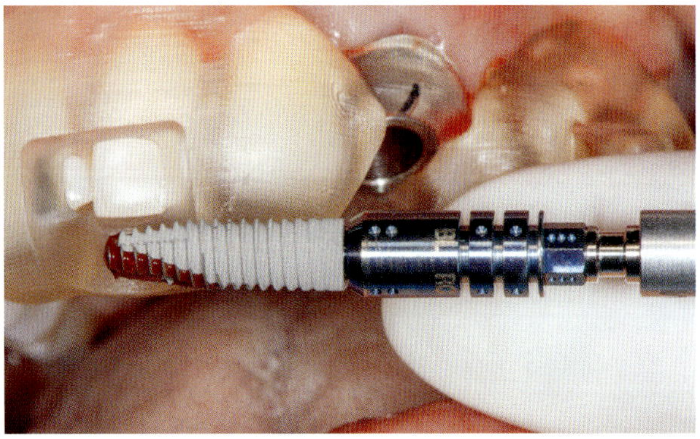

Fig 23 The implant with its preinstalled guided adapter before installation.

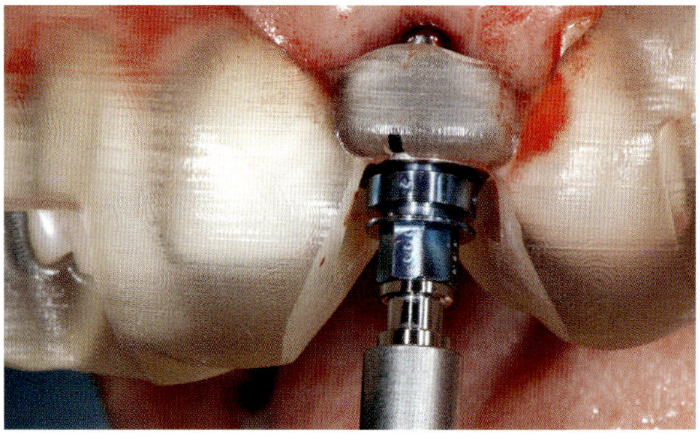

Fig 24 The H4 depth stop was the reference for the insertion depth of the implant.

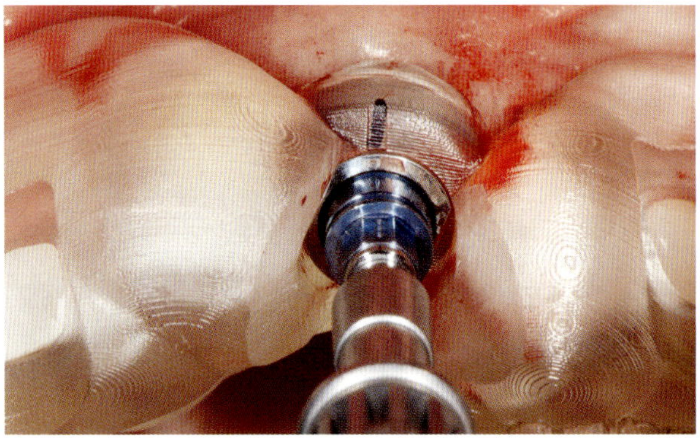

Fig 25 The index position was achieved by aligning the dots of the carrier abutment with the black index marks on the guide.

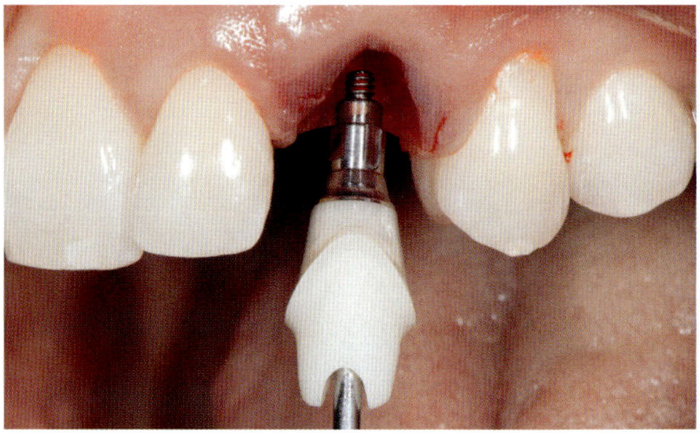

Fig 26 Insertion of the hybrid abutment.

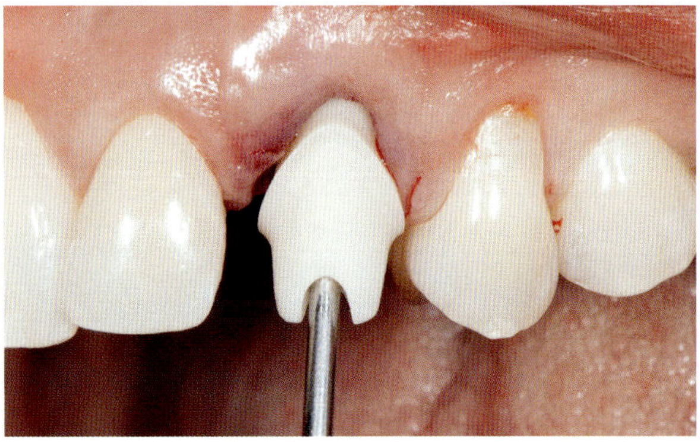

Fig 27 Scalloped design of the abutment following the soft tissue contour.

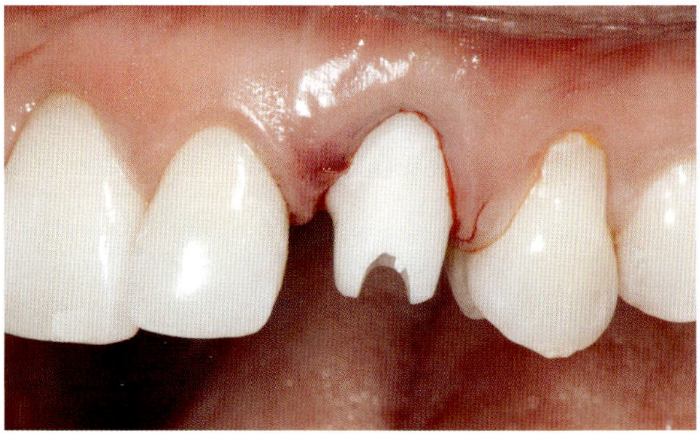

Fig 28 Abutment margin 0.5 to 1.0 mm below the soft tissue margin.

The osteotomy was performed with guided surgery instruments in a flapless approach, following the surgical protocol document created in the coDiagnostiX software.

The implant (BLT SLA Roxolid RC, diameter 4.1 mm, length 14 mm; Institut Straumann AG, Basel, Switzerland) was prepared for insertion (Fig 23).

To minimize implant deviation during insertion, the implant was placed through the guide. The depth of the insertion was indicated by the H4 depth stop (Fig 24), achieving its index position by aligning the dots on the carrier abutment with the black index marks on the guide (Fig 25). A final torque of 38 Ncm was achieved, as measured by the surgical unit.

After removing the guide and implant carrier, the optimum implant platform position was verified. The space between the implant and vestibular plate was filled with xenograft material (cerabone; Botiss Biomaterials, Zossen, Germany) to preserve the soft and hard tissue architecture.

After the augmentation, the hybrid abutment was inserted (Figs 26 and 27).

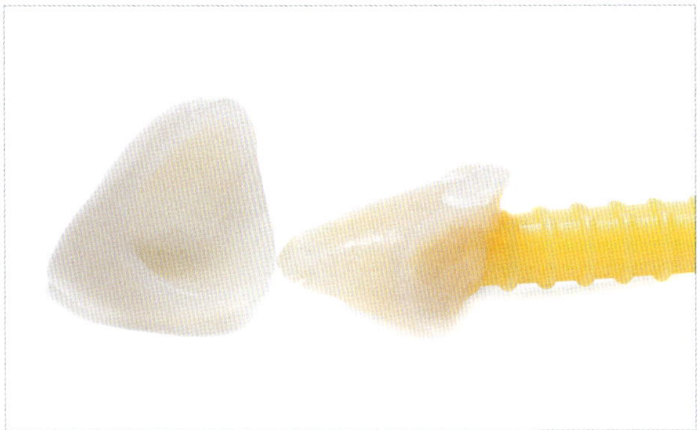

Fig 29 Temporary crown and custom abutment analog created with bis-acryl composite.

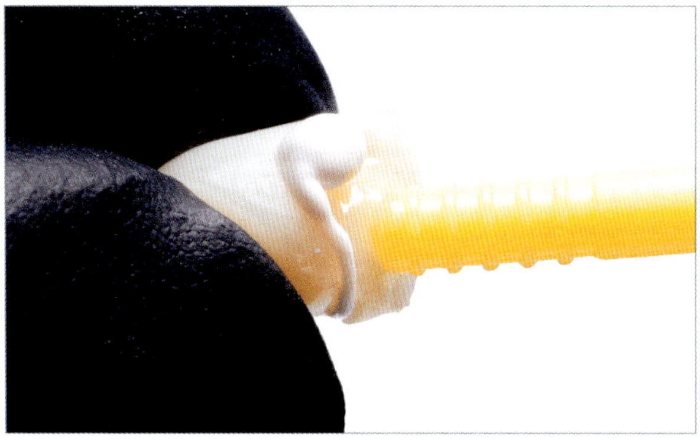

Fig 30 Excess temporary cement removed with a custom abutment analog.

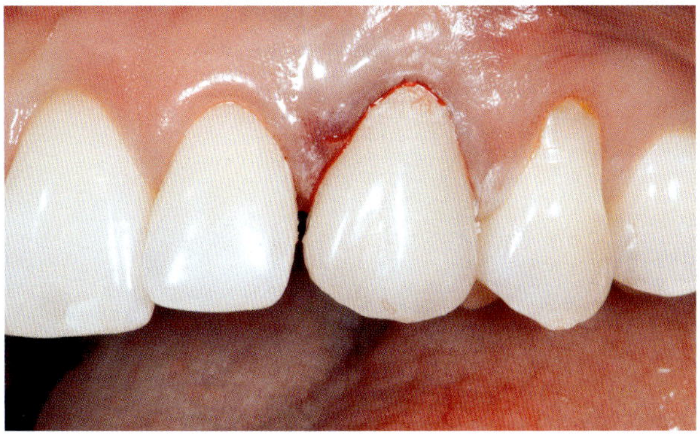

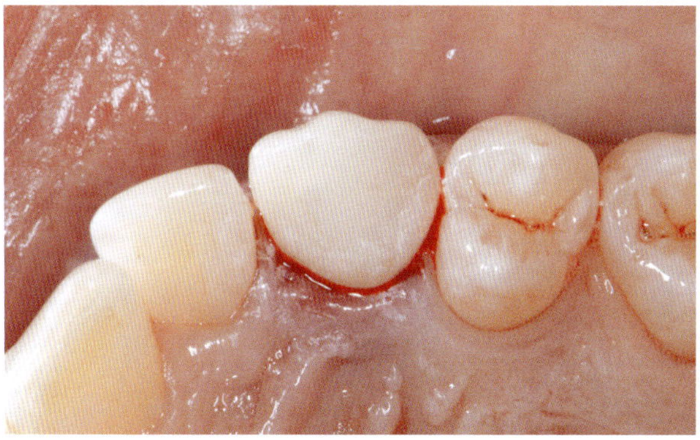

Figs 31 and 32 Thorough removal of temporary cement residue.

The abutment was tightened to a torque of 30 Ncm. The abutment shoulder was placed 0.5 to 1.0 mm below the soft tissue margin (Fig 28). The screw access channel of the abutment was closed with PTFE tape (USA Dental Tape; Milledgeville, GA, USA).

TEMPORARY RESTORATION

After surgery, the temporary crown was cemented with temporary cement (Temp-Bond; Kerr Dental, Rastatt, Germany). To minimize the expression of excess cement into the wound, a custom abutment analog (Fig 29) was prepared with bis-acryl composite (Luxatemp; DMG, Hamburg, Germany).

After application of the temporary cement (Temp-Bond; Kerr), the abutment analog was pressed into the temporary crown to remove excess cement before intraoral cementation.

After cementation, the soft tissue socket was thoroughly cleaned of any remaining cement particles (Figs 31 and 32).

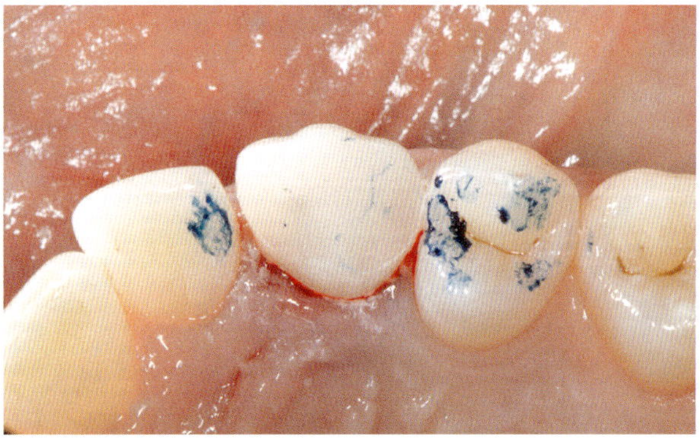

Fig 33 Temporary crown in infraocclusion.

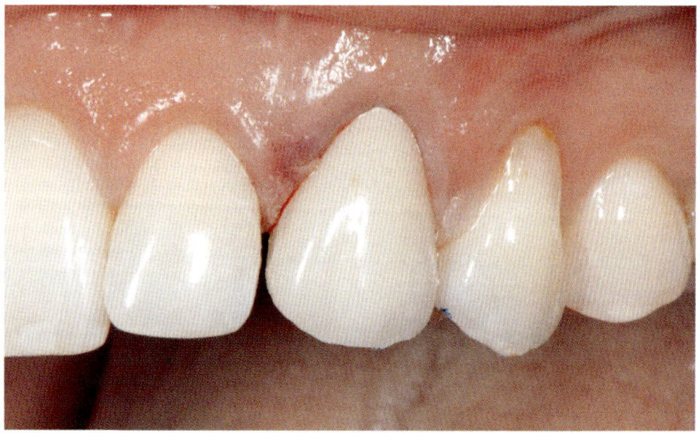

Fig 34 Soft tissue adaptation after surgery.

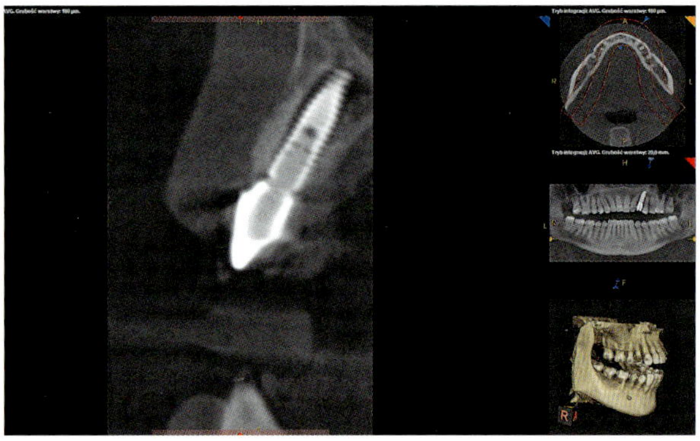

Fig 35 Postsurgical CBCT control.

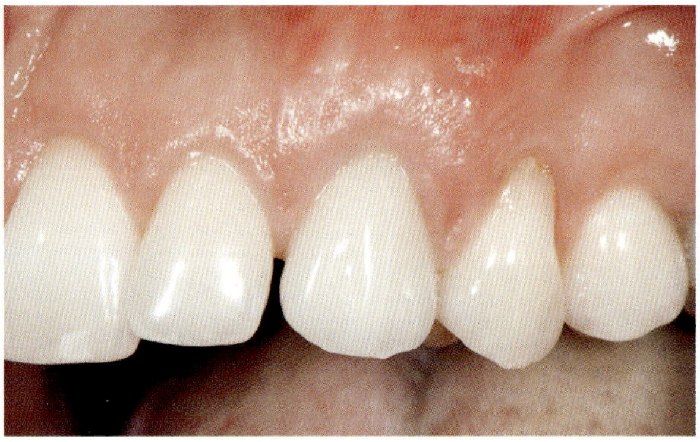

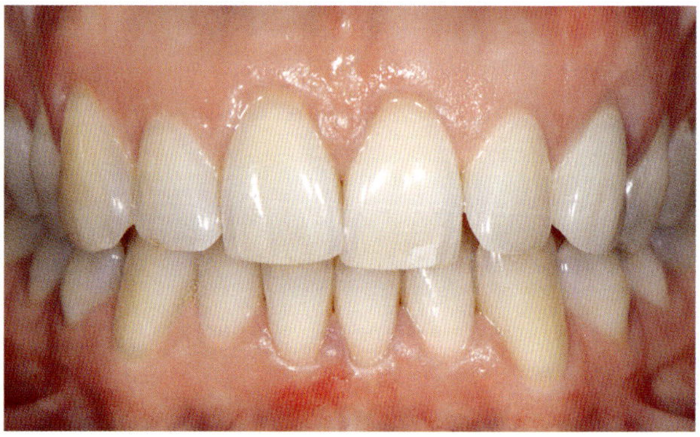

Figs 36 and 37 Soft tissue healing at two weeks.

The occlusal contact points were marked with 200-µm articulating paper (Bausch) during occlusal movements and were adjusted to avoid functional loading of the crown (Fig 33). The crown was also free of proximal contact points.

Immediately after placement, the soft tissue margins were nicely adapted (Fig 34).

After the surgery, the achieved 3D implant position was checked with an additional CBCT (Fig 35). The cross-sectional view showed the correct implant position and final hybrid abutment with the additional augmentation material in the post-extraction socket.

The healing process was evaluated at two weeks (Figs 36 and 37), two months (Figs 38 and 39), and four months (Figs 40 and 41).

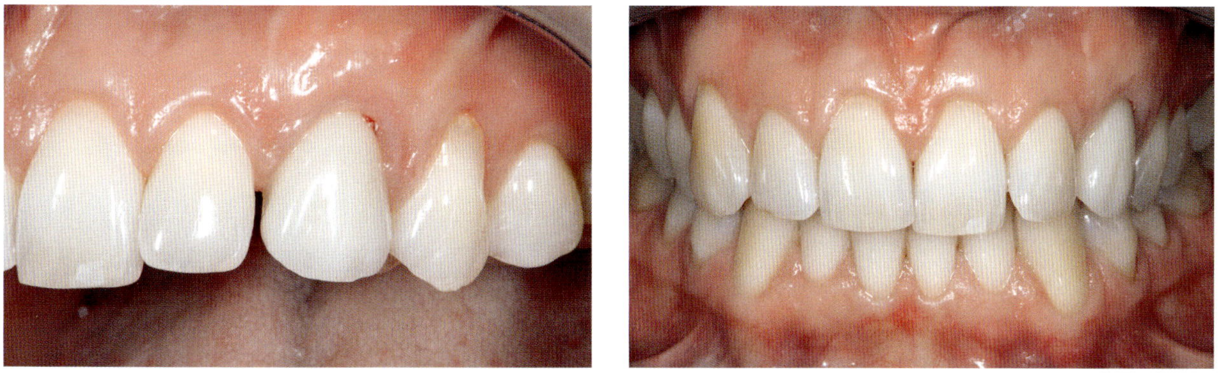

Figs 38 and 39 Soft tissue healing at two months.

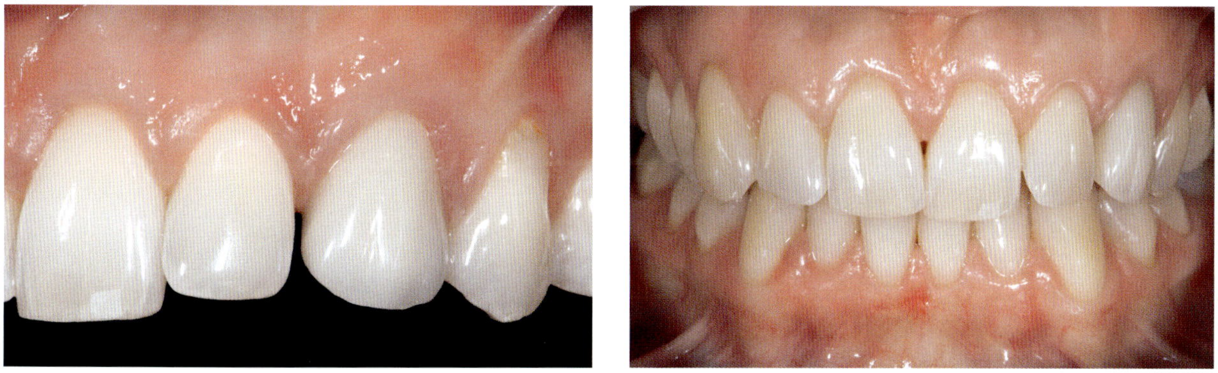

Figs 40 and 41 After four months of healing, the soft tissue looked very stable.

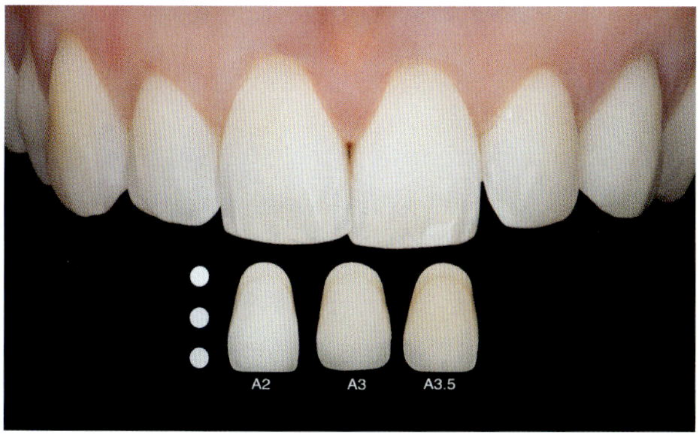

Fig 42 Shade transfer using reflected cross-polarized photography.

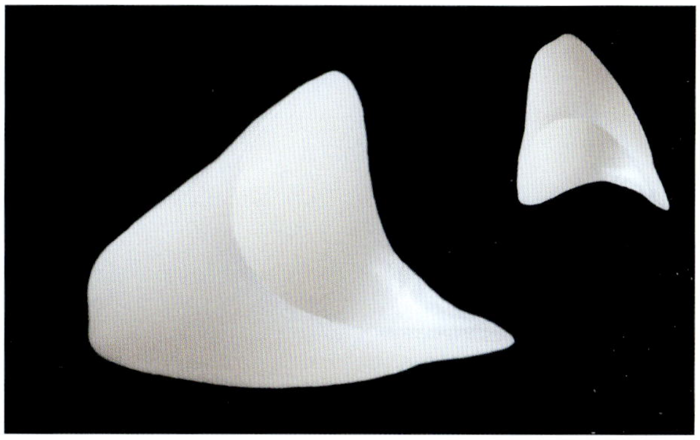

Fig 43 Zirconium oxide coping for the final crown.

DEFINITIVE RESTORATION

To achieve the best possible esthetic result, a shade reference photograph was taken (Fig 42) along with Vita Classical shade guide tabs (Vita Zahnfabrik, Bad Säckingen, Germany) using a reflected cross-polarized technique with dedicated polarizing filters (Polar Eyes; Emulation Lab, Freiburg im Breisgau, Germany).

The "one-abutment one-time" principle means installing the abutment once during the surgery and never removing it again. However, the abutment position needs to be transferred for the final crown production.

In the present case, a zirconium oxide coping of perfect fit for the abutment was designed, produced, and delivered before surgery (Fig 43).

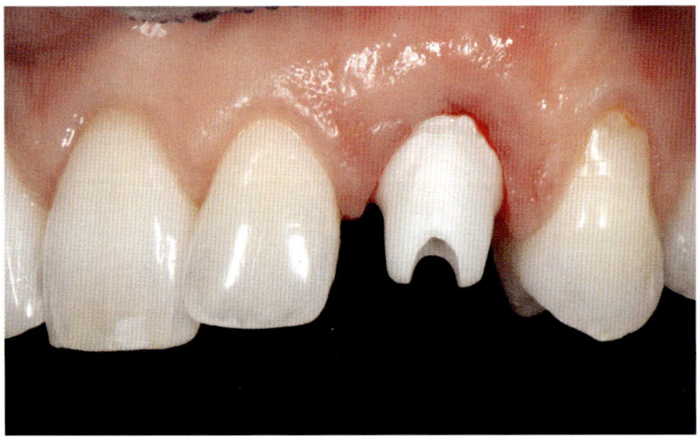

Fig 44 Soft tissue margin around the abutment before the impression.

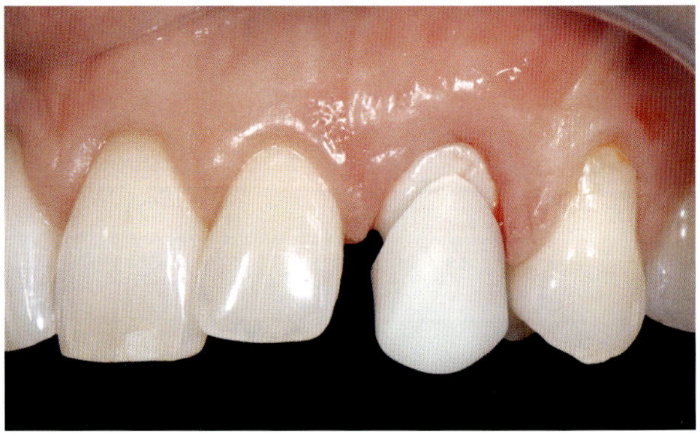

Fig 45 The coping margins follow the shape of the abutment.

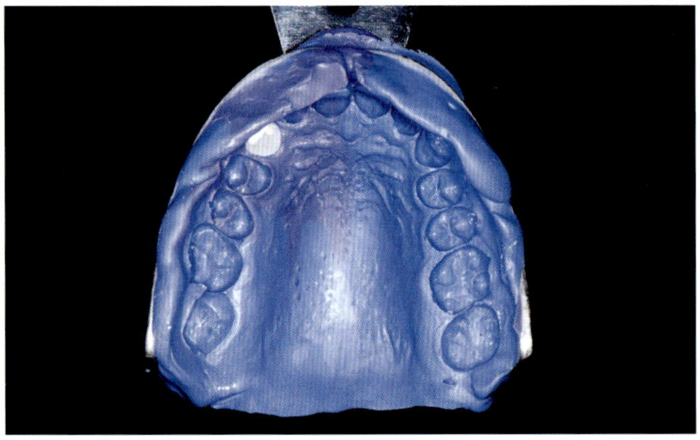

Fig 46 Silicone impression with coping in place.

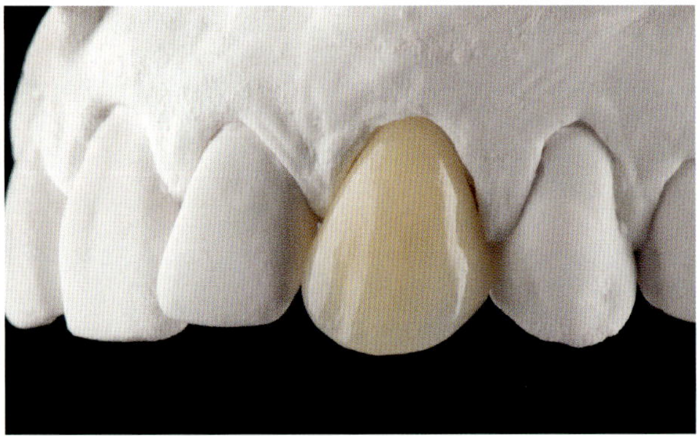

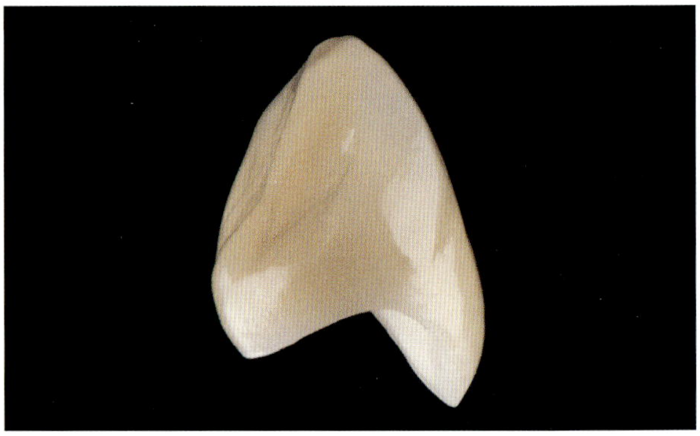

Figs 47 and 48 The final crown.

After removal of the temporary crown and residual temporary cement (Fig 44), the fit of the coping was checked (Fig 45).

The coping shape guaranteed an optimal transfer of the margins. Before taking the impression, it was important to avoid any soft tissue irritation. No retraction cords or other technical means were used to isolate or retract the soft tissue margins around the hybrid abutment. To avoid displacement of the coping during impression-taking, a small amount of temporary cement was used for fixation. A silicone impression was taken with a metal tray (Fig 46) and sent to the laboratory.

For veneering the framework, CZR ceramics in shade A2/A3 (Kuraray, Germany) was used and fired according to the manufacturer's instructions in a Dekema Austrat 624 furnace (Kulzer, Hanau, Germany) (Figs 47 and 48).

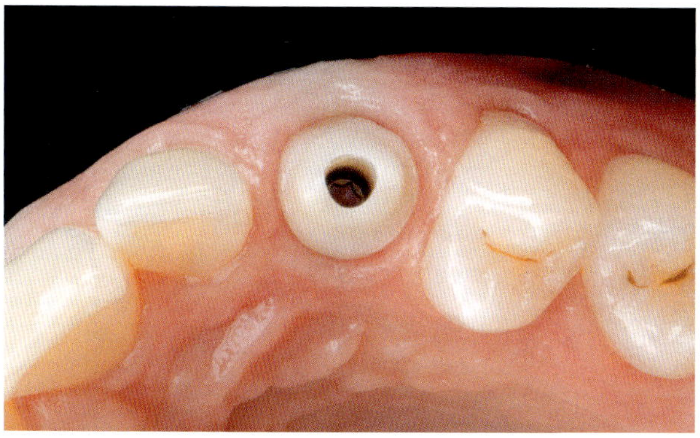

Fig 49 Abutment and soft tissue relation.

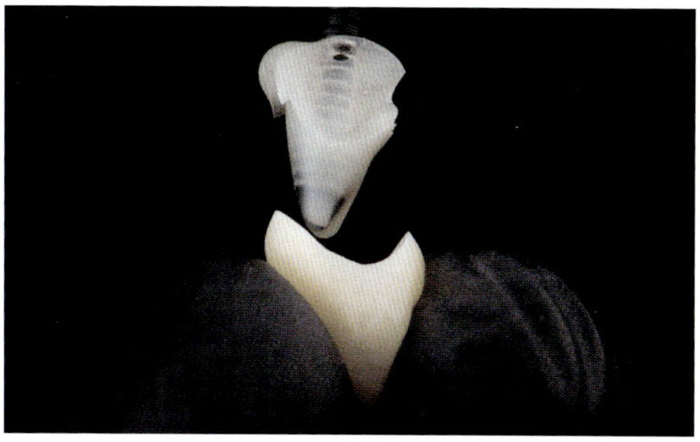

Fig 50 Custom abutment analog preparation.

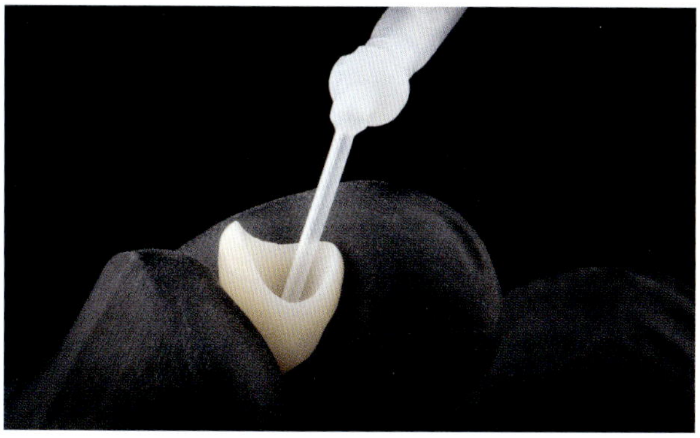

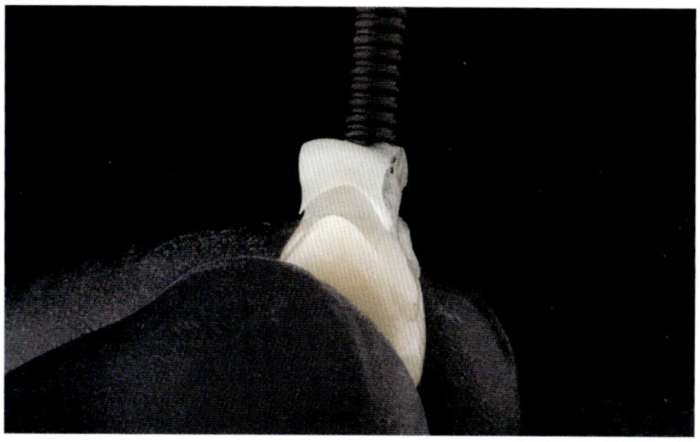

Figs 51 and 52 Resin cement application and excess removal with the custom abutment analog.

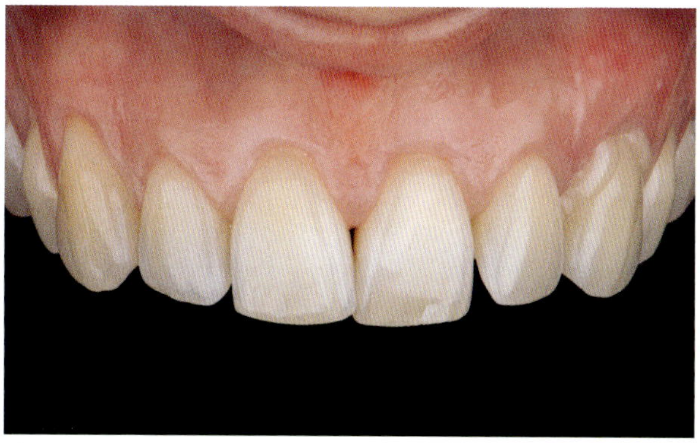

Fig 53 Resin cement above the sulcus.

Before the cementation of the final crown, the abutment was cleaned in situ (Fig 49). The surrounding soft tissue was healthy and stable without signs of inflammation. A new piece of PTFE tape (USA Dental Tape) was used to seal the screw access channel.

To control the cement when inserting of the crown, a new custom abutment analog was prepared (Fig 50).

The crown was definitely connected using dual-cure RelyX U200 Automix self-adhesive resin cement (3M Espe). This was applied with a thin cannula to avoid air bubbles (Fig 51). Any excess cement was removed with the prepared custom abutment analog (Fig 52).

When the crown was gently inserted, excess cement overspilled (Fig 53).

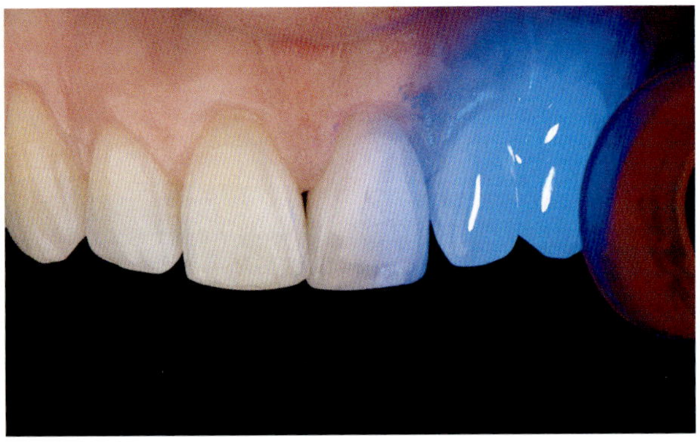

Fig 54 Light-curing the cement.

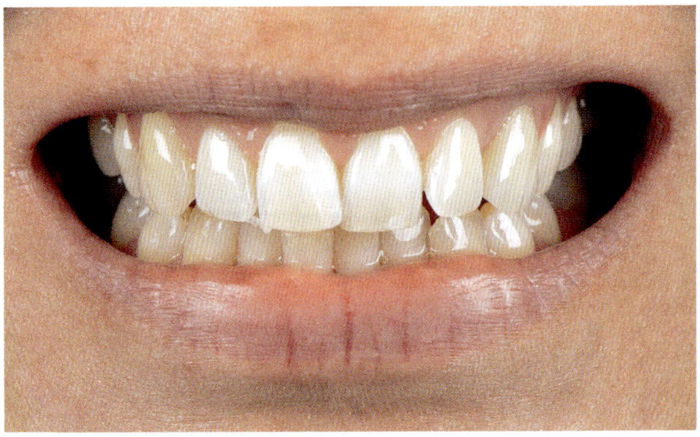

Fig 55 Intraoral situation after delivery of the final crown.

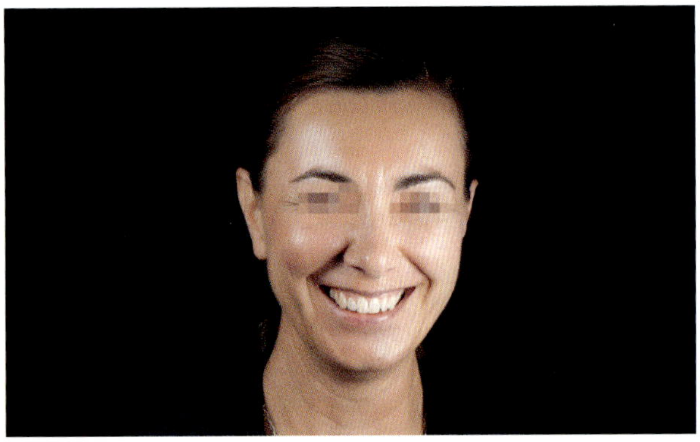

Fig 56 Final treatment result (facial view).

After brief exposure to a curing light, excess cement could be removed (Fig 54).

The close-up view shows that the implant-supported crown blends in perfectly within the oral cavity (Fig 55).

The final esthetic of the restoration and the favorable soft tissue situation represents a good result (Fig 56).

The CBCT shows stable bone levels four and five years after implant loading (Figs 57 and 58).

The intraoral photographs document stable soft tissue and acceptable esthetics of the final restoration three and five years after delivery of the final crown (Figs 59 and 60).

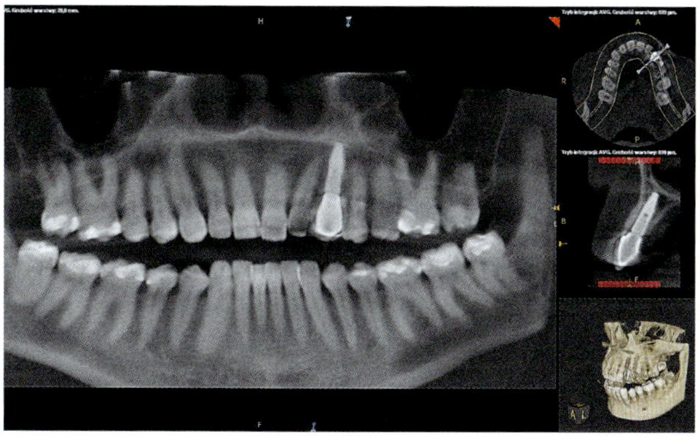

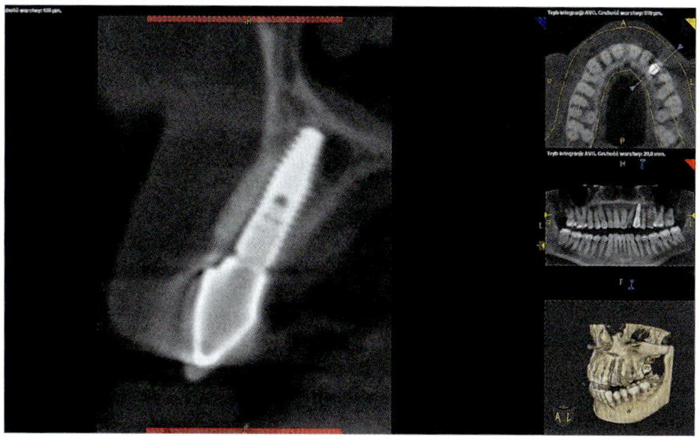

Figs 57 and 58 Stable bone situations four and five years after implant loading.

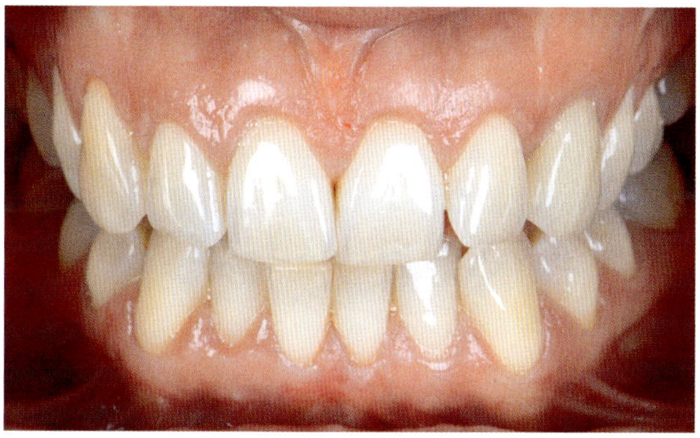

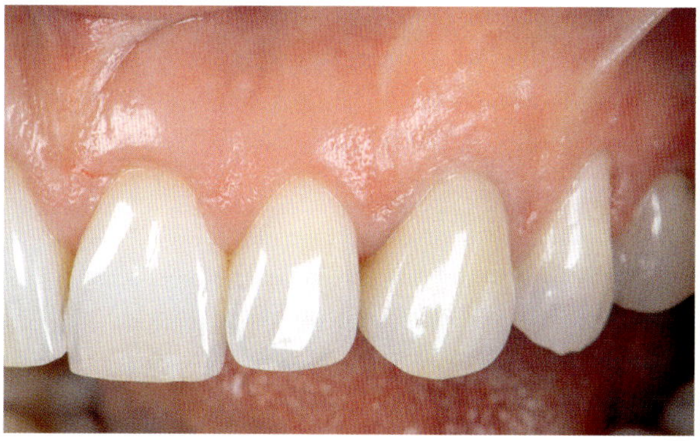

Figs 59 and 60 Stable esthetics at three and five years.

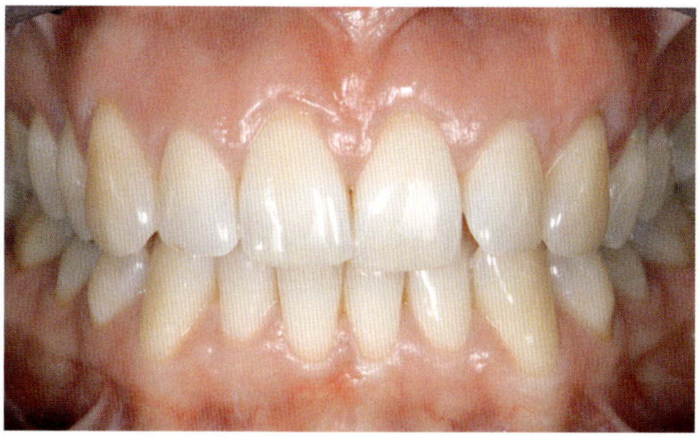

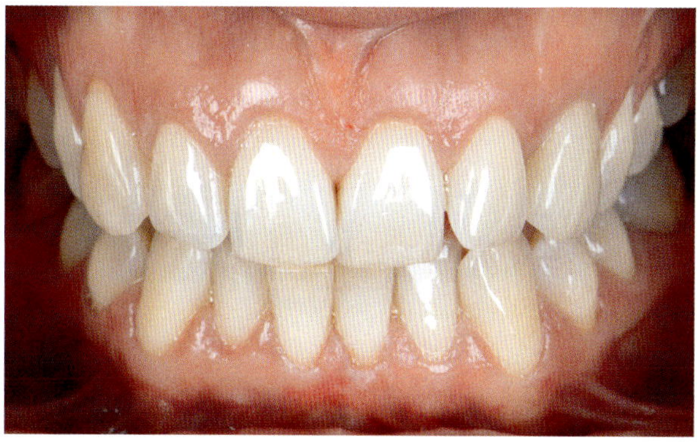

Figs 61 and 62 Comparison of the initial situation and the treatment result at five years.

The zenith and architecture of the soft tissue and interdental papilla remain stable when comparing the initial photo (Fig 61) to the situation almost five years later with the definitive crown 23 in situ (Fig 62).

At the follow-up visit in May 2021, an additional radiograph (RVG) was taken to further confirm the bone level at the contact points (Fig 63). The very stable result allows an optimistic forecast regarding the long-term treatment outcome.

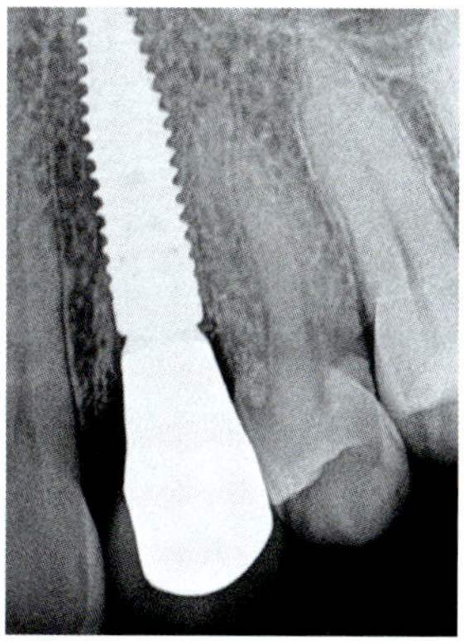

Fig 63 Stable bone levels at five years after the implant and final abutment were placed.

DISCUSSION

Immediate implant placement (Chen and Buser 2009; Chen and coworkers 2004; Hämmerle and coworkers 2004) is a well documented procedure. The present case represents immediate placement and immediate restoration/loading, which fulfills the classification criteria of Gallucci type 1A (Gallucci and coworkers 2018).

To enhance the peri-implant mucosal integration, a "one-abutment one-time" approach was selected. The purpose of this procedure is to avoid disturbing the peri-implant mucosal barrier interface at the point where the abutment connects with the implant. In a classic reconstruction procedure, we would disconnect the prosthetic elements from the implant multiple times before delivering the final crown. The definitive use of an abutment after implant placement seems to have a positive effect on the soft tissue response (Canullo and coworkers 2018).

Digital planning techniques and CAD/CAM now offer the ability to plan the optimal implant position and design the abutment shape to match the individual clinical situation. The basis for the success of the one-abutment one-time technique is that it provides the precise 3D position of the implant as previously planned, especially when a custom abutment is prepared.

The present treatment resulted in a pleasing esthetic outcome despite the initial clinical situation, which had been highly demanding esthetically. A high lip line with soft tissue exposure above the crown zeniths is an important risk factor in these cases.

The treatment plan for this patient included extraction and immediate implantation with guided surgery and a one-abutment one-time approach. One-time surgery with immediate implantation and immediate augmentation significantly reduced the treatment time and limited patient trauma.

The follow-up at five years documented three-dimensional stability of the soft and hard tissue volume around the prosthetic interface of the implant.

5.6 Guided Immediate Placement of a Ceramic Implant in a Maxillary Right Second Premolar and Immediate Restoration with a CAD/CAM-Fabricated Provisional Crown

A. Chen

Every tooth extraction initiates a cascade of continuous events that lead to hard and soft tissue volumetric and linear changes (Araújo and coworkers 2019; Grunder 2011).

In recent years, implant dentistry has aimed to understand the biology of alveolar socket/bone remodeling in order to minimize the impact on linear and volumetric parameters, with lower morbidity and fewer esthetic problems (Atieh and coworkers 2015).

Immediate implant placement is a treatment modality that, given an appropriate clinical indication, may mitigate most of these post-extraction alveolar changes (Tarnow and coworkers 2014).

One of the first metal oxides used and studied in the context of osseointegration was titanium dioxide (Brånemark and coworkers 1969). Recent patient demand for other types of implant materials have caused clinicians and researchers to seek alternative biomaterials that result in osseointegration, including ceramics (Miani and coworkers 1993; Akagawa and coworkers 1993).

In general, reports of overall survival rates for commercially available ceramic implants in randomized clinical trials (Balmer and coworkers 2020; Grassi and coworkers 2015) do not extend beyond five years. Systematic reviews and w-analyses have recorded implant survival rates of 98.3% and 97.2% at one and two years, respectively (Röhling and coworkers 2018a).

The recent growth in the field of ceramic implant technology has been driven by novel surface treatments and the development of microgeometrical topographies, resulting in improved biological and biomechanical properties.

As in titanium oxide, the passivation layer of ceramic materials facilitates osseointegration, providing bone-to-implant contact and other histomorphometric benefits similar to titanium implants, as was shown in preclinical (Röhling and coworkers 2019) and clinical (Röhling and coworkers 2018b) studies.

Due to its improved biomechanical features, yttria-stabilized zirconia (Y-TZP) is the most commonly offered ceramic implant material. Other materials such as ceria (cerium oxide, Ce_3O_4) are rapidly being introduced, potentially offering more promising mechanical results. (Miyazaki and coworkers 2013; Lopez-Píriz and coworkers 2017).

A number of clinical features may support the use of ceramic implants, such as a low inflammatory potential (Cionca and coworkers 2016) and the ability to reduce plaque accumulation (Röhling and coworkers 2017), which, along with enhanced spectrophotometric features of the final restoration (Thoma and coworkers 2016) and healing abutment (Pitta and coworkers 2020), have made ceramic materials a strong alternative for implant-supported rehabilitations.

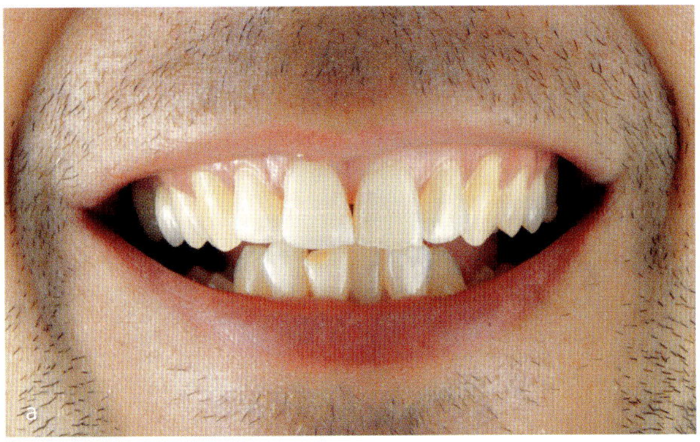

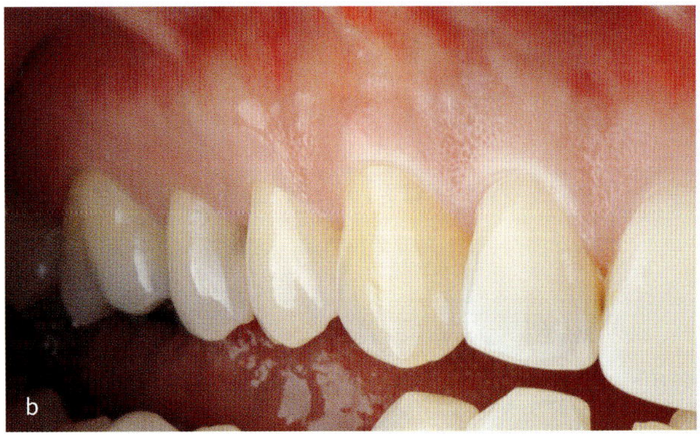

Figs 1a-b Initial intra- and extraoral situation.

Soft tissue response has always been regarded as one of the key factors for ceramic implants. While there is no sound evidence of superior results, some linear soft tissue parameters such as papilla height are at least broadly equivalent to titanium (Kniha and coworkers 2016). According to clinical studies, ceramics may behave more favorably, with faster maturation of peri-implant epithelial and connective tissues (Liñares and coworkers 2015), a significantly improved Jemt index score in peri-implant papilla formation (Spies and coworkers 2015), and improved attachment to gingival tissue (Shahramian and coworkers 2020). Some publications have reported a positive impact on the overall pink esthetic score (Fürhauser classification), which continued to improve even after two years (Payer and coworkers 2013; Payer and coworkers 2015).

In patients with titanium or general metal hypersensitivity, ceramic implants are considered a predictable and practical alternative. Patient demand for metal-free restorations has made this material a more popular option for implants.

CASE PRESENTATION

A 37-year-old male patient presented with pain in the maxillary right second premolar (tooth 15) associated with a large carious lesion. Following an endodontic consultation, he was diagnosed with a vertical fracture; the tooth was believed to have a hopeless prognosis. His medical history was unremarkable, showing no underlying conditions, alterations, or other significant findings, no chronic or acute medication, and no known allergies. His blood pressure (125/60 mmHg) and pulse rate (58 bpm) at rest were within normal limits, and there were no parafunctional habits such as smoking, alcohol abuse, or other substance issues. The patient's expectations were high. Extraoral analysis showed a high smile line with exposure of the papillae and cervical tooth contours (Figs 1a-b).

The periodontal status showed a healthy and disease-free dentition. Periodontal probing of teeth 16, 15 and 14 showed probing depths not exceeding 4 mm, and bone-crest levels were well maintained, providing a decent potential for soft tissue support (Figs 2a-c).

Full-mouth bleeding on probing was below 25% (Ainamo and Bay 1975). The gingival phenotype was recorded as medium-thick, medium-scalloped, with triangular teeth.

The periodontal anatomical contours were clinically maintained. The adjacent teeth had direct restorations, with a class I occlusal amalgam filling on tooth 16 and a distal composite on tooth 14 (Figs 2a-c).

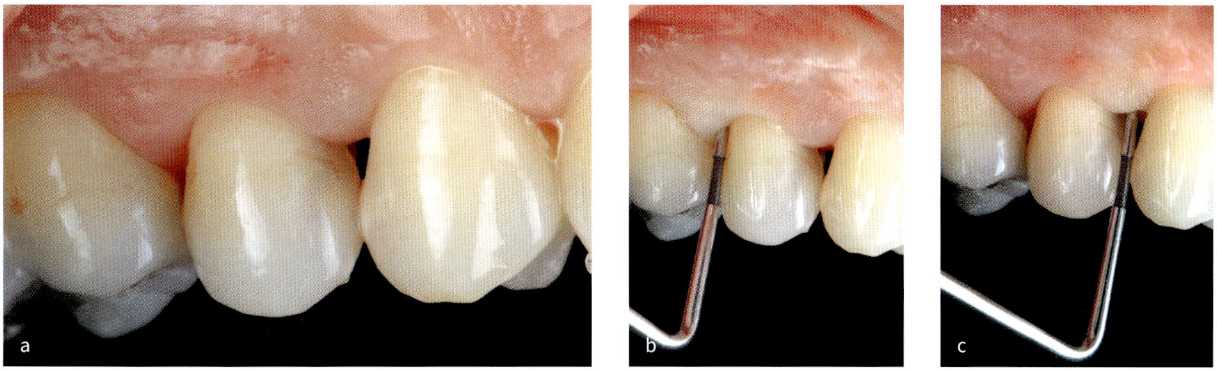

Figs 2a-c Intraoral exam, periodontal examination.

IMAGING AND AUXILIARY DIAGNOSTICS

An intraoral scanner (IOS) was used to produce a Standard Tessellation Language (STL) file for 3D printing (Formlabs 2; Formlabs, Somerville, MA, USA), yielding the initial study models.

The radiographic examination (cone-beam computed tomography, Romexis; Planmeca, Helsinki, Finland) showed all the cortical plates (buccal, lingual, and interproximal) to be present and intact, with no signs of acute or chronic periapical disease (Figs 3a-c).

The DICOM files from the CBCT were merged with the IOS STL files for implant-supported rehabilitation planning (Implant Studio: 3Shape, Copenhagen, Denmark) and anatomical assessment (Figs 4a-d).

Once all anatomical and clinical parameters were accounted for, an immediate implant was planned for immediate loading. The provisional restoration was designed with no occlusal contacts in centric or eccentric positions, provided that primary stability in the order of 30 Ncm of insertion torque could be achieved and the restoration would be provided.

The suggested treatment plan was discussed with the patient. He did not want a titanium or any other metallic implant. He was therefore presented with the option of a ceramic implant, which he agreed to and signed the informed consent and medical forms for implant placement.

The treatment plan proposed a cementable restoration on a monotype (one-piece) zirconia implant with an abutment height of 4 mm (Pure Ceramic Monotype ZLA, diameter 3.3 mm, length 12 mm; Institut Straumann AG, Basel, Switzerland).

The decision to use a monotype implant was based on the fact that it has no two-piece metal interface and indeed does not contain any metal.

A one-piece implant makes it more difficult to attain the perfect prosthodontic position and may create problems in the medium and long term. In terms of biomechanical options, it does not offer the possibility of compensating for a misaligned axis with an intermediate or angled cemented abutment. This would require a bulkier crown on the palatal or buccal aspect or a reduced abutment, which is far from ideal.

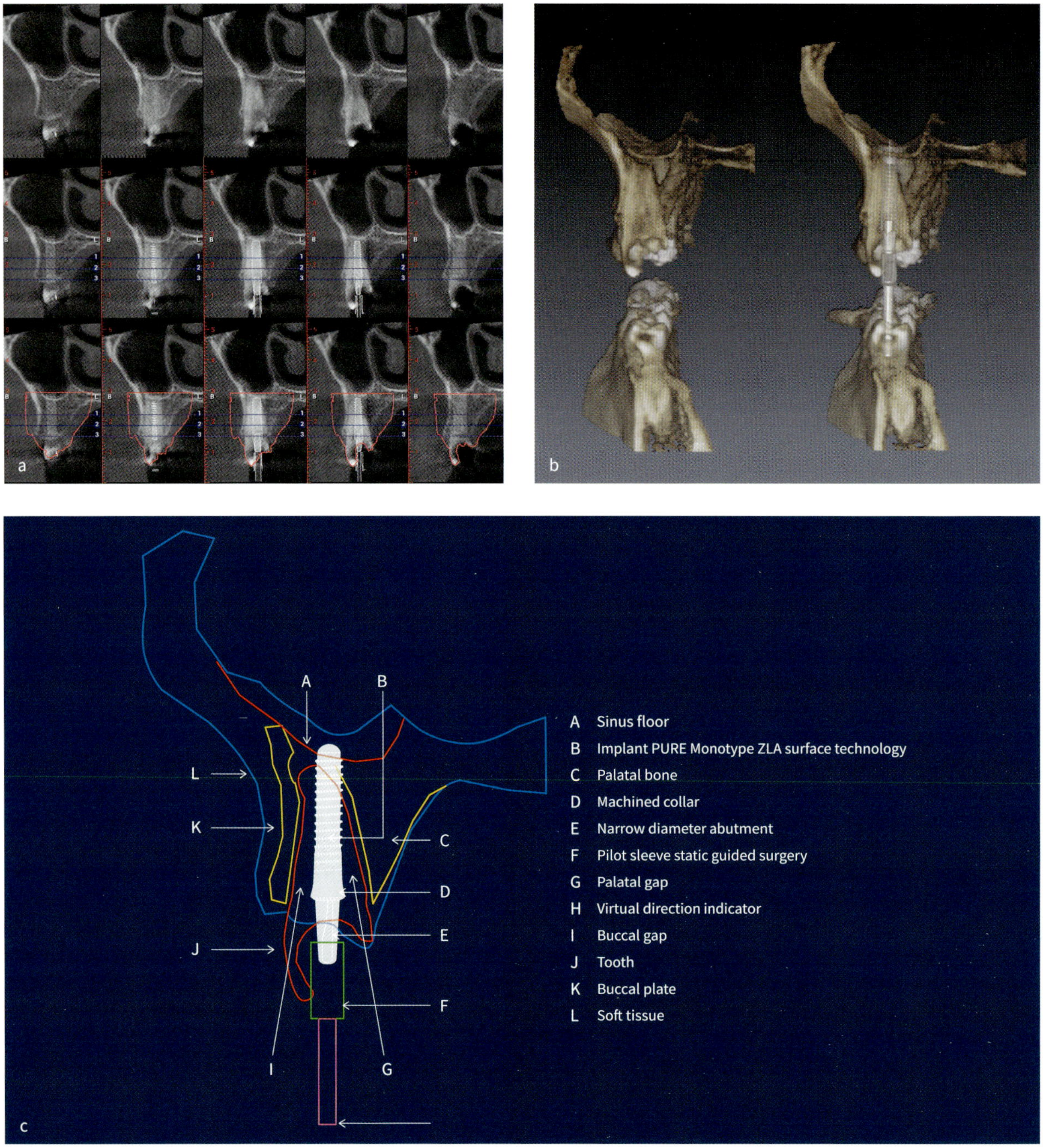

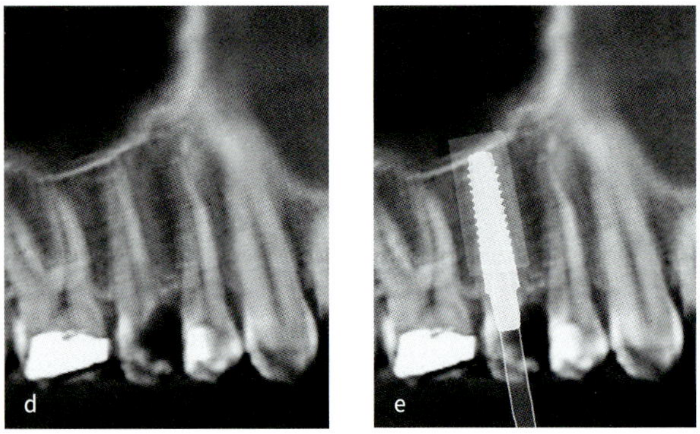

Figs 3a-e CBCT with merged STL evaluation (a), a 3D image diagnostic tool for implant planning (b), and an illustration of the 3D plan for an immediate ceramic implant (c). Interproximal bone and implant position on lateral cuts (d and e)

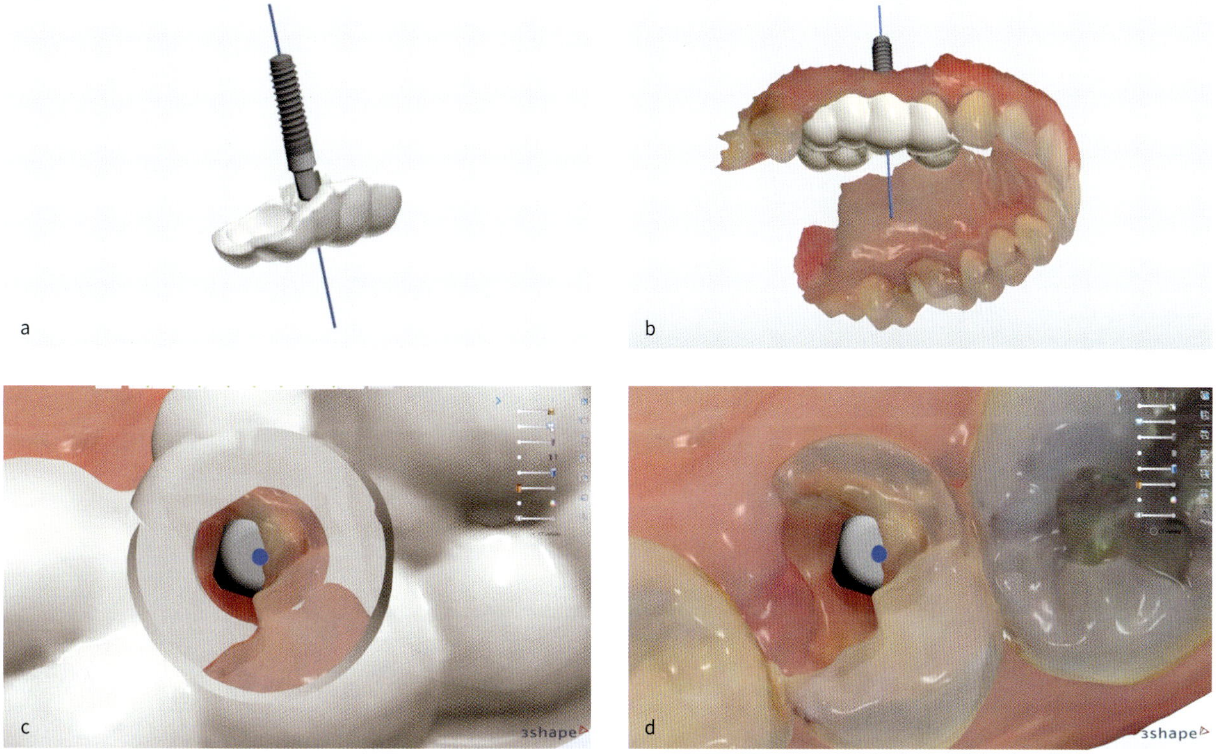

Figs 4a-d Merging STL files with DICOM for virtual patient assessment and for planning the implant-supported rehabilitation.

On the biological level, implants with an incorrect three-dimensional position may adversely affect hard and soft tissue remodeling during healing; apical migration of attached mucosa may occur if its position is too far buccal, which may create an esthetically undesirable outcome.

The implant type was selected, its optimal position was determined, and a surgical guide was created in the software environment (Fig 5).

After obtaining a clear medical history and evaluation of the case, the Risk Assessment Table for immediate implant placement and immediate restoration/loading in single-tooth sites was used to define the complexity of the treatment (Tables 1 and 2).

The case was categorized as “low risk.” The STL file on which the surgical guide was designed was sent to a 3D printer (Formlabs 2; Formlabs) to be fabricated.

The case was planned to include pilot drill-guided surgery/semi-guided static surgery. The provisional restoration was created by CAD/CAM (Coritec, Imes-Icore, Eiterfeld, Germany) inserted on a peek prefabricated component and left reduced on the buccal part for adhesive connection of the buccal remnant of the patient’s tooth for esthetic purposes (Fig 6).

Table 1 Risk assessment for immediate implant placement in single-tooth sites

	Low risk	Medium risk	High risk
Preoperative assessment			
Patient-related			
Medical status	Healthy, uneventful healing		Compromised healing
Esthetic risk	Low/medium esthetic risk	High esthetic risk	Significant esthetic compromise expected
Site-related			
Gingival-margin position	No recession	Minor gingival recession	Gingival recession ≥ 2 mm
Soft tissue quality	Thick gingival phenotype	Thin gingival phenotype or limited keratinized gingiva	No keratinized gingiva
Bone anchorage	Sufficient bone anchorage to achieve primary stability		Lack of bone anchorage to achieve primary stability
Facial bone wall	≥ 1 mm facial bone thickness	Facial bone plate < 1 mm thickness, or small fenestration or dehiscence defect	Significant fenestration or dehiscence of facial bone
Need for a mucoperiosteal flap	Sufficient alveolar bone for a flapless approach		Need for flapped bone augmentation
Socket position within alveolar envelope	Socket within the alveolar bone envelope		Socket and facial bone wall protruding out of the bone envelope
Presence of endodontic infection	No infection	Chronic periapical infection	Acute infection
Presence of periodontal disease	Periodontally healthy	Controlled periodontal disease	Active periodontal disease
Planning implant position	Ideal three-dimensional position with axis exiting through the cingulum or incisal edge		Facially positioned or over-angulated implant or excessive implant depth
Gap between buccal bone and planned implant position	≥ 2 mm	1–2 mm	< 1 mm
Intraoperative assessment			
Extraction	Minimally invasive tooth extraction	Damage to surrounding soft tissue, including severed/detached papillae	Significant damage to soft tissue and surrounding bone
Primary implant stability	Primary stability achieved		Lack of primary stability
Final implant position	Ideal three-dimensional position achieved		Facially positioned or over-angulated implant or excessive implant depth

Table 2 Risk assessment for immediate loading of an immediately placed single implant

	Low risk	Medium risk	High risk
Preoperative assessment			
Patient-related			
Occlusal scheme	No direct occlusal contacts	Minimal occlusal contact and/or shared guidance	Main determinant of anterior guidance
Occlusal parafunction	Absent		Present
Site-related			
Bone anchorage	Sufficient bone anchorage to resist loading forces		Insufficient bone anchorage to resist loading forces
Tooth position	Incisor, premolars	Canine	Molars
Intraoperative assessment			
Primary implant stability	30–45 Ncm insertion torque	20–30 Ncm insertion torque	< 20 Ncm insertion torque

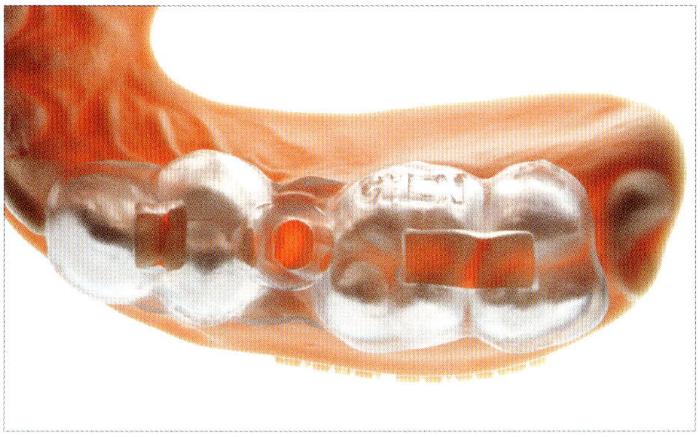

Fig 5 Virtual planning, taking implant and tooth positions into account.

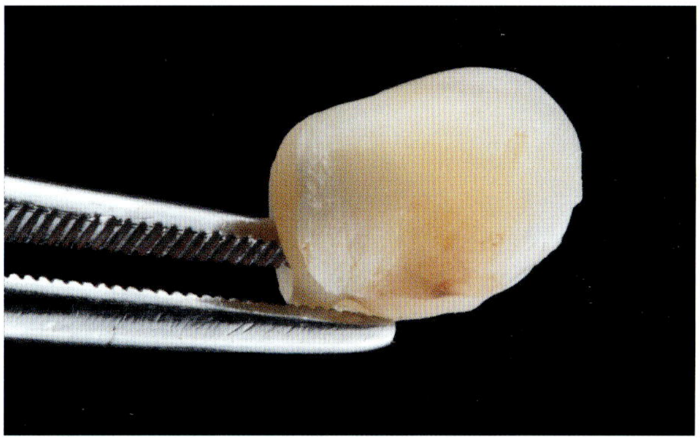

Fig 6 Fabrication of the provisional crown.

SURGICAL PROCEDURES

Use this QR code to view a highlight video of the surgical procedure.

On the day of surgery, under sterile conditions, a minimally invasive extraction (Figs 7a-b) was performed to preserve the buccal bone and the soft tissue contours. A surgical guide was placed, and implant preparation performed according to the manufacturer's instructions, following the protocol for static guided pilot-drill surgery (Straumann Pure Ceramic Drilling Protocol) (Figs 8a-d).

Primary stability is dependent on three main factors: native bone quality and quantity, the drilling protocol, and implant microgeometry.

Immediate implants are restricted to the available bone, which can be limited. Different strategies are used to achieve primary stability. In the present case, anchorage was achieved in the apical/palatal 0,75 mm of residual bone, engaging the cortical bone of the maxillary sinus and the mesial and distal walls. Due to the conical shape of the premolar root, the 3.3 mm parallel-walled implant engaged well, and primary stability was achieved.

The implant bed was prepared with a 2.8 mm drill, that is, slightly underprepared for a ceramic implant 3.3 mm in diameter. A torque of 35 Ncm was achieved.

A zirconia implant 3.3 mm in diameter generally offers good primary stability when all the above factors are carefully addressed. But in type IV residual bone, this may not be enough to achieve sufficient insertion torque. Where possible, an increased implant diameter may be the preferred choice for improved apical engagement.

In certain situations, there may not be enough residual bone for primary stability; in this case, changing the treatment approach to a delayed implant placement may be preferable.

The implant was torqued to 35 Ncm and the buccopalatal position was confirmed using the surgical guide (Fig 9).

The buccal gap was filled with deproteinized bovine bone mineral (DBBM, Bio-Oss; Geistlich, Wolhusen, Switzerland) (Fig 10), and the provisional restoration was prepared by removing the buccal aspect of the tooth and attaching it to the CAD/CAM acrylic provisional restoration (Figs 11a-b).

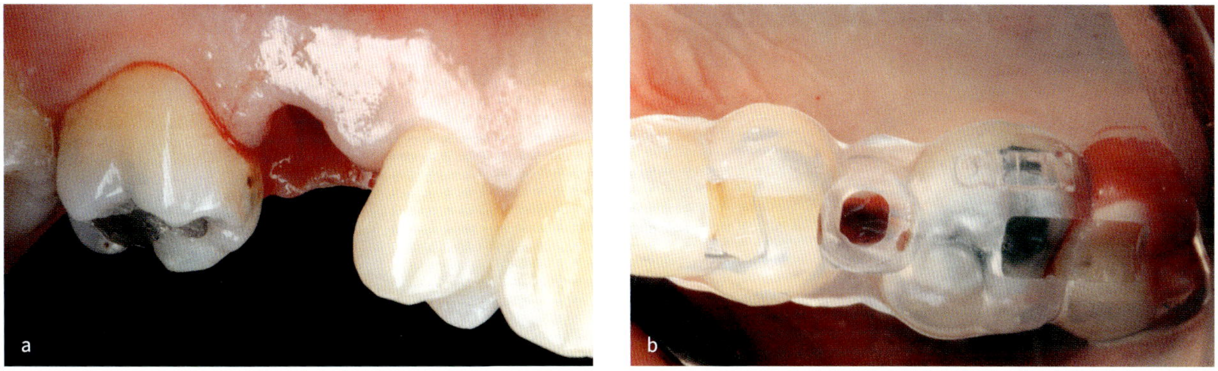

Figs 7a-b Minimally invasive extraction for periodontal contour maintenance and surgical guide try-in.

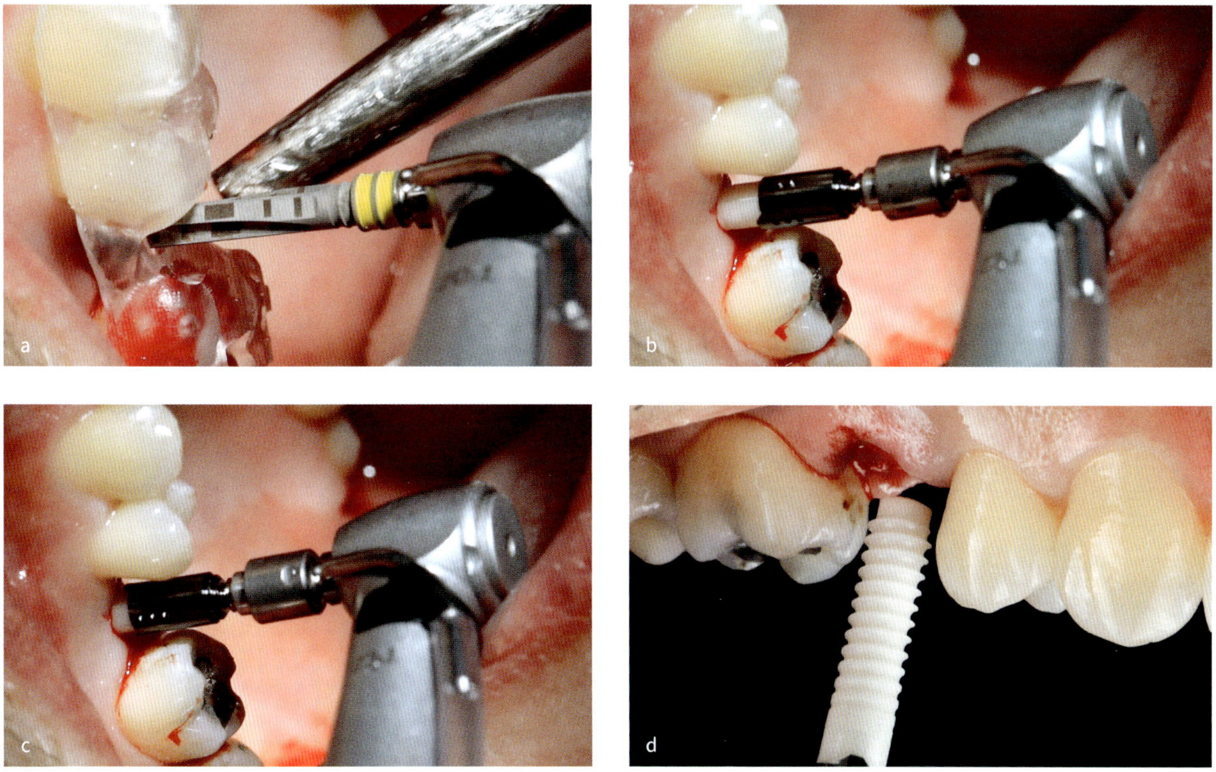

Figs 8a-d Implant bed preparation for pilot-guided surgery and implant placement.

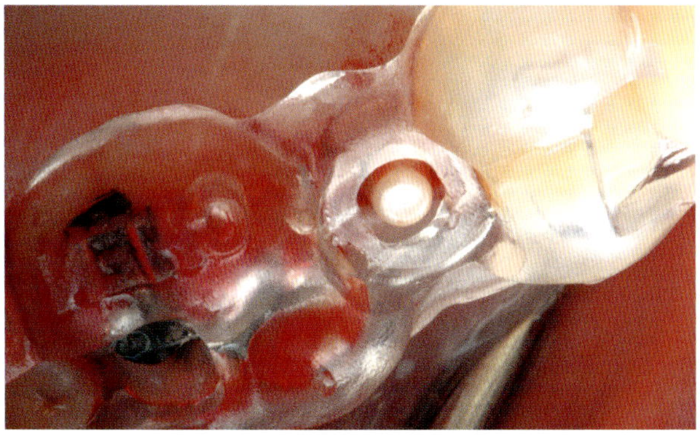

Fig 9 Implant placement confirmed with a guided pilot-drill surgical guide.

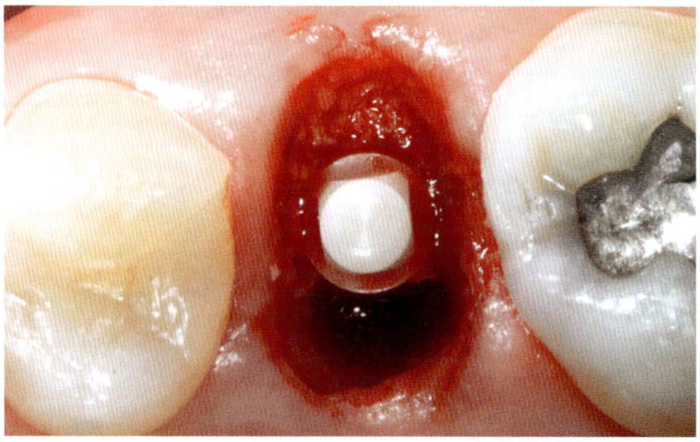

Fig 10 Implant position, with the gap filled with inorganic hydroxyapatite.

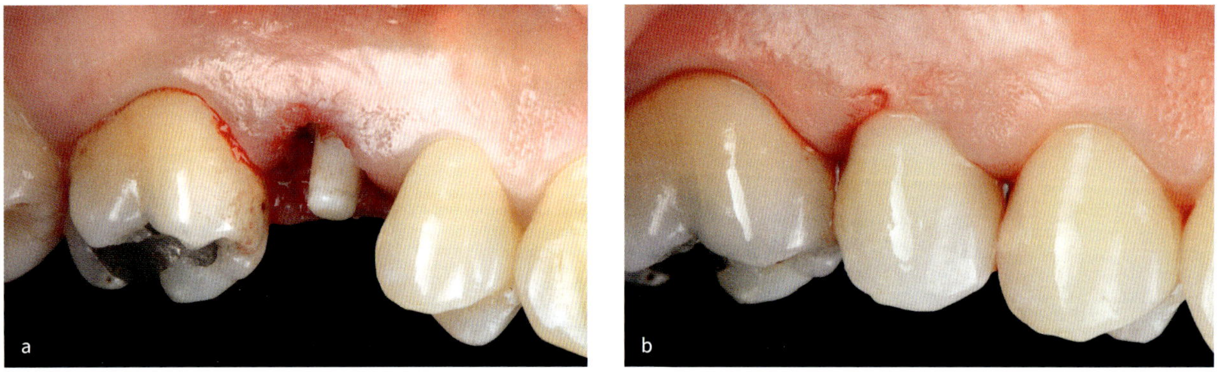

Figs 11a-b Implant position and cemented provisional rehabilitation.

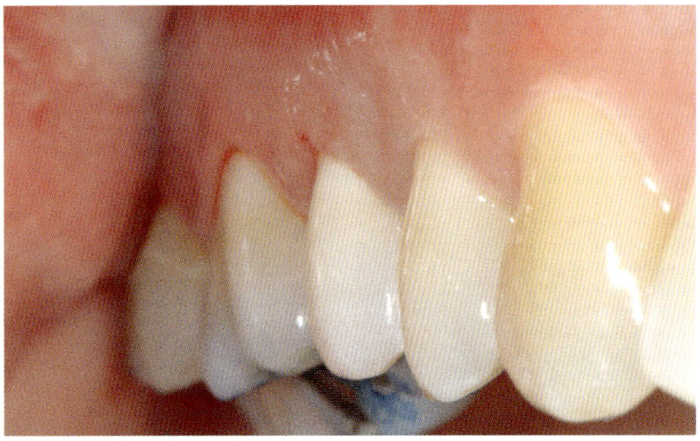

Fig 12 Result after completed surgery and occlusal adjustment.

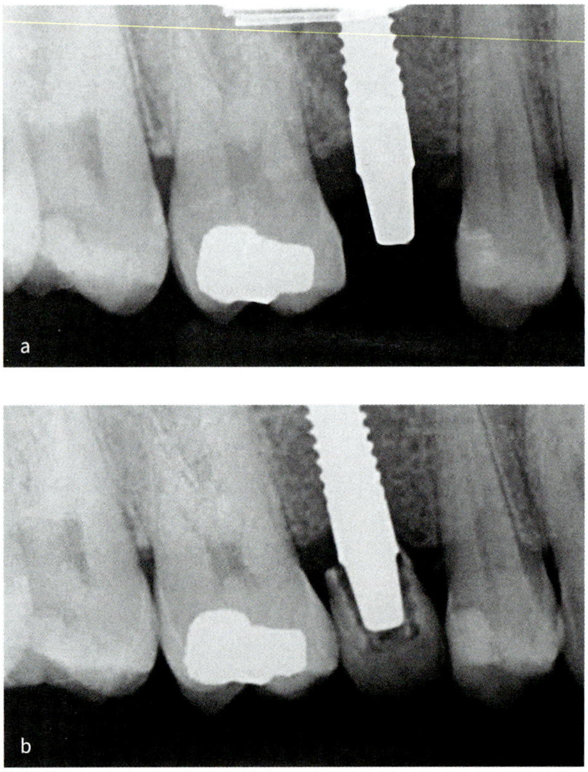

Fig 13a-b Radiographic situation on completed surgery. PEEK abutment with the CAD/CAM provisional.

The provisional was cemented with provisional zinc oxide-eugenol cement (Temp Bond; Kerr, Orange, CA USA) while ensuring that all cement residue was removed (Fig 12). The occlusion was checked to ensure that there were no occlusal or eccentric contacts during any jaw movements.

The patient was medicated with 2 g of amoxicillin one hour prior to surgery and instructed to take 1 g of paracetamol every 8 hours. A postoperative intraoral periapical radiograph was taken (Figs 13a-b).

PROSTHODONTIC PROCEDURES

Use this QR code to view a highlight video of the prosthodontic procedure.

Three months following implant placement (at the end of the osseointegration period), the soft tissue and bone contours had healed uneventfully (Figs 14a-c).

A final intraoral impression was taken with an IOS (Trios; 3Shape) and sent to the 3D printer for model fabrication and abutment preparation. The implant was digitally scanned, and the abutment margin was defined and customized in the laboratory software (Dental Design; 3Shape) (Figs 15a-d).

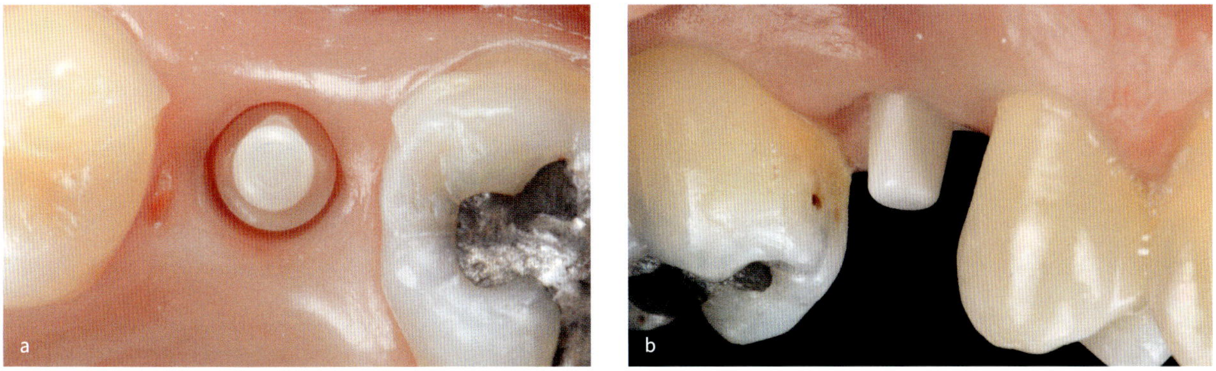

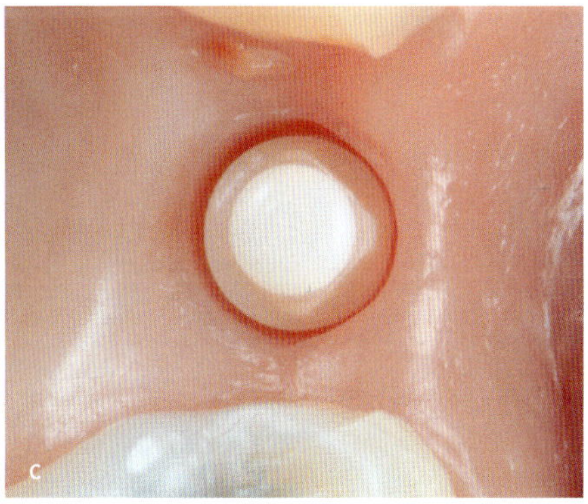

Figs 14a-c Clinical situation three months after placement.

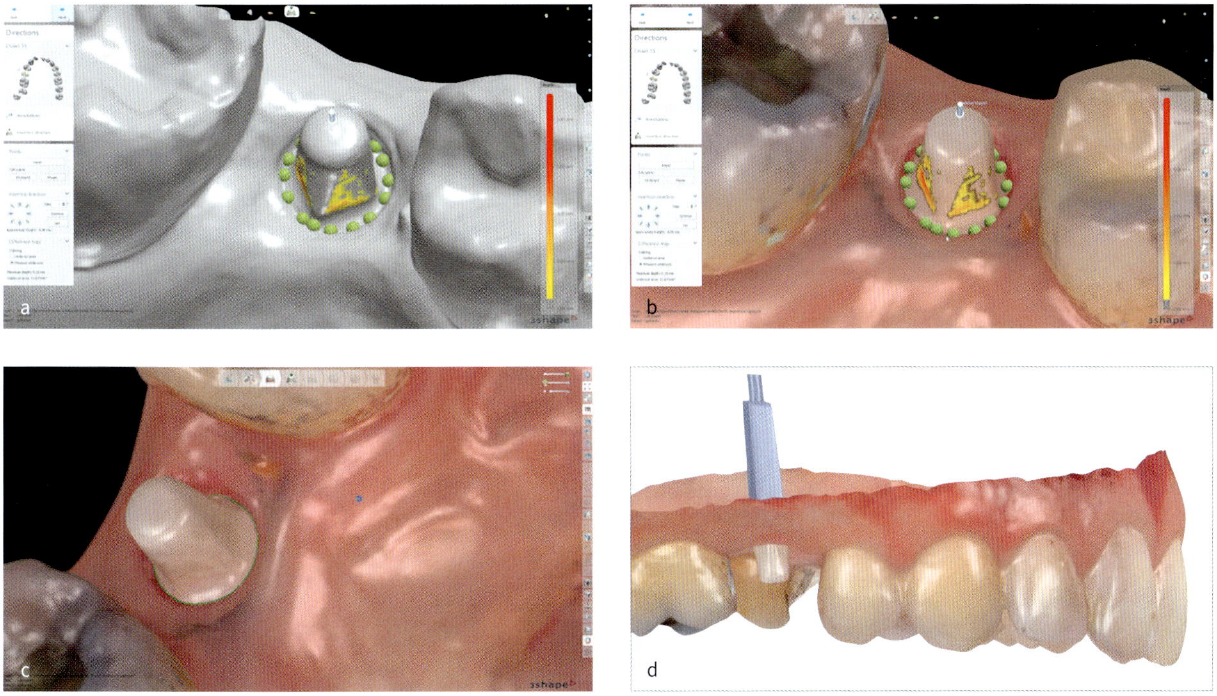

Figs 15a-d Planning the final rehabilitation in 3D.

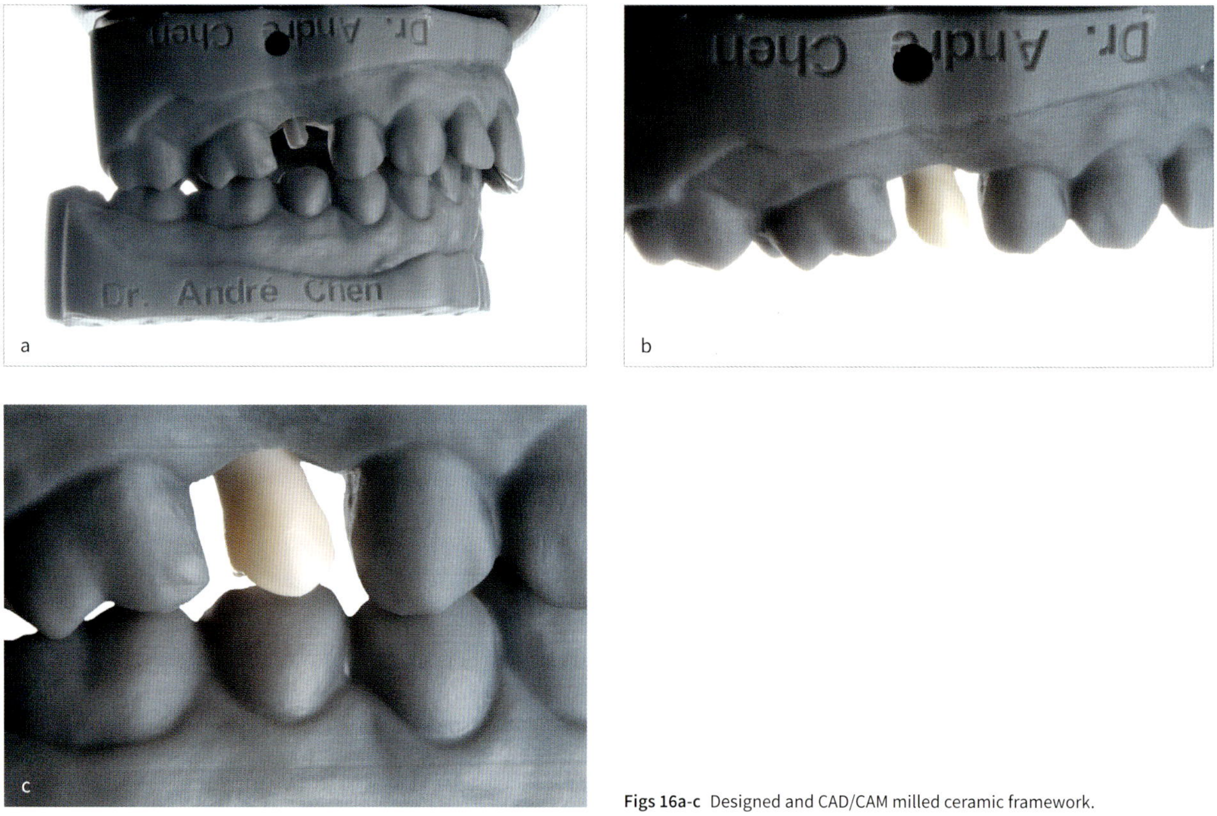

Figs 16a-c Designed and CAD/CAM milled ceramic framework.

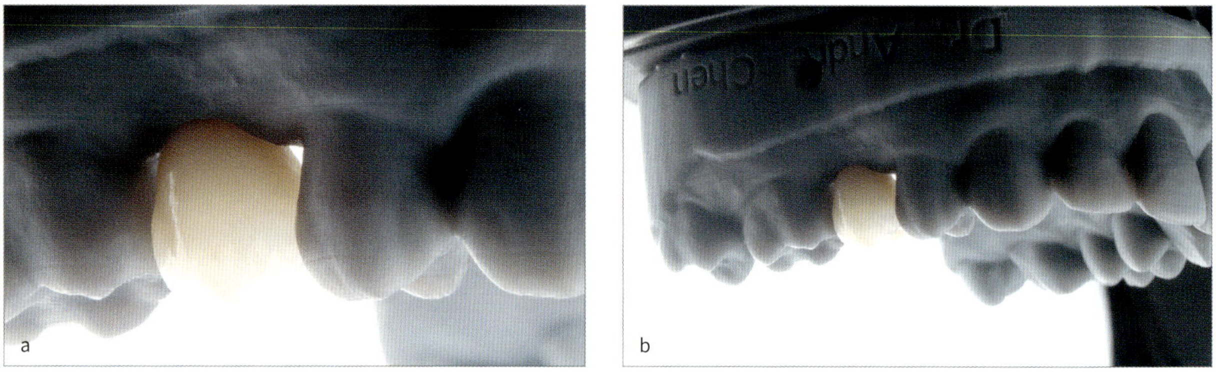

Figs 17a-b Fabrication of the framework and final veneering.

Since no digital library for the Pure Ceramic Monotype was available at that time, an external STL post-production program was used to customize the analog from the model. Both resulting STL files (for the model and for the implant analog) were sent for 3D impressions (Formlabs 2; Formlabs) (Figs 16a-c).

A CAD/CAM framework (Coritec; Imes-Icore) was designed on the computer by copying the contralateral premolar and adjusted it on the model. Finally, a lab technician provided a feldspathic veneer (Figs 17a-b).

The restoration was inserted and cemented with definitive glass ionomer cement (Ketac Cem; 3M, St. Paul, MN, USA) (Figs 18a-c).

A final periapical radiograph was taken for control purposes (Fig 19).

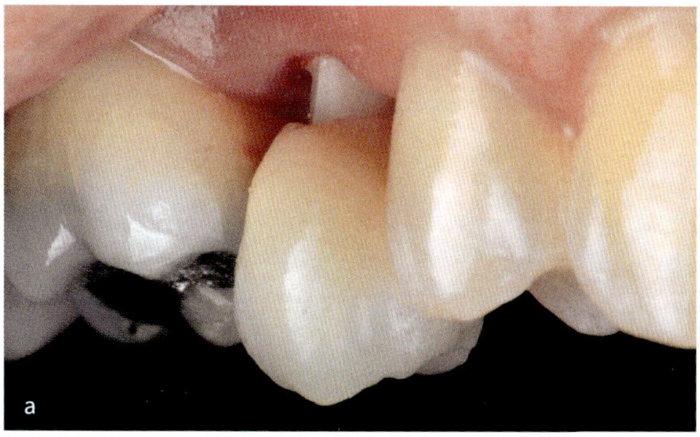

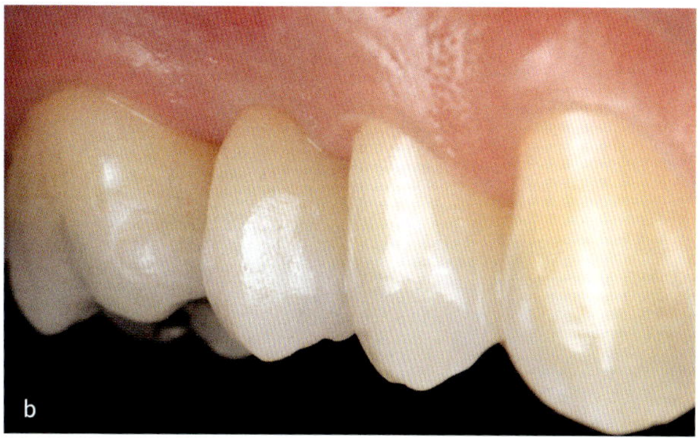

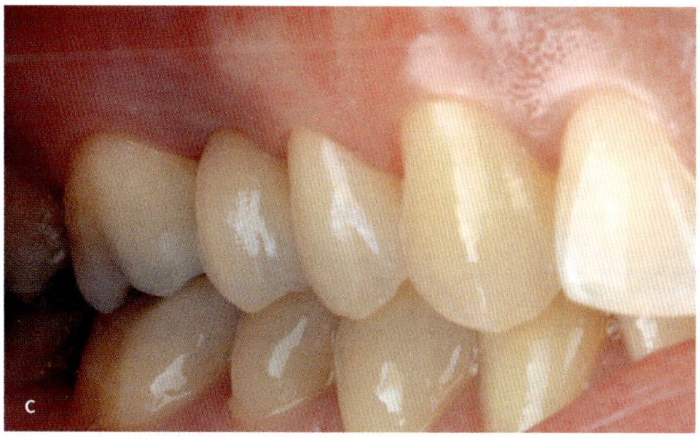

Figs 18a-c Cementing of zirconia-ceramic crown (a) and final zirconia-ceramic crown (b and c).

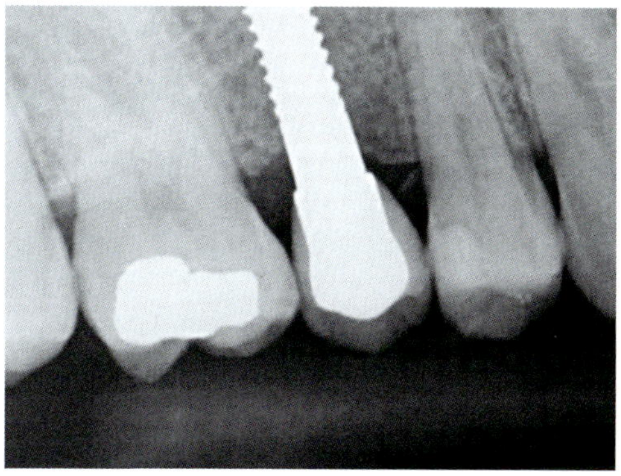

Fig 19 Final zirconia-ceramic radiographic confirmation.

FOLLOW-UP

The patient was placed on an individualized preventive maintenance program and recalled on a yearly basis. At the four year follow-up, an IOS impression and localized CBCT were taken for routine control purposes. The CBCT images demonstrated a very stable bone response to the ceramic implant (Figs 20a-d).

The clinical examination confirmed that the implant-supported rehabilitation was stable (Figs 21a-b).

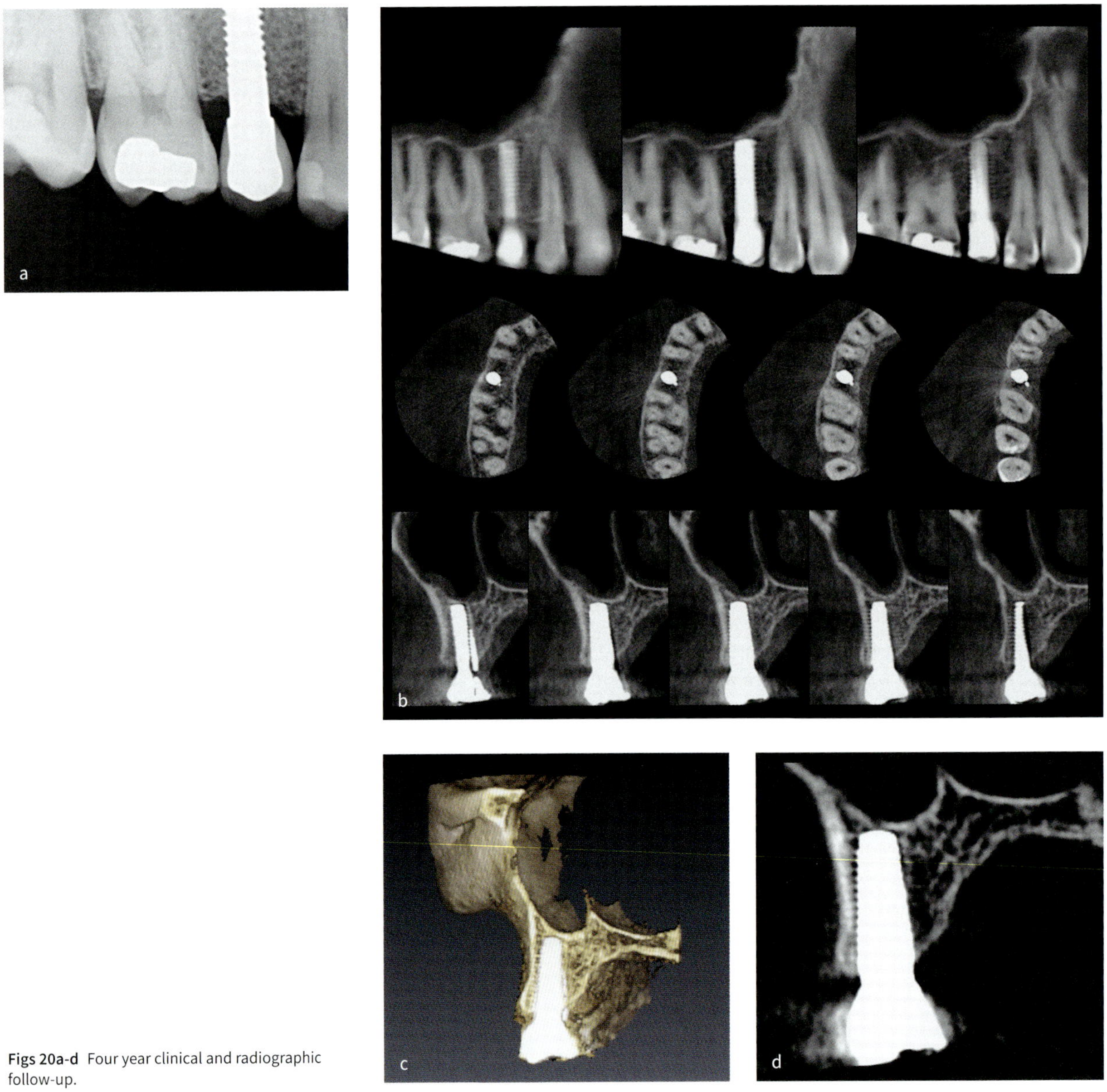

Figs 20a-d Four year clinical and radiographic follow-up.

DISCUSSION

This case and its four years of follow-up data demonstrate the performance of a monotype ceramic implant placed immediately in a single-tooth situation.

Recent studies have shown that factors such as implant design, loading protocol, simultaneous bone augmentation, and type of prosthetic reconstruction did not significantly influence the survival rate of ceramic implants (Röhling and coworkers 2018a). We therefore believe that, while this case included a number of confounding variables, the clinical choice was a good one. Immediate implant placement is a well-established technique with high survival rates and good predictability when a titanium implant is used.

This case was classified as Gallucci type 1A (immediate placement and immediate restoration/loading) (Gallucci and coworkers 2018).

The implant chosen in this case was based on a patient preference that was confirmed by the dentist and supported by evidence-based data. Ceramic implants in healed ridges exhibit proven biocompatibility and osseointegration patterns in terms of bone-to-implant contact (Pieralli and coworkers

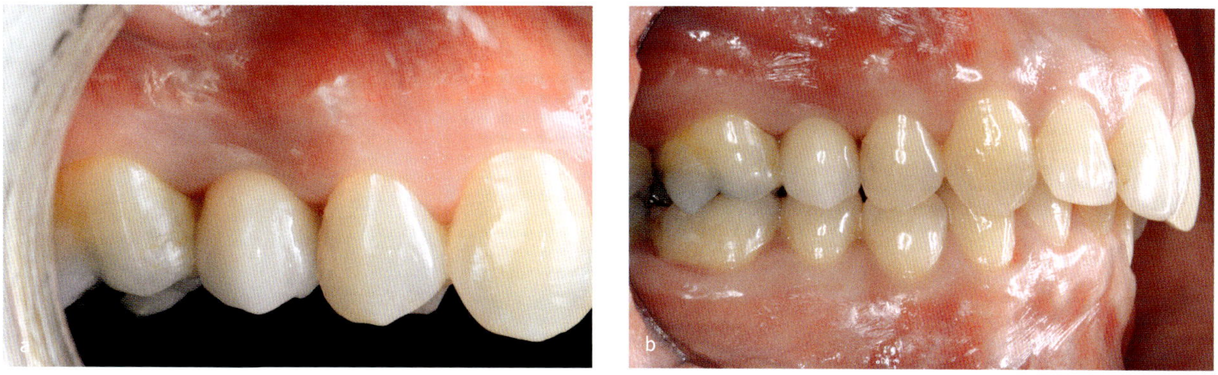

Fig 21a-b Four year clinical follow-up showing stable hard and soft tissues.

2017; Röhling and coworkers 2019), but immediate ceramic implants ranked lower than titanium in evidence-based research; for some clinical parameters there is no medium or long-term follow-up available as yet.

The osseointegration of immediate ceramic implants has a favorable record in terms of histological parameters, tending to perform at least as well as titanium implants in preclinical studies (Calvo-Guirado and coworkers 2014), but being prone to the same limitations and complications.

Marginal bone remodeling around monotype ceramic implants in healed ridges was studied in a systematic review including 11 publications with observation periods of up to seven years, showing a mean bone loss of 0.98 mm (Haro Adánez and coworkers 2018). This level was confirmed in 19 publications in a second review (Borges and coworkers 2020).

Successful immediate implants require several clinical steps: a minimally invasive extraction (keeping the alveolar socket as well as the buccal plate and soft tissue intact) in a flapless intervention (Fickl and coworkers 2008), the correct three-dimensional apicocoronal and buccolingual position, primary stability, and a correct emergence profile from the outset (Gallucci and coworkers 2018).

The success and predictability of implant-supported rehabilitations depends on the correct three-dimensional positioning of the implant. One-piece implants have biological advantages—no microgap, no implant-abutment interface—but placing them in the correct position from a prosthodontic point of view is still a challenge.

To master this challenge, a surgical guide was used to transfer the best virtual implant position determined in the software, accurately to the clinical field.

Another factor that is independent of the material is primary stability. This may be a problem with one-piece immediate implants and forms a risk as it as the implant cannot be placed in a submerged position.

The apical or lateral bone anchorage is critical when undertaking an immediate implant in ensuring primary stability. Not only does the clinician have to place the implant in the bone, ensuring that the proper prosthodontic position has been achieved, but also sufficient insertion torque to allow immediate loading must be achieved. In order to reach the correct torque, the drilling protocol is crucial and, in this case, an insertion torque of 35 Ncm allows for the placement of a provisional restoration.

Immediate provisionalization of immediate implants is regarded as one of key clinical steps that may mitigate (but not prevent) soft tissue volume changes. Although the esthetic advantages of immediate provisionalization have been disputed in the literature, when using one-piece implants, immediate provisionalization has been suggested to be a common procedure (Chan and coworkers 2019; Kan and coworkers 2018; van Nimwegen and coworkers 2018; Wang and coworkers 2020).

In this type of one-piece cemented restoration, the apicocoronal position of the implant is crucial—not only from a biological point of view but also in terms of cementing and the ability to properly remove excess cement. The implant must never be placed too deeply, as this would create oral hygiene problems and a greater susceptibility to peri-implant pathology, and also problems related to the emergence profile (Sailer and coworkers 2012).

General prosthodontic guidelines should be applied when ceramic implants are immediately loaded with no occlusal contacts in a centric or eccentric position. Proper patient instruction and education are essential to facilitate undisturbed osseointegration and healing. When these guidelines are followed, the literature states that immediate placement plus immediate restoration/loading as a clinically documented protocol has a survival rate of 98% (Gallucci and coworkers 2018).

Emergence profiles can be a limitation in the case of one-piece implants, irrespective of the implant material; it is important to choose the right abutment aspect of the monotype implant. The second premolar in the present case had a slim mesiodistal emergence profile, so a narrow-diameter implant was indicated. However, if a central incisor were to have been replaced, a wider abutment would have to be chosen for esthetic, biological, and cleaning reasons.

Immediate ceramic implants have been reported to yield good short term outcomes compared to titanium (Kniha and coworkers 2017), but with low evidence for the medium term results. The standard of care would probably require the use of a titanium implant, but evidence-based dentistry also requires respecting two other aspects: patient needs and expectations, and clinical expertise. In the present case, the patient had explicitly requested a non-metallic, ceramic-based rehabilitation with a ceramic implant and a ceramic crown.

Zirconia, or zirconium dioxide (ZrO_2), is sometimes confused with the metal zirconium (Zr), a metal directly below titanium (Ti) in the periodic table of elements. Dental zirconia can be derived from zirconium(IV)silicate ($ZrSiO_4$) by several different techniques, resulting in a ceramic material that is very different from either metals or metal alloys.

The two main features that will influence the biomechanical and biological behavior are an ionic bond (as opposed to a metallic bond) where, as no electrons are released from the material structure, undesirable interactions such as corrosion are absent.

Whether or not to fill the space e between the buccal wall of the extraction socket and the immediately placed implant when using ceramic implants has also been a matter discussion; less literature data is available on biomaterial selection and outcomes than when using titanium implants. Whether or not to fill the gap is a question discussed in the context of the physiology of extraction socket healing. Although some reports show good healing and bone-to-implant contact in type 1 sockets without specific socket management efforts (Tarnow and Chu 2011), most publications (systematic reviews and consensus proceedings) show post-extraction tissue remodeling (bone and soft tissue) that can lead to esthetically unfavorable outcomes (Chen and Buser 2014; Hämmerle and coworkers 2004).

In the present case, a 3.3 mm ceramic implant left a gap between the implant and the buccal bone.

The healing pattern of inorganic hydroxyapatite placed in socket gaps next to titanium implants is predictable and reduces post-extraction tissue remodeling in anterior, single-root teeth (Tarnow and coworkers 2014) and on posterior, multi-rooted teeth (Ragucci and coworkers 2020).

The biomaterial selection in this case was based on the (admittedly scant) available evidence. In animal models with immediate zirconia implants, a good volumetric outcome was reported when xenografts are placed in the gap between the implant and the buccal wall, supplying additional hard tissue (Alves and coworkers 2021).

Nevertheless, at the four year follow-up there was a slight loss of buccal contour immediately apical to the cervical margin of the crown, but with no clinical impact on the patient. We attribute this loss to buccal bone remodeling (thick phenotype) after the delivery of the crown. Two other factors may have contributed to this outcome: some xenograft particles that may have become embedded in the connective tissue were lost over the four year period, and the abutment diameter of the one-piece implant was very narrow.

The biomechanical properties of ceramic implants presented limitations in the past, but thanks to novel biomaterials and technologies, zirconia implants now feature improved mechanical properties. Compared to other oxide ceramics (such as aluminum oxide), zirconium dioxide exhibits high bending strength and fracture toughness, and a low modulus of elasticity. These improved properties are responsible for the fact that zirconia implants offer good resistance to masticatory forces in the oral cavity (Christel and coworkers 1989; Andreiotelli and Kohal 2009; Silva and coworkers 2009; Monzavi and coworkers 2020; Bethke and coworkers 2020).

Manufacturing and surface technologies also have a positive impact on the frequency of ceramic implant fractures (Gahlert and coworkers 2012; Osman and coworkers 2013).

The combination of these two factors has resulted in ceramic implants, and zirconia implants in particular, now having similar fractures rates to titanium implants, improving from 3.4% to 0.2% between 2004 and 2017 (Röhling and coworkers 2018b).

Aging or phase transformation in ceramic materials is a concern for most implant manufacturers. Incorrect processing causes a shift from less (tetragonal phase) to more (monoclinic phase) susceptibility to breakage. This is not always avoidable, but manufacturers have developed new surface technologies and more stringent production processes. resulting in ceramic implant products that remain stable over time (Monzavi and coworkers 2020).

Titanium-based implantology is not free from problems in terms of late outcomes, such as mucositis and peri-implant pathology. Scientific studies have cited incidence rates of 43% for mucositis and 22% for peri-implantitis (Derks and Tomasi 2015).

The choice of a ceramic implant was not dictated by immediate outcome parameters such as osseointegration or immediate soft tissue response (which we know are similar) but by the potential this therapy offers for lowering long-term peri-implantitis rates. This becomes apparent on the sagittal CBCT, showing that the bone and soft tissue next to the ceramic implant showed optimal performance after four years.

Once a rehabilitation on a ceramic implant has passed the early-outcome tests, its further fate will depend on factors that will influence marginal bone resorption, bone breakdown, and tissue infection.

All parameters identified in the literature that have led to pathologies such as plaque accumulation, inflammatory patterns, ion release, or interleukin expression seem to favor ceramics over titanium. Even in the case of active infection, peri-implant disease seems to progress differently on ceramic implants than on titanium implants (Röhling and coworkers 2019).

CONCLUSION

This case report shows the good compliance of the ceramic implant in an immediate extraction model.

Ceramic implants have introduced new concepts and new levels of clinical performance to the world of implant dentistry—such as low inflammatory patterns, low bacterial counts, and improved esthetics, all of which may constitute key important biological advantages over titanium.

Evidence-based clinical procedures involving immediately placed ceramic implants are a viable alternative to titanium implants. Short-term data already support this, but more clinical evidence is needed, particularly in the medium term (e.g., five year) data.

5.7 Replacement of a Mandibular Central Incisor with an Immediately Placed Monotype Zirconia Implant

S. Röhling, T. Borer

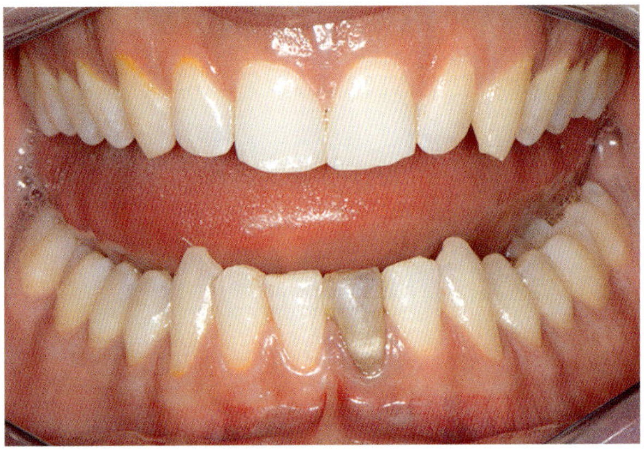

Fig 1 Initial clinical situation before oral hygiene instruction and plaque removal. Before implant placement, the patient received basic oral hygiene instruction and periodontal treatment was performed to remove plaque until a BPE score of 0 was achieved.

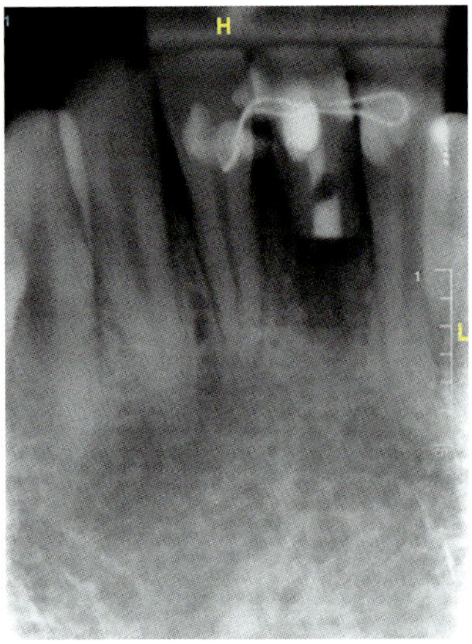

Fig 2 Initial radiographic situation.

A 25-year-old male patient had suffered a traumatic loss of tooth 31 as a child. He was a light smoker (less than 10 cigarettes per day) and in good general health, with an otherwise unremarkable medical history.

Tooth 31 had been immediately re-implanted but not endodontically treated, resulting in external root resorption. Later, the tooth did receive endodontic treatment; the apical part of the root was resected, and the crown was stabilized with composite and attached to the neighboring teeth with a wire.

Because of the provisional fixation and the discoloration of the tooth, the patient was dissatisfied with the clinical situation and asked to have the tooth replaced by an implant to guarantee proper function and to improve his esthetic appearance. He had previously learned about ceramic implants from his dentist and explicitly wanted to receive a zirconia implant.

The clinical examination showed a complete maxillary and mandibular dentition. At the time point of the first clinical examination, plaque was visible around single teeth, however, no pathological probing depths were detectable (BPE score 2) (Fig 1). Tooth 31 was stable but showed an obvious discoloration (Fig 1). The gingiva around tooth 31 did not exhibit any clinical signs of inflammation; the adjacent teeth were naturally healthy, whereas the incisors of the maxilla and mandible showed wear facets. Apically to the crown, there was 3–4 mm of attached gingiva with a medium-thick phenotype and a medium scallop height. Tooth 31 and the adjacent teeth revealed no pathological probing depths, their gingiva showing no recession or other soft tissue defects. The periapical radiograph showed the resected apical root portion of tooth 31 with its wire attachment to the adjacent teeth. The vertical bone volume was sufficient, with no radiological signs of inflammation (Fig 2).

Table 1 Risk assessment for immediate implant placement in single-tooth sites

	Low risk	**Medium risk**	**High risk**
Preoperative assessment			
Patient-related			
Medical status	Healthy, uneventful healing		Compromised healing
Esthetic risk	Low/medium esthetic risk	High esthetic risk	Significant esthetic compromise expected
Site-related			
Gingival-margin position	No recession	Minor gingival recession	Gingival recession ≥ 2 mm
Soft tissue quality	Thick gingival phenotype	Thin gingival phenotype or limited keratinized gingiva	No keratinized gingiva
Bone anchorage	Sufficient bone anchorage to achieve primary stability		Lack of bone anchorage to achieve primary stability
Facial bone wall	≥ 1 mm facial bone thickness	Facial bone plate < 1 mm thickness, or small fenestration or dehiscence defect	Significant fenestration or dehiscence of facial bone
Need for a mucoperiosteal flap	Sufficient alveolar bone for a flapless approach		Need for flapped bone augmentation
Socket position within alveolar envelope	Socket within the alveolar bone envelope		Socket and facial bone wall protruding out of the bone envelope
Presence of endodontic infection	No infection	Chronic periapical infection	Acute infection
Presence of periodontal disease	Periodontally healthy	Controlled periodontal disease	Active periodontal disease
Planning implant position	Ideal three-dimensional position with axis exiting through the cingulum or incisal edge		Facially positioned or over-angulated implant or excessive implant depth
Gap between buccal bone and planned implant position	≥ 2 mm	1–2 mm	< 1 mm
Intraoperative assessment			
Extraction	Minimally invasive tooth extraction	Damage to surrounding soft tissue, including severed/detached papillae	Significant damage to soft tissue and surrounding bone
Primary implant stability	Primary stability achieved		Lack of primary stability
Final implant position	Ideal three-dimensional position achieved		Facially positioned or over-angulated implant or excessive implant depth

The data from the clinical and radiographic examination were assessed to perform a risk assessment for immediate implant placement and immediate loading (Tables 1 and 2). Additionally, an esthetic risk assessment was performed according to previously published criteria (Buser and coworkers 2017b). Regarding immediate implant placement, most parameters were assessed to be "low risk." A "high risk" assessment applied to the position of the socket within the al-

Table 2 Risk assessment for immediate loading of an immediately placed single implant

	Low risk	Medium risk	High risk
Preoperative assessment			
Patient-related			
Occlusal scheme	No direct occlusal contacts	Minimal occlusal contact and/or shared guidance	Main determinant of anterior guidance
Occlusal parafunction	Absent		Present
Site-related			
Bone anchorage	Sufficient bone anchorage to resist loading forces		Insufficient bone anchorage to resist loading forces
Tooth position	Incisor, premolars	Canine	Molars
Intraoperative assessment			
Primary implant stability	30–45 Ncm insertion torque	20–30 Ncm insertion torque	< 20 Ncm insertion torque

veolar envelope (since the clinical investigation had shown that the socket and the facial bone protruded) and for the gap between the buccal bone wall and the planned implant position (expected to be smaller than 2 mm, based on the narrow socket configuration of tooth 31) (Table 1). However, it should be noted that this assessment is more applicable to large extraction sockets, whereas in a mandibular incisor position with a much narrower socket, this risk may not be as significant as the regenerative potential will be greater from the interproximal bone. Regarding immediate loading, a "high risk" assessment applied for patient-related factors since the patient suffered from occlusal parafunction identified by wear facets of the upper and lower anterior teeth (Fig 1). In addition, a deep overbite as a main determinant of anterior guidance was present (Fig 20). Regarding site-related factors, a "low risk" assessment applied to all parameters (Table 2).

Based on the clinical and radiological findings (Figs 1 and 2), it was decided to extract tooth 31. Various treatment options were discussed with the patient, who categorically refused treatment with a resin-bonded Maryland bridge. In addition, this treatment option was inadvisable because of the retroclined position of the upper incisors, the deep overbite, and the visible wear facets (Figs 1 and 20). Since he wanted a fixed prosthesis and given the presence of naturally healthy adjacent teeth, it was planned to close the gap with an implant-supported single crown. As the patient had high esthetic expectations, an all-ceramic zirconia implant was recommended for optimal white and pink esthetics. Based on the narrow gap, it was planned to use a reduced diameter monotype zirconia implant.

The patient was informed of the treatment plan, and the surgical and prosthetic procedures. Because sufficient bone volume was available, immediate implant placement and an immediate provisional prosthetic reconstruction—Gallucci type 1A (Gallucci and coworkers 2018)—was planned. However, the patient was informed that an immediate prosthetic reconstruction with a laboratory-fabricated provisional crown would be possible only if the implant were to show sufficient primary stability after placement. Because of the complexity of the clinical situation, the case was surgically and restoratively classified as "Advanced" according to the ITI SAC classification.

Before implant surgery, the patient received basic oral hygiene instructions, and periodontal treatment was performed to remove plaque until a BPE score of 0 was achieved.

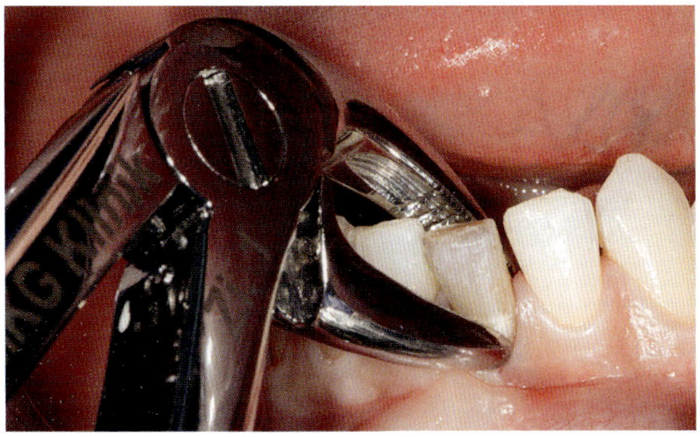

Fig 3 Tooth extraction.

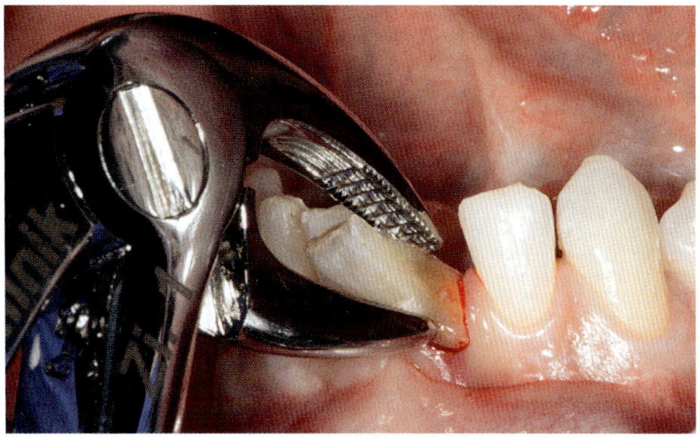

Fig 4 Tooth extraction.

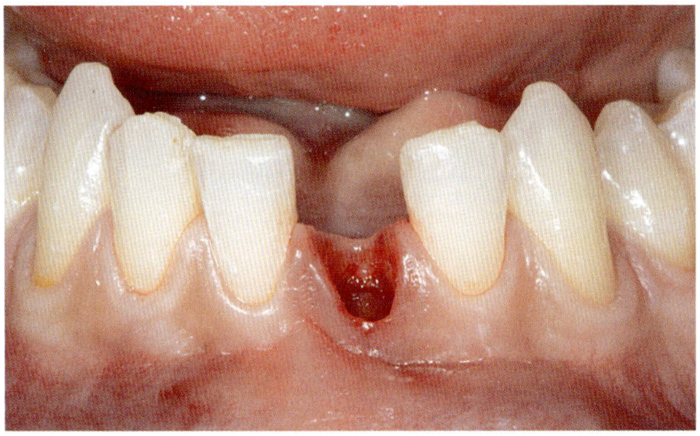

Fig 5 Extraction socket immediately after tooth extraction.

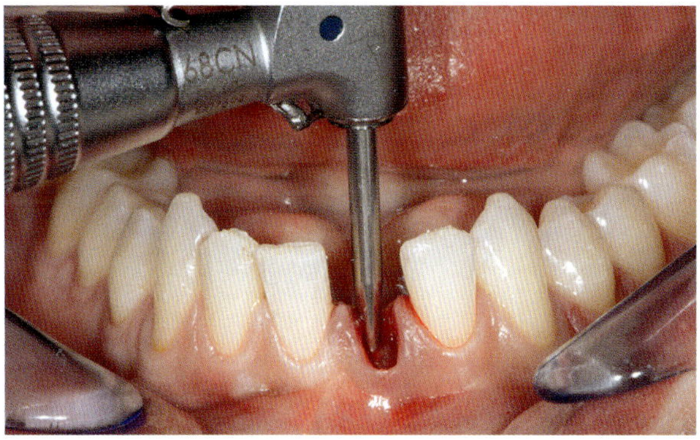

Fig 6 Marking of implant position using round bur.

Also prior to the surgery, a surgical template was fabricated for guidance during implant placement. Since tooth 31 was in the clinically correct position, a mandibular impression was taken and the surgical template produced at the laboratory. When placing implants—particularly with immediate placed implant placement and monotype implants—a surgical stent can be very helpful in assuring the correct three-dimensional implant positioning.

At the beginning of the surgical procedure, the wire/composite splint that stabilized tooth 31 was removed. Under local anesthesia, tooth 31 was carefully extracted with forceps (Figs 3 and 4), the extraction socket was curetted, and the granulation tissue was removed. Clinically, the bone walls of the extraction socket were intact; no bone defect was detected, and the soft tissue was not damaged (Fig 5). During tooth extraction and implant placement, a mucoperiostal flap was not elevated in order to guarantee an unimpeded blood supply to the peri-implant soft tissue.

The implant position was marked with a round bur (Fig 6). This step is particularly important in fresh extraction sockets to ensure a stable position of the twist drills. The preparation of the osteotomy began with 2.2 mm and 2.8 mm twist drills, followed by a check of the implant position and angulation using position indicators (Figs 7 to 10). Because of the narrow gap, it was decided to place a reduced-diameter all-ceramic implant; hence, no additional twist drills were necessary to prepare the osteotomy.

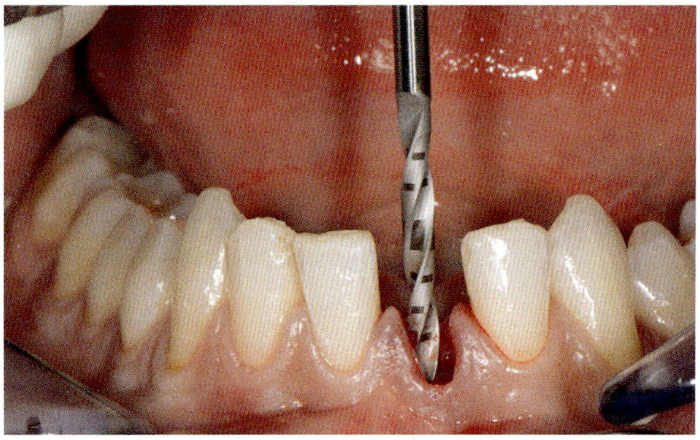

Fig 7 Osteotomy preparation using a 2.2 mm twist drill.

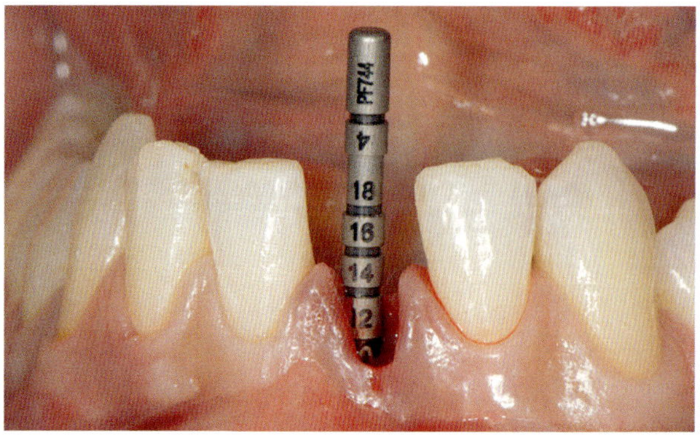

Fig 8 Checking the implant position using a position indicator.

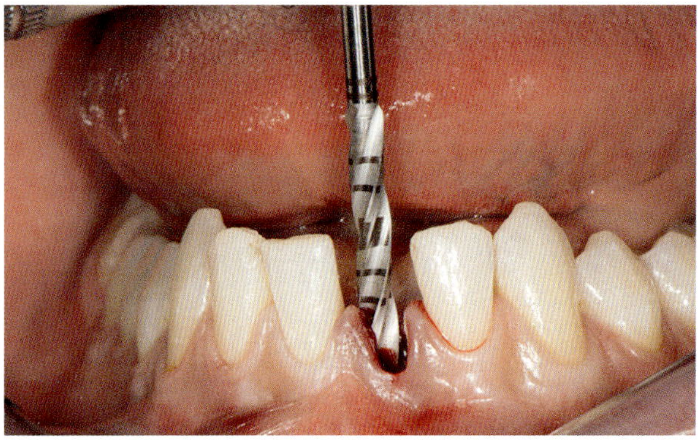

Fig 9 Osteotomy preparation using a 2.8 mm twist drill.

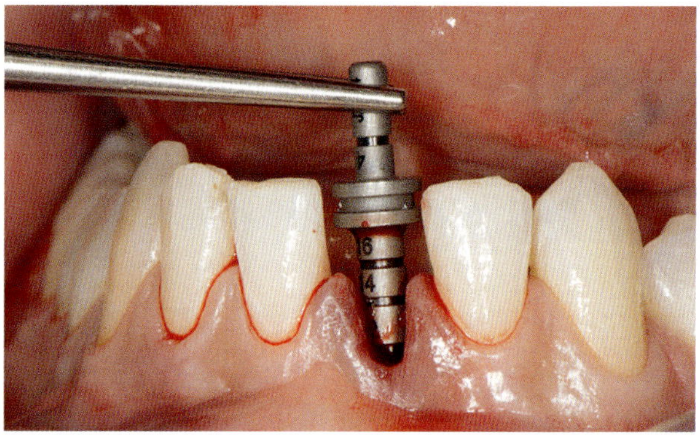

Fig 10 Checking the implant position using a position indicator.

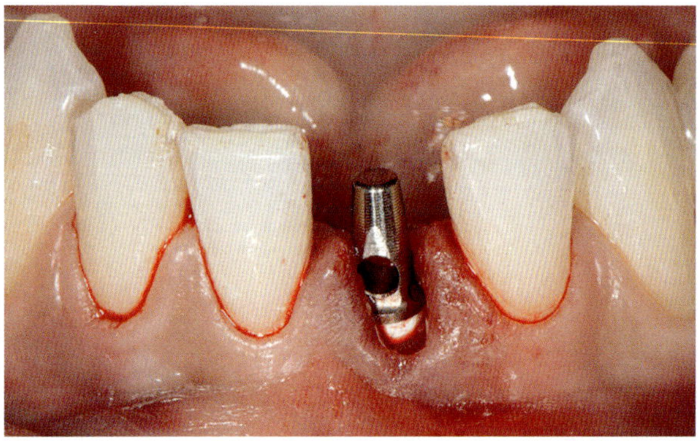

Fig 11 Checking the implant position using a monotype position indicator with an abutment height of 5.5 mm (vestibular view).

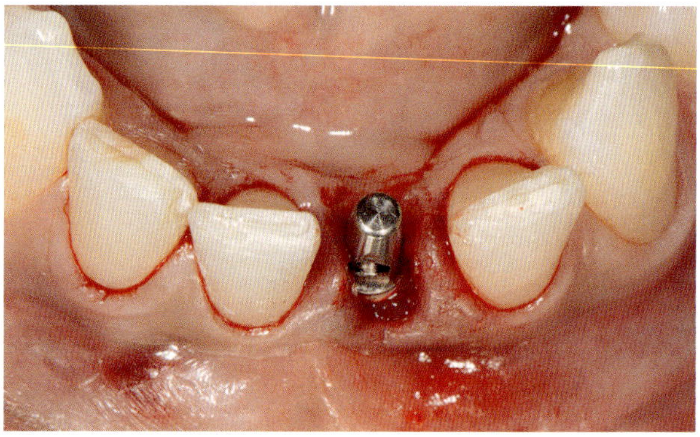

Fig 12 Checking the implant position using a monotype position indicator with an abutment height of 5.5 mm (occlusal view).

To select the correct abutment height (4.0 or 5.5 mm) of the monotype ceramic implant—which depends on the interocclusal distance—and to finalize the correct implant position and angulation, a specific monotype position indicator was inserted (Figs 11 and 12). In this case, the 5.5 mm abutment had the right height for the existing interocclusal distance and the design of the planned all-ceramic restoration. The final step of the osteotomy preparation was performed using a 3.3 mm profile drill (Fig 13). As current zirconia implants have a conical intraosseous design, the profile drill must be used regardless of bone quality, to guarantee the correct implant position.

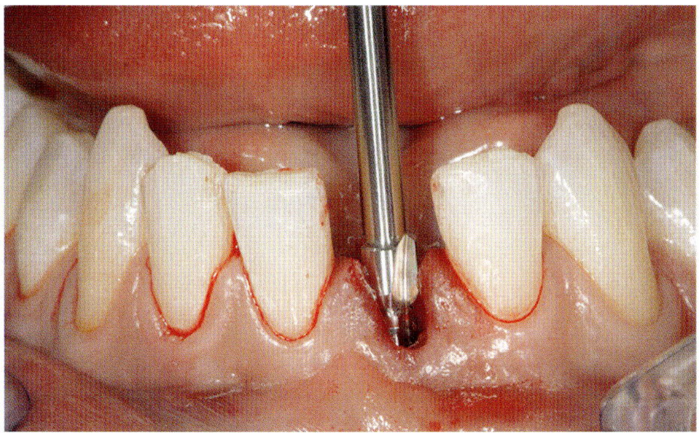

Fig 13 Osteotomy preparation using a 3.3 mm profile drill.

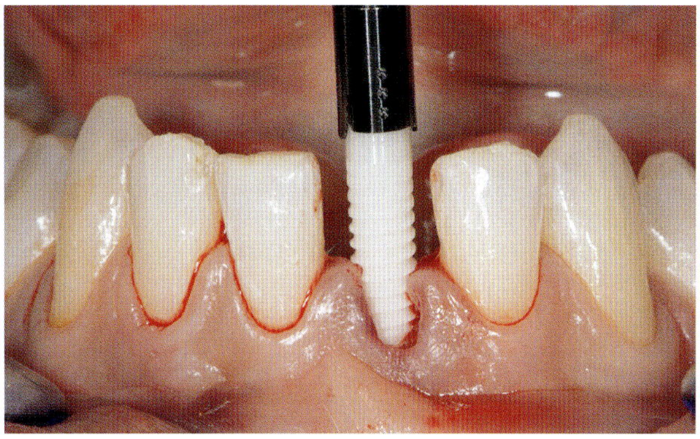

Fig 14 Insertion of a 3.3 mm monotype zirconia implant.

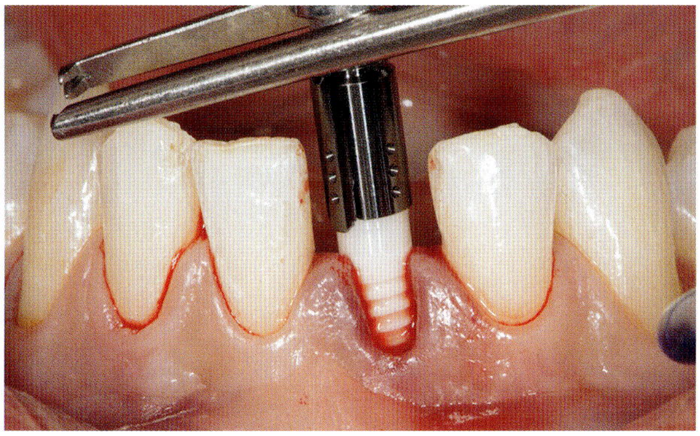

Fig 15 Insertion of a 3.3 mm monotype zirconia implant.

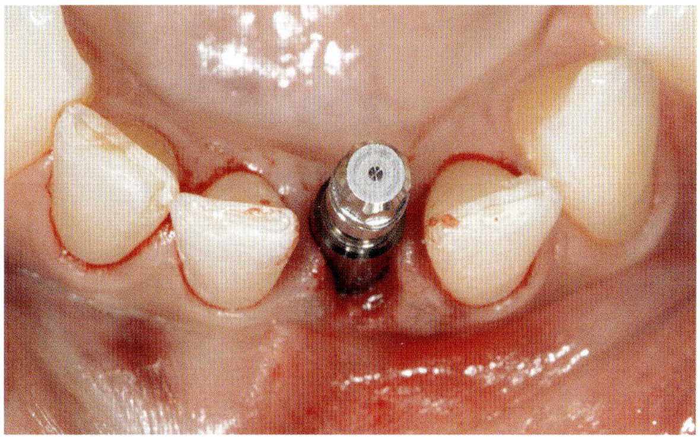

Fig 16 Inserted monotype zirconia implant with insertion tool (occlusal view).

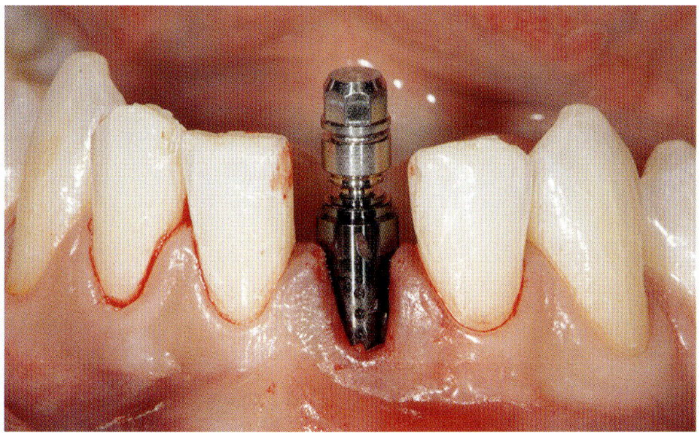

Fig 17 Inserted monotype zirconia implant with insertion tool (vestibular view).

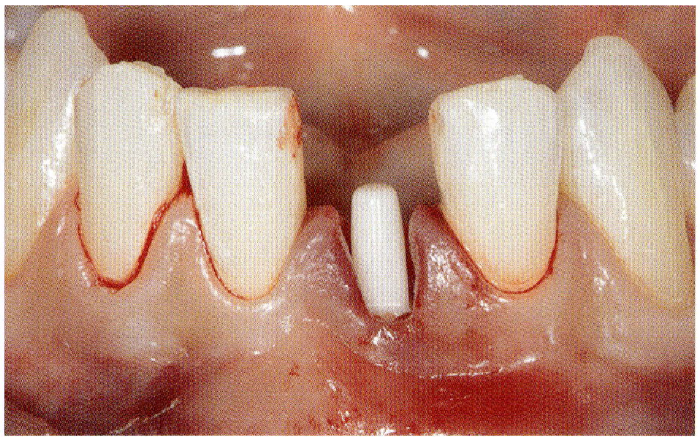

Fig 18 Inserted 3.3 mm monotype zirconia implant with an abutment height of 5.5 mm (vestibular view).

A monotype all-ceramic implant (PURE Ceramic Implant, diameter 3.3 mm, length 10 mm, abutment height 5.5 mm; Institut Straumann AG, Basel, Switzerland) was placed in an optimal three-dimensional, prosthetically driven position (Figs 14 to 20) with high primary stability of more than 35 Ncm. The implant shoulder was placed approximately 1.5 mm apical to the expected gingival margin of the final restoration. Because of the narrow single root extraction socket and the undamaged and stable facial bone plate, simultaneous bone augmentation was not indicated.

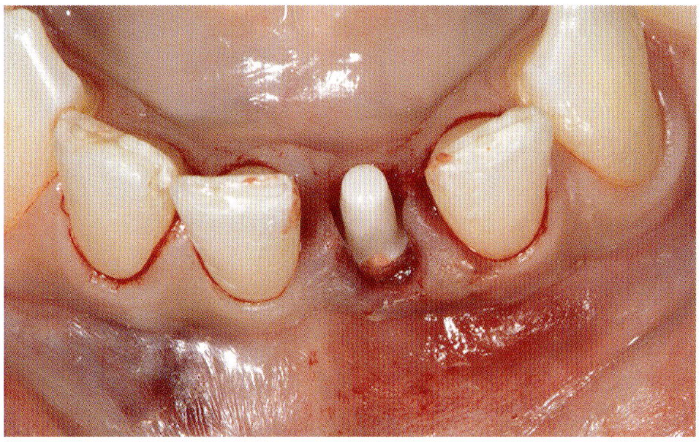

Fig 19 Inserted zirconia implant (occlusal view).

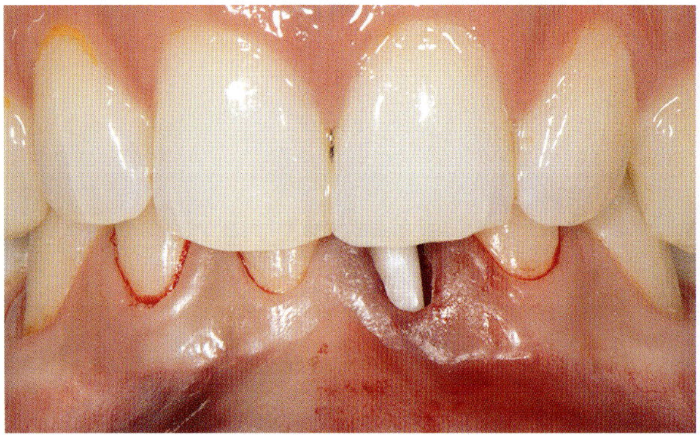

Fig 20 Inserted zirconia implant.

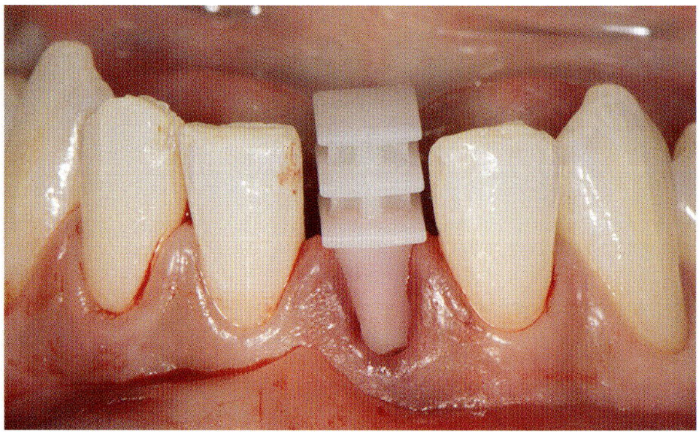

Fig 21 Inserted prefabricated impression cap is snapped onto the implant abutment and shoulder.

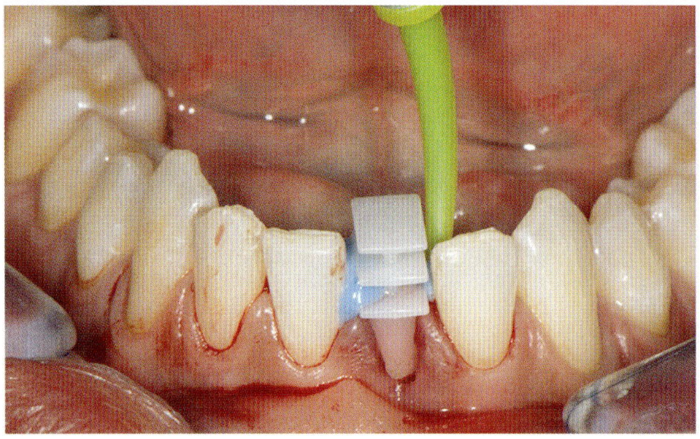

Fig 22 Impression-taking directly after implant placement.

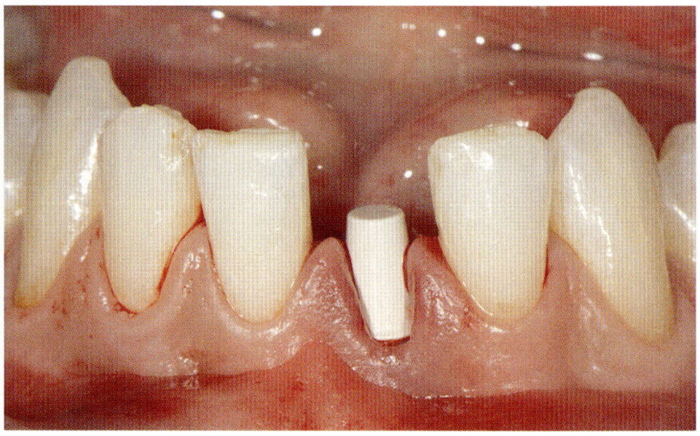

Fig 23 Inserted zirconia implant with protective cap to avoid adherence of soft tissue to the implant shoulder.

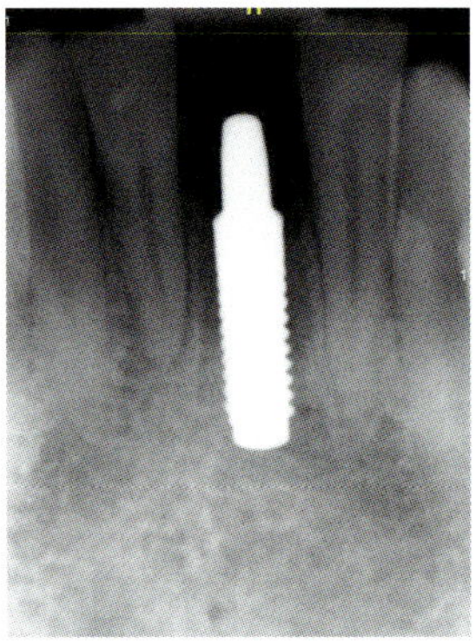

Fig 24 Radiographic investigation directly after implant placement.

At the end of the surgery, a prefabricated impression cap was snapped onto the implant abutment and shoulder (Fig 21). A conventional impression was taken using silicone (Fig 22) and a laboratory-made custom tray. Finally, a protective cap was snapped onto the implant abutment to avoid adherence of soft tissue to the implant shoulder (Fig 23). A periapical radiograph was also taken (Fig 24).

Two days after implant placement, uneventful healing and irritation-free peri-implant soft tissues were observed (Figs 25 and 26). The protective cap was removed and a laboratory-made acrylic provisional crown with a cement vent on the lingual side was delivered with temporary cement (Temp-Bond; Kerr, Biberach, Germany) without occlusal contact (Figs 27 to 30). The lingual cement vent (Fig 28) served to avoid cement residue in the peri-implant mucosa.

After three months of uneventful healing, the implant showed no clinical signs of mobility; the peri-implant mucosa was free of irritation (Figs 31 and 32). During the osseointegration period, the laboratory-made temporary acrylic crown had been regularly adapted with acrylic filling material to shape the peri-implant mucosa (emergence profile) and to simulate the final esthetic outcome. The temporary crown was removed (Fig 32), and once more a prefabricated impression cap was snapped onto the implant abutment and shoulder (Fig 33).

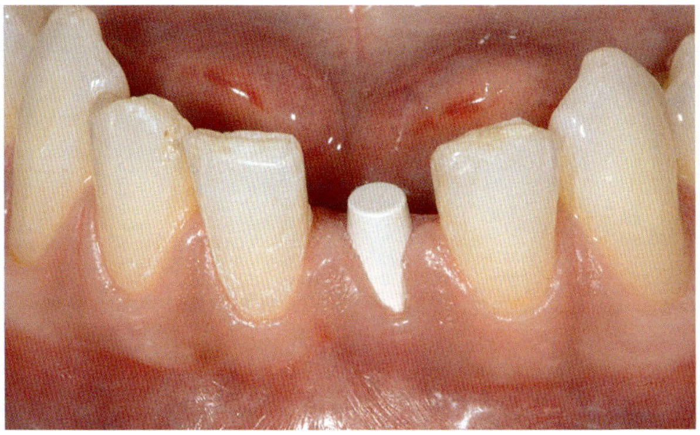

Fig 25 Two days after implant placement. Zirconia implant with protective cap.

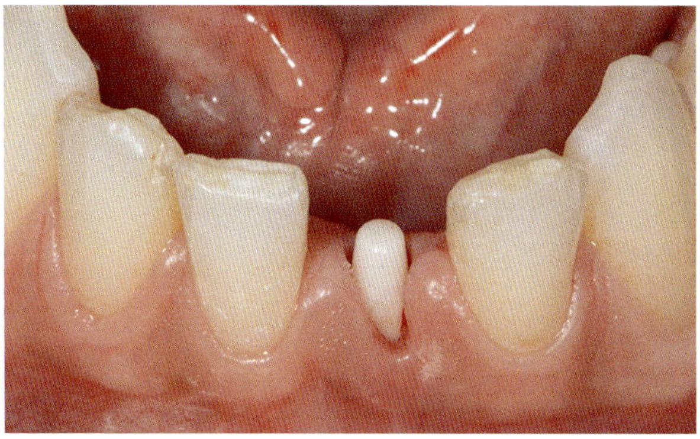

Fig 26 Two days after implant placement.

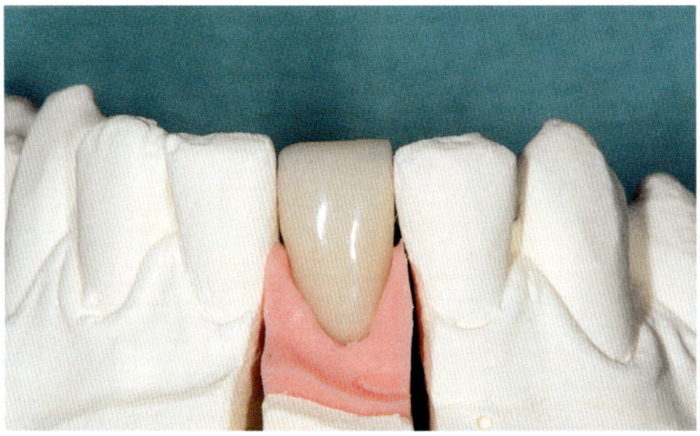

Fig 27 Provisional laboratory-made acrylic crown two days after implant placement (vestibular view).

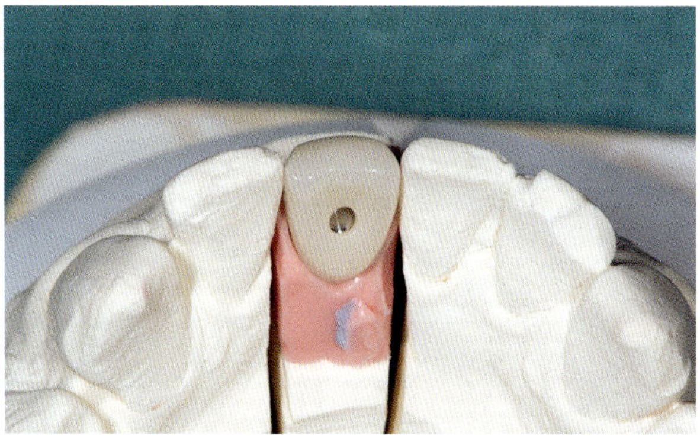

Fig 28 Laboratory-made provisional acrylic crown with vent for cementation (occlusal view).

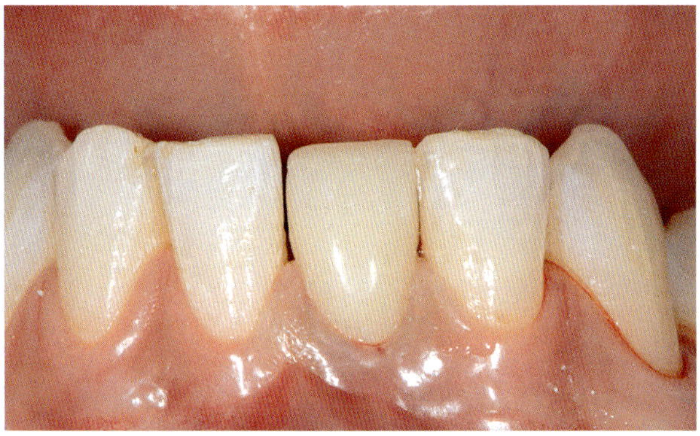

Fig 29 Laboratory-made provisional acrylic crown cemented with Temp-Bond. No occlusal contact.

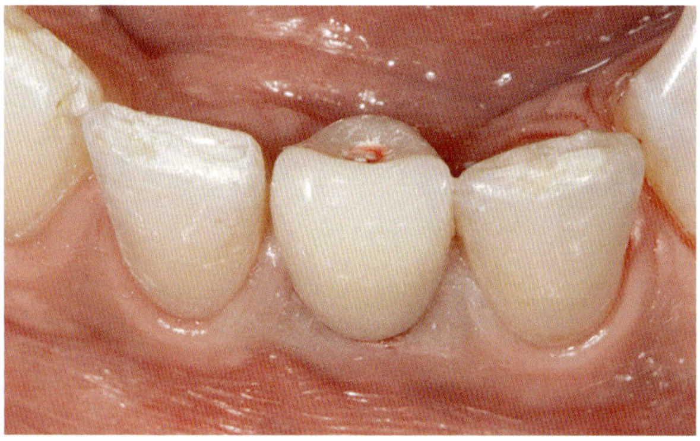

Fig 30 Laboratory-made provisional acrylic crown cemented with Temp-Bond.

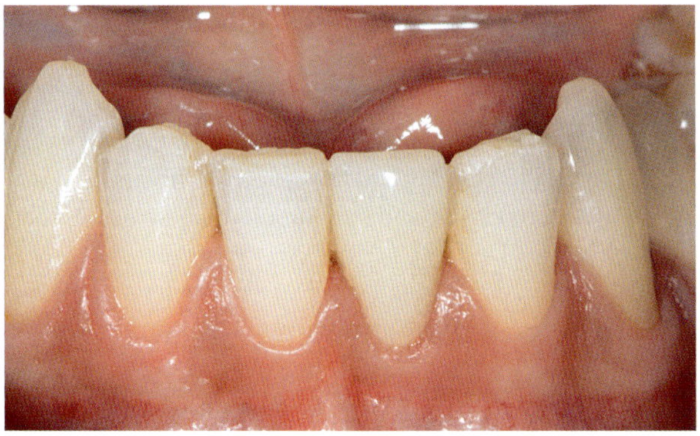

Fig 31 Three months after implant placement (vestibular view).

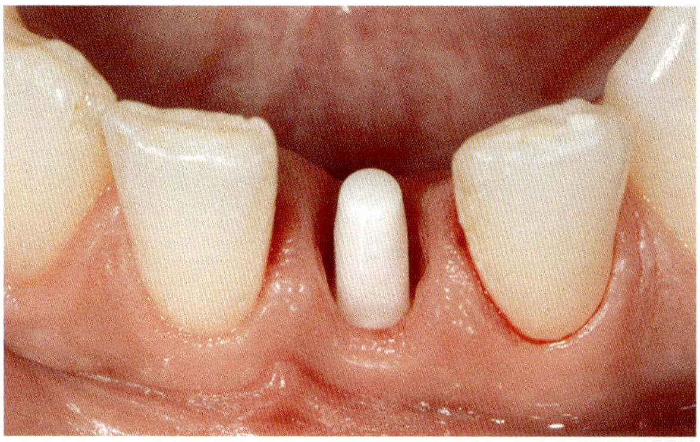

Fig 32 Three months after implant placement. Zirconia implant without provisional crown.

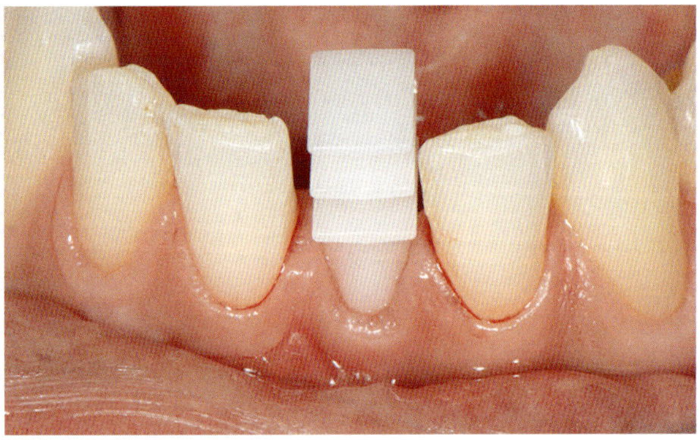

Fig 33 Impression-taking for the definitive ceramic crown.

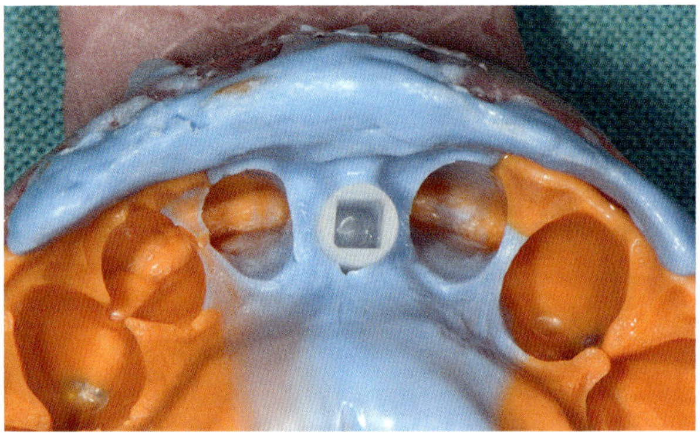

Fig 34 Impression-taking for the definitive ceramic crown.

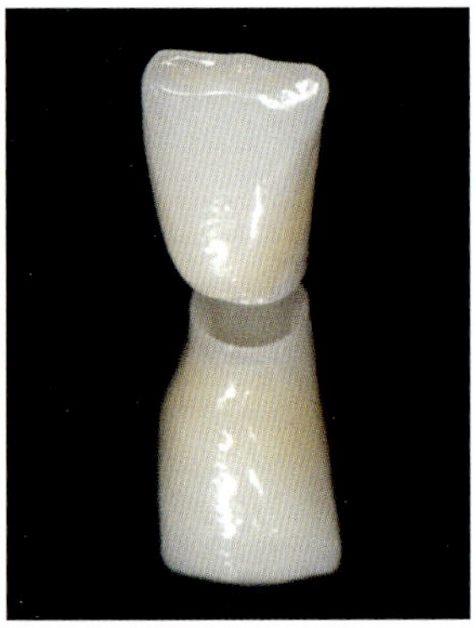

Fig 35 Definitive all-ceramic crown.

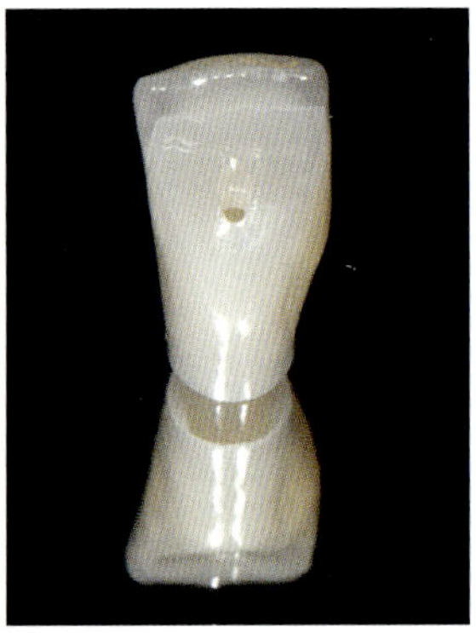

Fig 36 Definitive all-ceramic crown with vent for cementation.

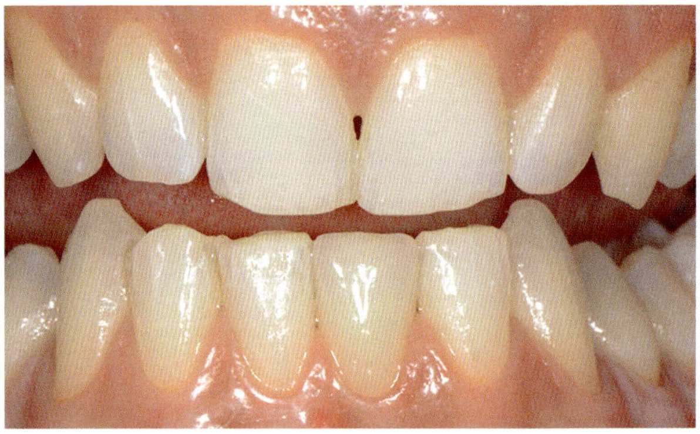

Fig 37 Two years after implant placement.

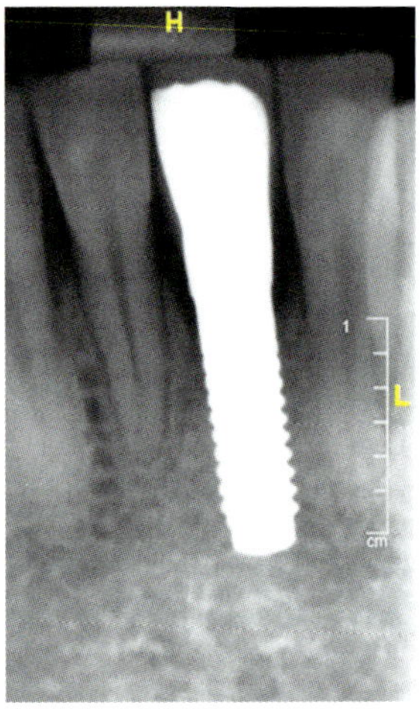

Fig 38 Radiograph two years after implant placement.

Another conventional impression was taken using silicone in a laboratory-made custom tray (Fig 34). During the three-month osseointegration period, the provisional was regularly adapted with acrylic filling material to shape the peri-implant mucosa and to simulate the final esthetic outcome.

Next, an all-ceramic crown was fabricated (Figs 35 and 36). To avoid excess cement during cementation, the ceramic crown was designed with a cement vent on the lingual side. The crown was cemented following a defined cementation protocol, which included a moderate/thin application of the glass-ionomer cement (Ketac Cem; 3M, Neuss, Germany) with a small dental brush. Additionally, during cement curing , submarginal excess cement was removed with specific dental floss (Superfloss; Procter & Gamble, Schwalbach am Taunus, Germany).

Two years after implant placement, the clinical and radiographic investigation showed completely irritation-free and stable peri-implant soft and hard tissues (Figs 37 and 38).

DISCUSSION

The correct timing of implant placement has become an important issue in implant dentistry during the last twenty years. Immediately placed implants can reduce the overall treatment time—an attractive option for patients as well as for clinicians.

The longer the period after tooth extraction, the more extensive the possible ridge dimension alterations. This can result in an overall reduction in bone volume that might complicate implant therapy (Buser and coworkers 2017a). However, immediate implant placement is a complex clinical procedure that should only be performed by experienced clinicians and when ideal anatomic conditions are present. As defined by the ITI, these conditions are characterized by fully intact socket walls with a facial/buccal bone wall thickness of at least 1 mm, a thick gingival phenotype, no acute infection at the extraction site, and sufficient bone volume apical and coronal to the extraction site to allow implant placement in the correct three-dimensional position with sufficient primary stability (Buser and coworkers 2017a; Morton and coworkers 2014).

For predictable esthetic outcomes in immediate implant placement without flap elevation, the ITI recommends correct three-dimensional positioning of the implant platform, including positioning the implant in the extraction socket with a minimum distance of 2 mm between the implant platform and the inner surface of the buccal socket wall (Morton and coworkers 2014).

In the past two decades, zirconia implants have become a reliable and attractive treatment option. Relevant milestones included optimized manufacturing processes and the development of fracture-resistant zirconia implants with a micro-roughened surface. Experimental studies have shown that the soft and hard tissue integration of micro-roughened zirconia implants is comparable to that of established titanium implants (Gahlert and coworkers 2009; Janner and coworkers 2018; Röhling and coworkers 2019b).

Clinical studies have reported survival rates of 95% and more for follow-up periods of up to five years or more for commercially available zirconia implants (Balmer and coworkers 2020; Bormann and coworkers 2018; Röhling and coworkers 2018). In addition, a meta-analysis found a mean two year survival rate of 97.2% for zirconia implants; potentially confounding factors such as implant design, loading and implant placement protocols, simultaneous bone augmentation, or the type of prosthetic reconstruction did not significantly influence the reported survival rates (Röhling and coworkers 2018). Consequently, based on the available evidence, the 6th ITI Consensus Conference stated that monotype ceramic implants can be used as a clinical alternative to titanium implants (Morton and coworkers 2018; Röhling and coworkers 2018).

A critical aspect of zirconia implants is that evidence-based clinical data have not been available for all zirconia implant systems.

In the present case, immediate implant placement according to type 1A of the Gallucci classification (Gallucci and coworkers 2018) was performed to reduce the treatment time and to provide the patient with a fixed implant-supported prosthetic reconstruction directly after implant placement. Monotype zirconia implants with a tissue-level design offer a reliable and safe treatment option for experienced clinicians (Röhling and coworkers 2018). Based on accurate planning, and provided that the implants are adequately placed, zirconia implants may be considered as a treatment option, especially in esthetically challenging indications.

5.8 Immediate Replacement of Four Mandibular Anterior Teeth with a Conventionally Loaded Implant-Supported Fixed Dental Prosthesis

G. O. Gallucci, A. Hamilton, T. C. Sun

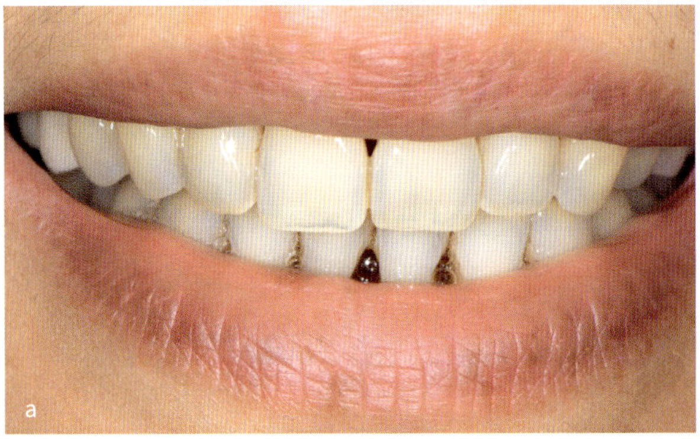

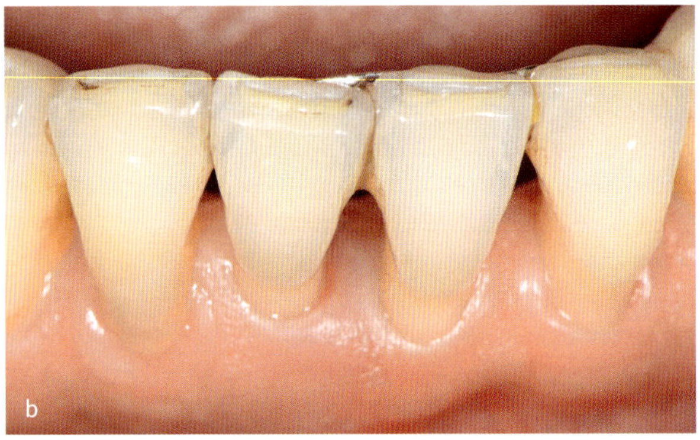

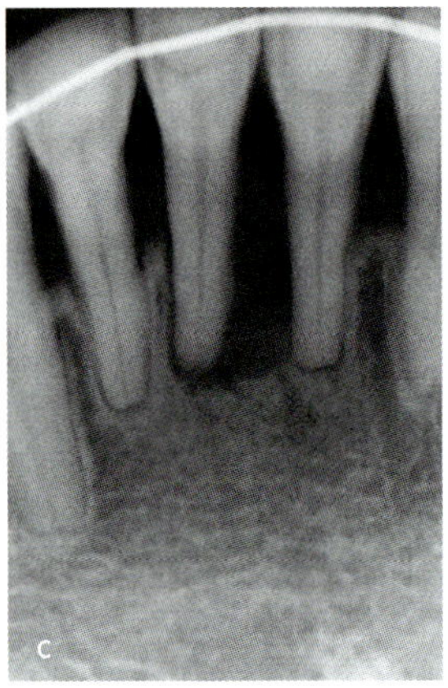

Figs 1a-c Initial clinical situation: extraoral smile view (a), intraoral view (b), and radiograph (c).

A 63-year-old female patient was referred by a periodontist for consultation and assessment with regard to implant rehabilitation of the mandibular incisors. The patient presented in good health with no history of smoking or significant medical history. The patient's chief complaint was mobility of the mandibular anterior dentition. She had a history of periodontal disease, which had been treated and followed by a periodontist with regular maintenance every four months over the previous ten years. The patient demonstrated excellent home care with full mouth plaque score and bleeding score less than 20%. She presented with an overall healthy reduced periodontium with probing depth within normal limits, except for localized deep pockets located in the mandibular anterior dentition. As part of her periodontal management, her mandibular incisors had previously been splinted to the adjacent canines for additional support.

A detailed interdisciplinary clinical and radiographic examination (Figs 1a-c) was made to evaluate the prognosis of her mandibular anterior dentition and to establish a proper treatment plan. Residual periodontal pockets greater than 5 mm were present on teeth 31 and 41 after a lengthy periodontal maintenance phase. There was extensive bone loss between teeth 31 and 41, with the bony defect extending to the root apex of tooth 31. Although the sites did not present with pockets deeper than 4 mm, gingival recession, the loss of the interdental papilla, and more than 50–60% of horizontal bone loss on teeth 32 and 42 demonstrated an extensive loss of periodontal attachment. Mobility greater than grade II was present on all four mandibular incisors.

According the 2017 World Workshop on the Classification of Periodontal and Peri-Implant Diseases and Conditions, the periodontal diagnosis was periodontitis, localized, stage III, grade A. Based on the McGuire and Nunn Periodontal Prognosis Classification System (1991, 1996, 1999), teeth 31 and 41 were classified as hopeless, while teeth 32 and 42 met the criteria of a questionable prognosis. After we had discussed the situation with the patient, she opted for removal of the periodontally compromised teeth and replacement with an implant-supported fixed restoration. Considering the implant-prosthetic design, a four-unit bridge supported by two implants was a favorable option over two adjacent implants in the lower incisor area, where the space was very restricted and the long term-outcome can be compromised.

An assessment was made to decide on the implant placement and loading protocol (Buser and coworkers 2017a; Gallucci and coworkers 2018). A risk assessment was also completed, based on the Risk Assessment Table for immediate implant placement in single tooth sites. Except for two site-related risk factors (minor gingival recession and controlled periodontal disease), which were categorized as medium risk, the risk assessment indicated a generalized low risk for immediate implant (Table 1).

Together with the Risk Assessment Table for immediate loading of an immediately placed single implant (Table 2), the following factors were also taken into consideration while performing the risk assessment for the loading protocol:

- The mandibular anterior dentition provides anterior guidance—the main determinant for a higher risk for immediate loading
- Presence of a suitable alternative, a fixed provisional restoration, so immediate loading was not critical
- While analyzing implant survival based on the placement and loading protocol for implants placed in various locations, the anterior mandible was the least reported site (Zhou and coworkers 2021) with clinically insufficient documentation to support a type 1A protocol in the anterior mandible for short-span implant-supported prostheses
- Possible staged extraction of multiple adjacent teeth, providing the potential benefit of maintaining interproximal bone levels and soft tissue architecture (Khoury and coworkers 2020; Al-Askar and coworkers 2013)

A disadvantage of the selected protocol (type 1C) is the need for a second surgical procedure, which requires extra treatment time.

Therefore, based on the periodontal prognosis, anatomical assessment, implant-prosthetic design, and the patient's chief complaint, immediate placement with a conventional loading protocol (type 1C) was selected, and the following treatment steps were planned:

- Extraction of teeth 32 and 42 and immediate implant placement using computer-guided surgery at sites 32 and 42
- Natural teeth 32 and 42 bonded to the adjacent dentition as a provisional restoration
- Implant-supported provisional restoration created with the crowns of the patient's extracted natural teeth
- Definitive restoration with a four-unit implant-supported bridge

DATA ACQUISITION, IMPLANT PLANNING, AND DESIGN OF THE SURGICAL GUIDE

Digital diagnostic impressions were taken with an intraoral scanner (iTero Element; Align Technology, Rotkreuz, Switzerland), and a cone-beam computed tomography (CBCT) image was acquired (i-CAT; Imaging Science, Hatfield, PA, USA) for treatment planning (Figs 2a-d). The uncompressed DICOM file from the CBCT examination was imported into virtual implant planning software (coDiagnostiX; Dental Wings, Montreal, Canada). Following the software workflow, the patient coordinate system was aligned and a panoramic curve defined. The threshold volume was properly adjusted to best display the three-dimensional rendering, and the DICOM dataset was segmented to create a digital model of the mandibular bone and the teeth. The Standard Tessellation Language (STL) file of the digital diagnostic impressions was then imported and superimposed, based on corresponding landmarks, on both the digital model and the STL file.

Table 1 Risk assessment for immediate implant placement in single-tooth sites

	Low risk	Medium risk	High risk
Preoperative assessment			
Patient-related			
Medical status	Healthy, uneventful healing		Compromised healing
Esthetic risk	Low/medium esthetic risk	High esthetic risk	Significant esthetic compromise expected
Site-related			
Gingival-margin position	No recession	Minor gingival recession	Gingival recession ≥ 2 mm
Soft tissue quality	Thick gingival phenotype	Thin gingival phenotype or limited keratinized gingiva	No keratinized gingiva
Bone anchorage	Sufficient bone anchorage to achieve primary stability		Lack of bone anchorage to achieve primary stability
Facial bone wall	≥ 1 mm facial bone thickness	Facial bone plate < 1 mm thickness, or small fenestration or dehiscence defect	Significant fenestration or dehiscence of facial bone
Need for a mucoperiosteal flap	Sufficient alveolar bone for a flapless approach		Need for flapped bone augmentation
Socket position within alveolar envelope	Socket within the alveolar bone envelope		Socket and facial bone wall protruding out of the bone envelope
Presence of endodontic infection	No infection	Chronic periapical infection	Acute infection
Presence of periodontal disease	Periodontally healthy	Controlled periodontal disease	Active periodontal disease
Planning implant position	Ideal three-dimensional position with axis exiting through the cingulum or incisal edge		Facially positioned or over-angulated implant or excessive implant depth
Gap between buccal bone and planned implant position	≥ 2 mm	1–2 mm	< 1 mm
Intraoperative assessment			
Extraction	Minimally invasive tooth extraction	Damage to surrounding soft tissue, including severed/detached papillae	Significant damage to soft tissue and surrounding bone
Primary implant stability	Primary stability achieved		Lack of primary stability
Final implant position	Ideal three-dimensional position achieved		Facially positioned or over-angulated implant or excessive implant depth

Table 2 Risk assessment for immediate loading of an immediately placed single implant

	Low risk	**Medium risk**	**High risk**
Preoperative assessment			
Patient-related			
Occlusal scheme	No direct occlusal contacts	Minimal occlusal contact and/or shared guidance	Main determinant of anterior guidance
Occlusal parafunction	Absent		Present
Site-related			
Bone anchorage	Sufficient bone anchorage to resist loading forces		Insufficient bone anchorage to resist loading forces
Tooth position	Incisor, premolars	Canine	Molars
Intraoperative assessment			
Primary implant stability	30–45 Ncm insertion torque	20–30 Ncm insertion torque	< 20 Ncm insertion torque

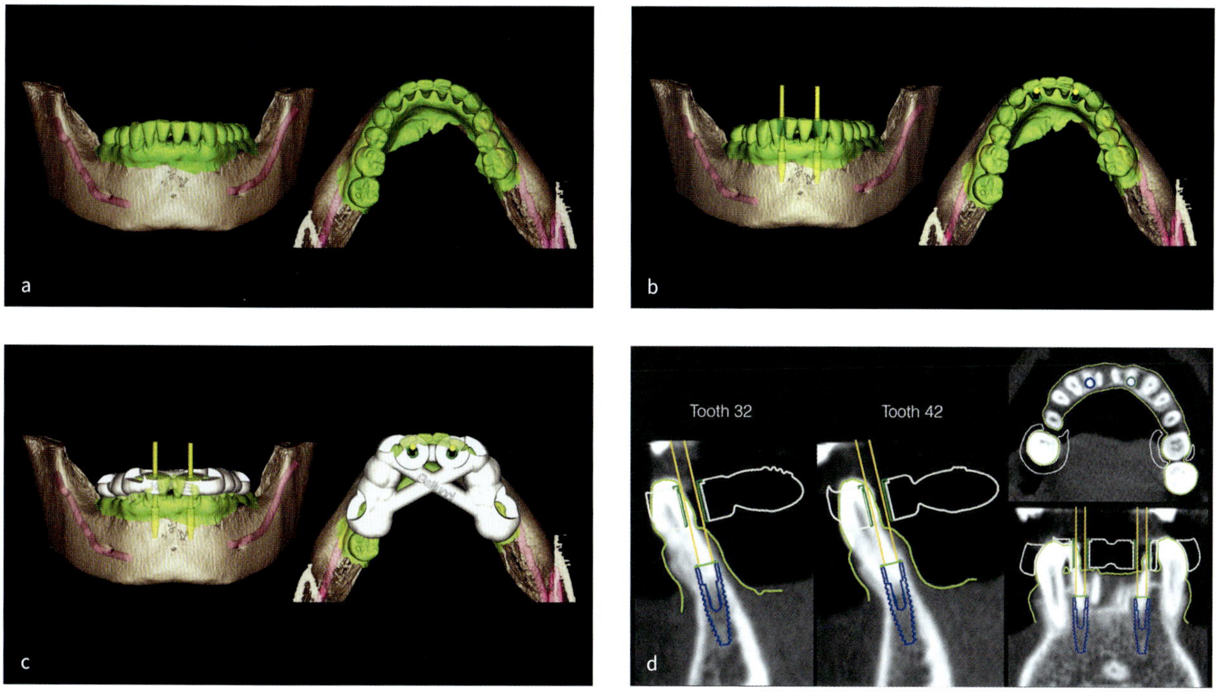

Figs 2a-d Prosthetically driven digital implant planning using CAD software.

Based on prosthetically driven optimal 3D implant positions for a screw-retained four unit implant-supported bridge, two implants (Bone Level Tapered, SLActive Roxolid, diameter 3.3 mm, length 12 mm; Institut Straumann AG, Basel, Switzerland) were planned for immediate implant placement after extraction of teeth 32 and 42. The pre-extraction intraoral digital scan served as a diagnostic tooth reference for the planned implant positions.

The surgical guide for static guided implant surgery was designed in the planning software. The occlusal support extended from the mandibular right first molar to the mandibular left first molar to provide structural stability with two cross-arch bars and four inspection windows equally distributed across the anterior and posterior region.

Due to the limited space available for the mandibular anterior teeth, 5 mm guide sleeves could not be inserted, so the surgical guide was designed for 2.8 mm guide sleeves. A STL file of the surgical guide was exported after completing the design and imported into 3D-printing software (Netfabb; Autodesk, San Rafael, CA, USA) for fabrication by means of additive manufacturing technology (Straumann P30+; Institut Straumann AG). The 3D-printed surgical template was post-processed and sterilized prior to the surgical procedure.

SURGICAL PROCEDURES

Based on the pre-surgical implant planning, the patient was eligible for flapless immediate implant placement at sites 32 and 42 (Figs 3a-f). The patient was anesthetized by facial and lingual local infiltration with 2% lidocaine hydrochloride and 1 : 100,000 epinephrine (Lignospan Standard; Septodont, Niederkassel, Germany).

The minimally traumatic extraction of tooth 32 and 42 was performed and the presence of an intact facial bone plate and surrounding soft tissues confirmed. The 3D printed surgical template was inserted and the fit was verified visually from the inspection windows.

The osteotomies were performed with Straumann Guided Surgical instruments following the manufacturer's guidelines. First, the 2.2 mm and 2.8 mm drills were used with full guidance for osteotomy preparation (Guided Surgical Kit; Institut Straumann AG) (Fig 3c). After removal of the surgical template, two implants (Bone Level Tapered, SLActive Roxolid, diameter 3.3 mm, length 12 mm; Institut Straumann AG) were successfully placed at sites 32 and 42 with an insertion torque of 25 Ncm. Primary stability was achieved at both implant sites.

Deproteinized bovine bone mineral (Bio-Oss; Geistlich, Wolhusen, Switzerland) was carefully placed into the gap between the buccal plate of the extraction socket and the implant. The healing abutments were connected and hand-tightened. The surgical wound was closed with 5-0 chromic gut resorbable suture material. The coronal aspects of the extracted teeth 32 and 42 were sectioned and shaped, and then bonded to the adjacent dentition to serve as a provisional restoration.

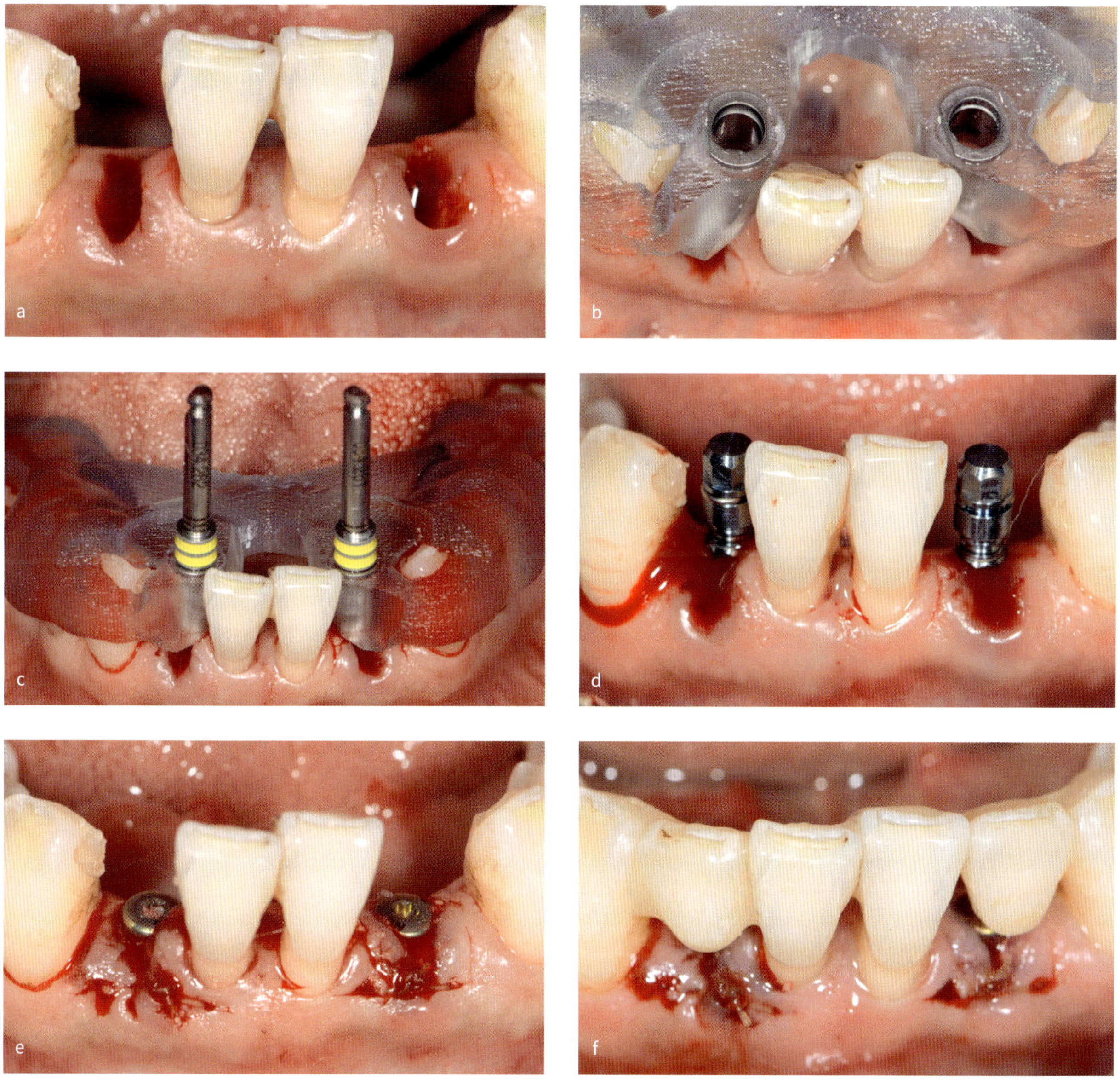

Figs 3a-f Immediate implant placement: Minimally traumatic extraction (a). Clinical assessment of the fit of surgical template through the inspection windows (b). Guided osteotomy (c). Implant placement, without a guide due to space restrictions (d). Wound closure (e). Natural teeth converted into a provisional bonded restoration (f).

IMPLANT-SUPPORTED PROVISIONAL RESTORATION

After ten weeks of healing, the transitional bonded restoration was removed. Straumann temporary abutments were placed on implants 32 and 42 and hand-tightened. A fixation wire was applied to cover the lingual surface of teeth 31 and 41, and further extended to connect two implants with flowable resin. The coronal aspects of teeth 32 and 42 were hollowed out from the lingual side and bonded to implant abutments 32 and 42. A thin layer of flowable composite resin (Filtek; 3M ESPE, St. Paul, MN, USA) was placed across the implant abutment and teeth 32 and 42 to connect the entire structure, successfully converting the natural teeth to an implant-supported provisional bridge.

The roots of teeth 31 and 41 were then sectioned and the remaining dental roots extracted using a minimally traumatic technique. The provisional bridge was removed and relined with composite resin. After polishing, the provisional bridge was delivered to support and develop the soft tissue contour in the area (Figs 4a-h).

The extraction wound was filled with deproteinized bovine bone mineral (Bio-Oss; Geistlich) and a resorbable collagen matrix and sutured with polytetrafluoroethylene suture material (Gore-Tex; W. L. Gore, Putzbrunn, Germany). The patient returned after two weeks for suture removal and a postoperative follow-up. The soft tissue appeared healthy and showed signs of uneventful healing.

DEFINITIVE RESTORATION

After six weeks of functional loading, the peri-implant soft tissue was found to be esthetic and healthy. The implant-supported provisional bridge was removed, and two digital impression posts (Mono scanbody; Institut Straumann AG) were inserted and hand-tightened. A final digital impression was acquired by intraoral scanning (iTero Element; Align Technology), providing a STL set of the articulated digital cast (Figs 5a-b). The maxillary and mandibular models were milled from the STL files with repositionable analogs to provide the dental technician with a set of working casts.

The final Implant-supported bridge was designed as a screw-retained restoration with a zirconia framework built up with feldspathic ceramics and bonded to two prefabricated titanium-base abutments (Variobase NC; Institut Straumann AG) (Figs 6a-b). Before delivery of the definitive restoration, the prothesis was tried in to assess the occlusion, marginal and interproximal fit, and esthetic outcome.

At the time of delivery of the definitive restoration (Figs 7a-d), the abutment screws were tightened to a controlled torque of 35 Ncm and protected by PTFE tape. The access channels were closed with composite. Oral hygiene instructions were reinforced to ensure the patient was able to perform adequate plaque control by using interdental brushes or dental floss (Oral-B Superfloss.; Procter & Gamble, Cincinnati, OH, USA).

With the immediate placement approach and the assistance of digital planning workflow, the patient was satisfied that the overall treatment time could be shortened for the final prosthesis to be ready within eighteen weeks.

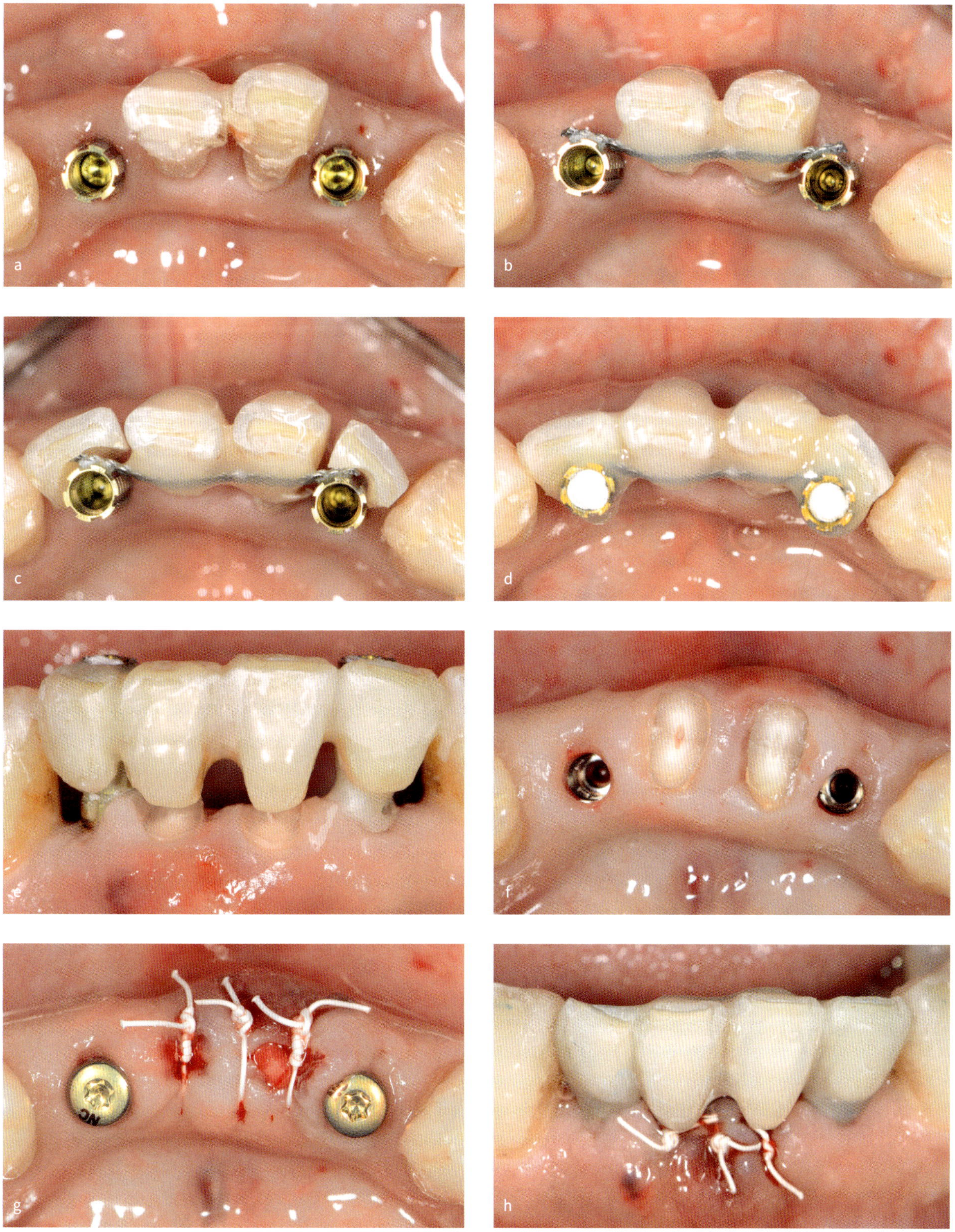

Figs 4a-h Soft tissue conditioning by the implant-supported provisional restoration converted from the patient's natural dentition.

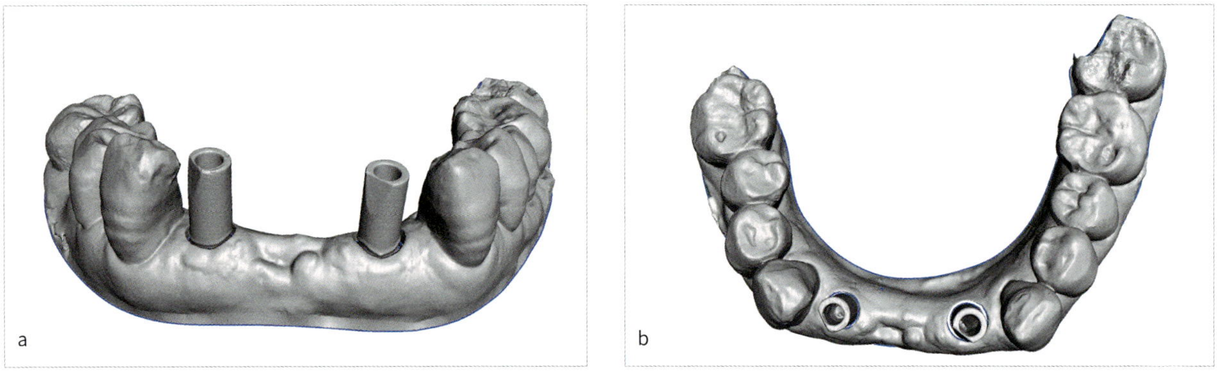

Figs 5a-b STL file based on the digital impression for fabrication of the final implant prosthesis.

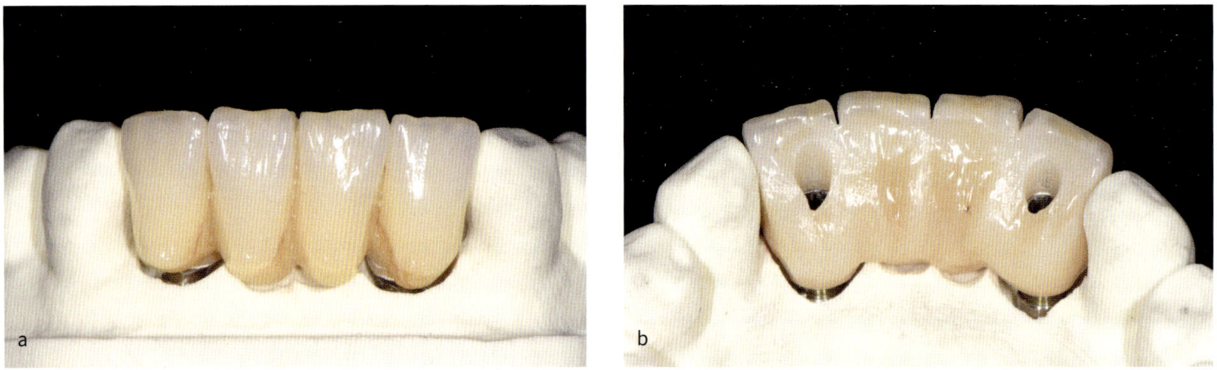

Figs 6a-b Definitive implant supported bridge. A screw-retained restoration with a milled zirconia framework, layered feldspathic ceramic, and bonded to two titanium-base abutments.

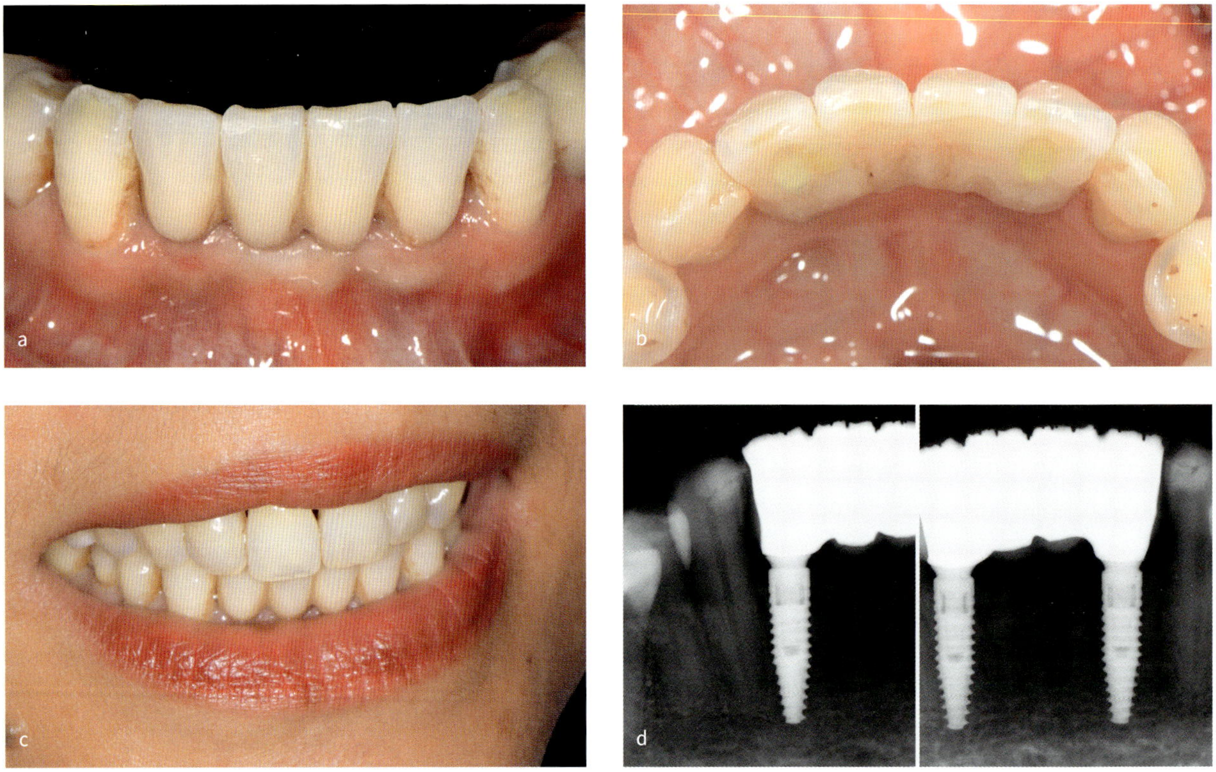

Figs 7a-d Final prosthesis at delivery. Intraoral frontal view (a), intraoral occlusal view (b), extraoral view (c), and radiographs (d).

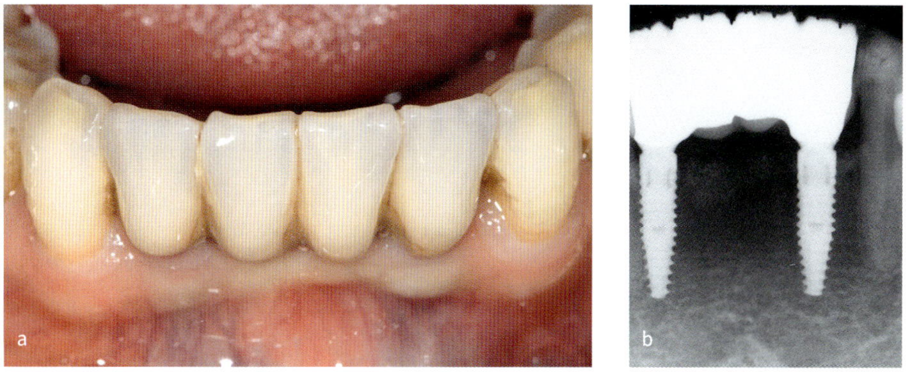

Figs 8a-b Three year follow-up.

FOLLOW-UP

The patient returned to her periodontist for maintenance care and presented to our clinic for the three year follow-up appointment (Figs 8a-b). The patient was satisfied with the esthetic and functional outcome. Radiographic examination showed stable interproximal bone levels and the peri-implant mucosa was healthy with no signs of inflammation, bleeding on probing, or gingival recession.

CONCLUSION

This case demonstrates the application of a digital workflow combined with risk assessment for the placement and loading protocol to determine the best possible treatment approach for replacing mandibular anterior teeth.

Anatomical, functional, and esthetic challenges are often present while placing dental implants in the anterior mandible. It is also the site that has been least covered in the literature with regard to the effect of implant placement and loading protocols on implant survival rates (Zhou and coworkers 2021). In the present case, virtual implant planning and guided implant surgery was highly valuable in facilitating preoperative treatment planning and intraoperative performance. A suitable fixed provisional restoration served as an appropriate alternative in order to avoid the risks of immediate loading; to ensure a successful outcome, conventional loading was chosen.

Further research is required to understand the possibility of different placing and loading protocols in the mandibular anterior position.

ACKNOWLEDGMENTS

Laboratory procedures

Yasu Kawabe – Oral Design Boston, Boston, MA, USA

5.9 Replacement of an Endodontically Compromised Mandibular Left First Molar with Immediate Implant Placement and a Sealing Socket Abutment (SSA)

G. Finelle

A 31-year-old woman was referred to our clinic by the endodontist for replacement of the mandibular left first molar (tooth 36) with a dental implant. The patient's medical history revealed no contraindications to dental implant therapy. According to the patient, tooth 36 was sensitive to heat and cold. The patient also reported discomfort and sensitivity during mastication, and mobility of tooth 36. The clinical examination showed no structural damage of the tooth crown or the surrounding soft tissue. The tooth was vital but sensitive to percussion. No signs of acute infection were noted at the clinical examination (Figs 1a-b). The radiographic evaluation showed a large radiolucency surrounding the pulp chamber of tooth 36 (Figs 2a-d), which was diagnosed as an irreversible external resorption; the tooth was therefore considered non-restorable.

It was decided to use a cone-beam computed tomography (CBCT) system (ProMax3D; Planmeca, Helsinki, Finland) to evaluate the anatomical situation in more detail. The three-dimensional imaging revealed (Figs 3a-b):

- A medium size interradicular septum at site 36
- Thick and intact buccal and lingual walls at site 36.
- Proximity of the root apices to the inferior alveolar nerve canal

A digital preoperative diagnostic impression was also taken before the extraction appointment to ensure that the anatomical information was properly captured and available to the lab technician for a potential future CAD/CAM restoration.

Based on the summary risk assessment for immediate placement, the case was classified as low risk, with no parameters in the high risk and 15 parameters in the low risk category (Table 1), which may represent a suitable case for immediate implant placement.

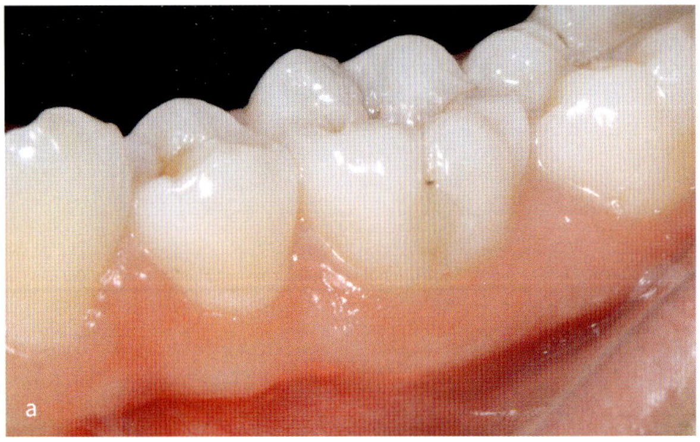

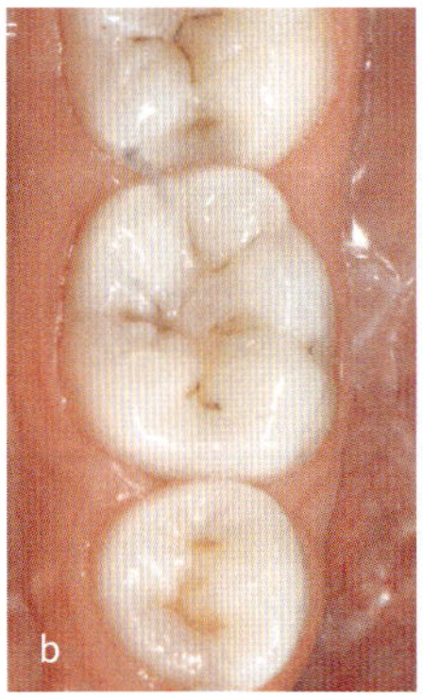

Figs 1a-b Initial clinical situation of a non-salvageable tooth 36 due to external root resorption.

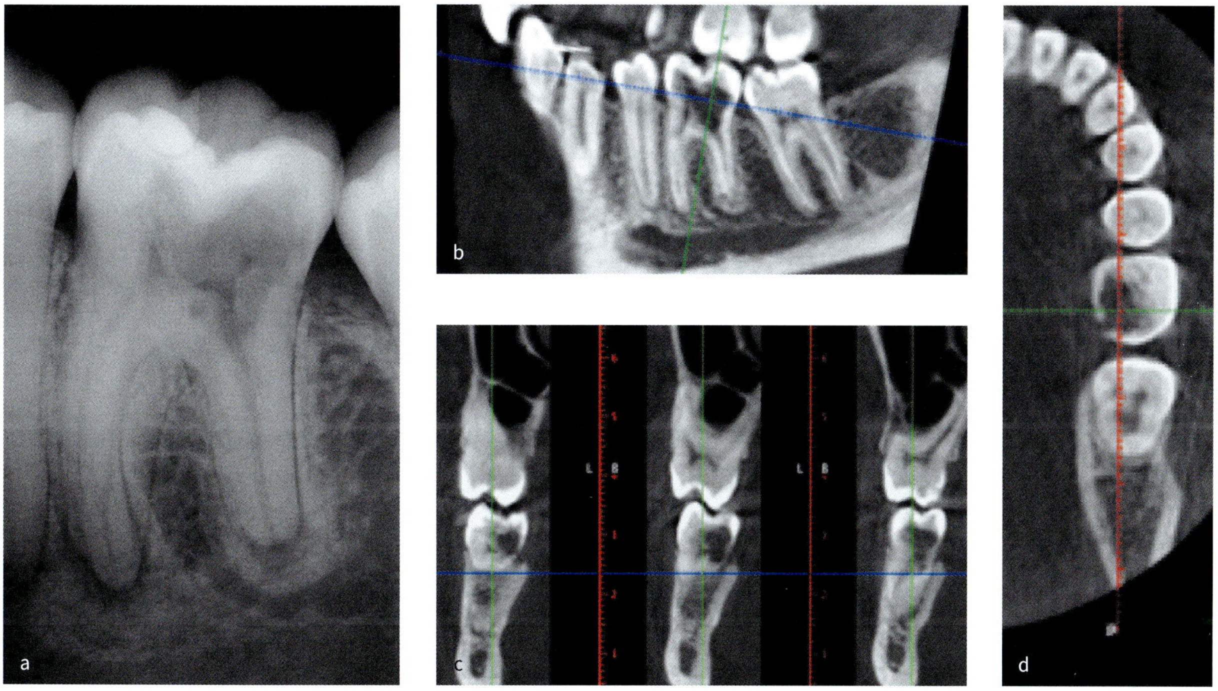

Figs 2a-d Periapical radiograph (a) and CBCT (b-d) showing irreversible external root resorption—an indication for tooth extraction.

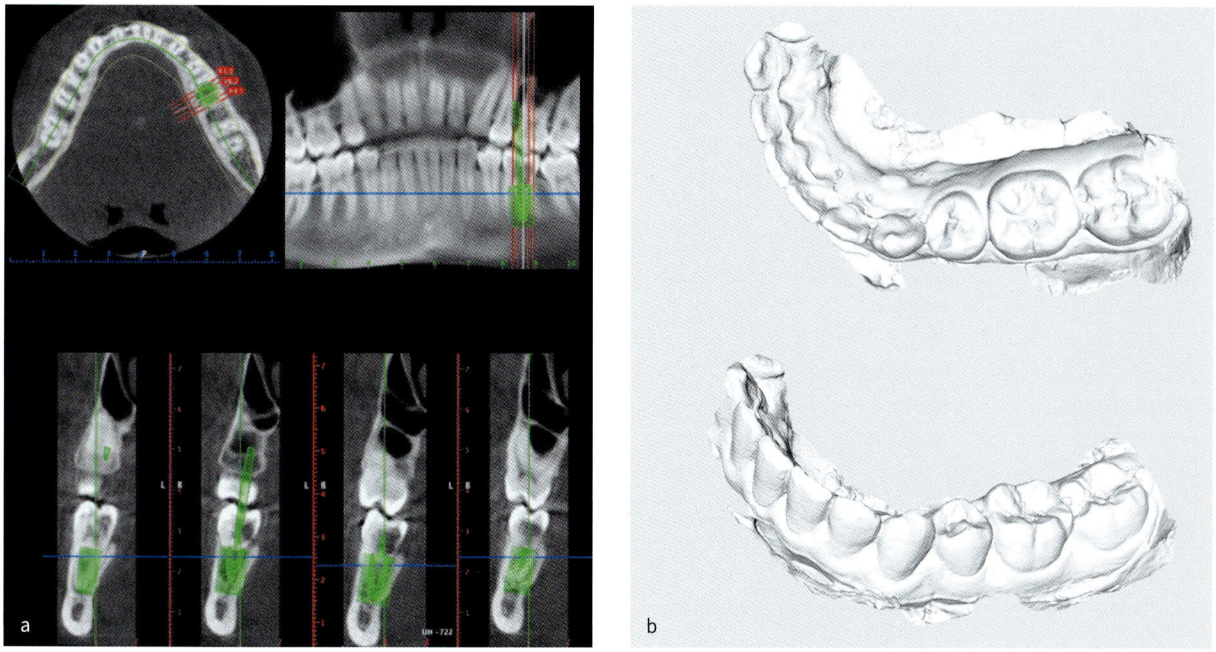

Figs 3a-b The digital diagnosis included digital planning of a Bone Level (BL) implant in an intraseptal position (a) and digital scanning of the initial situation with intact anatomical tooth structure (b).

Table 1 Risk assessment for immediate implant placement in single-tooth sites

	Low risk	Medium risk	High risk
Preoperative assessment			
Patient-related			
Medical status	Healthy, uneventful healing		Compromised healing
Esthetic risk	Low/medium esthetic risk	High esthetic risk	Significant esthetic compromise expected
Site-related			
Gingival-margin position	No recession	Minor gingival recession	Gingival recession ≥ 2 mm
Soft tissue quality	Thick gingival phenotype	Thin gingival phenotype or limited keratinized gingiva	No keratinized gingiva
Bone anchorage	Sufficient bone anchorage to achieve primary stability		Lack of bone anchorage to achieve primary stability
Facial bone wall	≥ 1 mm facial bone thickness	Facial bone plate < 1 mm thickness, or small fenestration or dehiscence defect	Significant fenestration or dehiscence of facial bone
Need for a mucoperiosteal flap	Sufficient alveolar bone for a flapless approach		Need for flapped bone augmentation
Socket position within alveolar envelope	Socket within the alveolar bone envelope		Socket and facial bone wall protruding out of the bone envelope
Presence of endodontic infection	No infection	Chronic periapical infection	Acute infection
Presence of periodontal disease	Periodontally healthy	Controlled periodontal disease	Active periodontal disease
Planning implant position	Ideal three-dimensional position with axis exiting through the cingulum or incisal edge		Facially positioned or over-angulated implant or excessive implant depth
Gap between buccal bone and planned implant position	≥ 2 mm	1–2 mm	< 1 mm
Intraoperative assessment			
Extraction	Minimally invasive tooth extraction	Damage to surrounding soft tissue, including severed/detached papillae	Significant damage to soft tissue and surrounding bone
Primary implant stability	Primary stability achieved		Lack of primary stability
Final implant position	Ideal three-dimensional position achieved		Facially positioned or over-angulated implant or excessive implant depth

Nevertheless, given the anatomical situations, immediate implant placement would present two challenges:

- Achieving primary stability is expected but can be compromised. Exclusively intraseptal stabilization is essential, as no apical anchorage is considered possible due to the superior position of the mandibular nerve. The CBCT (Figs 2b-d) showed a class B configuration (Smith and Tarnow 2013) of the septum; an implant may be stabilized but will not completely contained within the septal bone. Moreover, the availability of adequate apical bone volume would not allow for apical anchorage. This anatomical analysis indicated the possibility of an adequate three-dimensional prosthetic intraseptal implant position with sufficient insertion torque.
- Achieving socket protection using a sealing socket abutment (SSA), which is a customized anatomical healing abutment used to obturate the socket to properly stabilize the blood clot, prevent loss of bone augmentation materials, and prevent the collapse of the surrounding soft tissue (Finelle and Lee 2017).

Having discussed the situation and the considered combined immediate placement and SSA approach with the patient, the treatment plan was agreed on.

The tooth was extracted in a minimally invasive flapless procedure by removing the existing crown and roots (decoronation) (Fig 4) and then separating the supracrestal gingival fibers with periotomes. Careful attention was given to preserving the surrounding structures such as the buccal plate, interradicular septum, papillae, and gingival margin (Fig 5).

The alveolar socket was generously irrigated with sterile saline solution and cleaned with curettes to remove granulation tissue.

After the extraction, the alveolar socket was visually inspected to confirm the integrity of the gingival and bony structure. A BLT implant (BLT RC Roxolid SLA, diameter 4.8 mm, length 10 mm; Institut Straumann AG, Basel, Switzerland) was placed in accordance with the manufacturer's instructions. The osteotomy was prepared in the middle of the septum to match the prosthetically driven position as virtually planned at the diagnostic stage (Fig 6a). The insertion torque recorded was 28 Ncm.

Immediately postoperative periapical radiographs were taken to verify the proper position of the implant before proceeding to SSA fabrication.

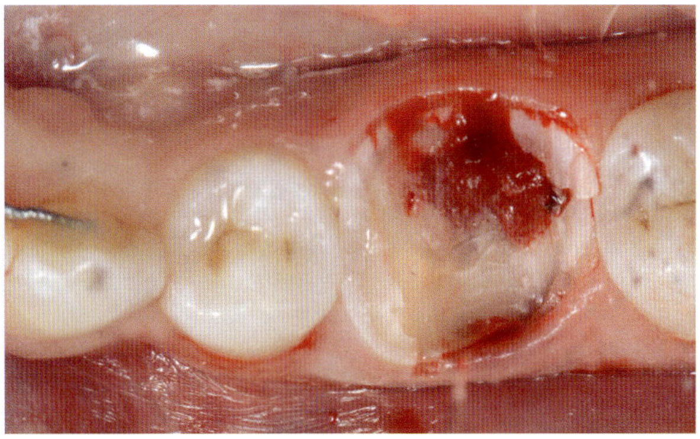

Fig 4 Clinical occlusal view of the active resorption, after coronal fragment removal.

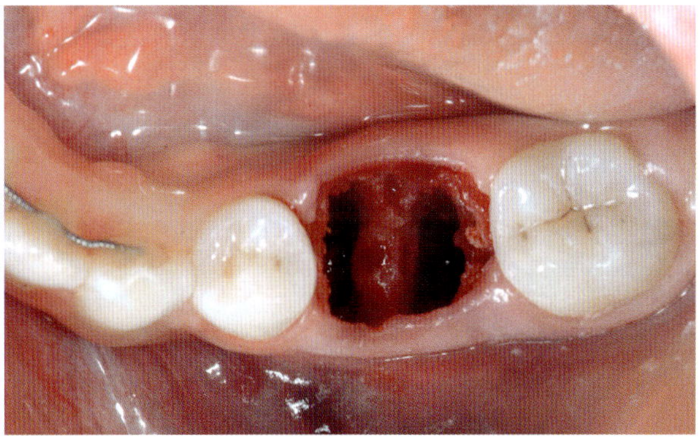

Fig 5 Occlusal view of the alveolar socket immediately after tooth extraction.

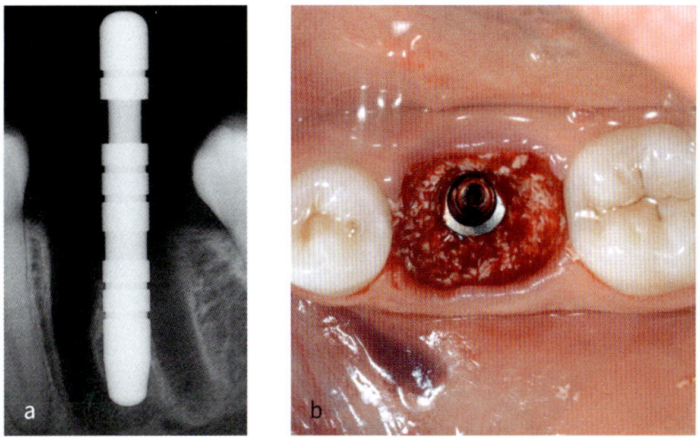

Figs 6a-b Placement of the implant, which was stabilized within the interradicular septum.

Autologous bone chips obtained from the drilling were mixed with a xenograft bone substitute (Bio-Oss Collagen, 0.5-g particles; Geistlich, Wolhusen, Switzerland) to fill the remaining socket surrounding the implant (Fig 6b). Biomaterials were placed to the level of the intact buccal bone.

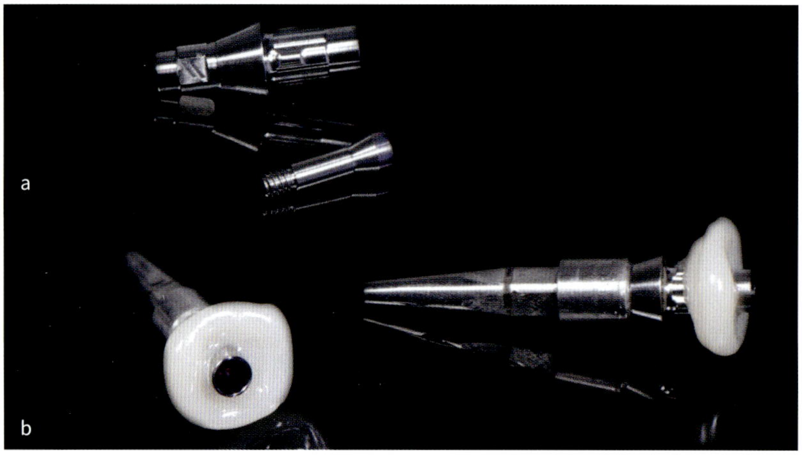

Fig 7a-b Selection of an appropriate prosthetic abutment (a). Extraoral customization of the SSA on the Ti-base (b).

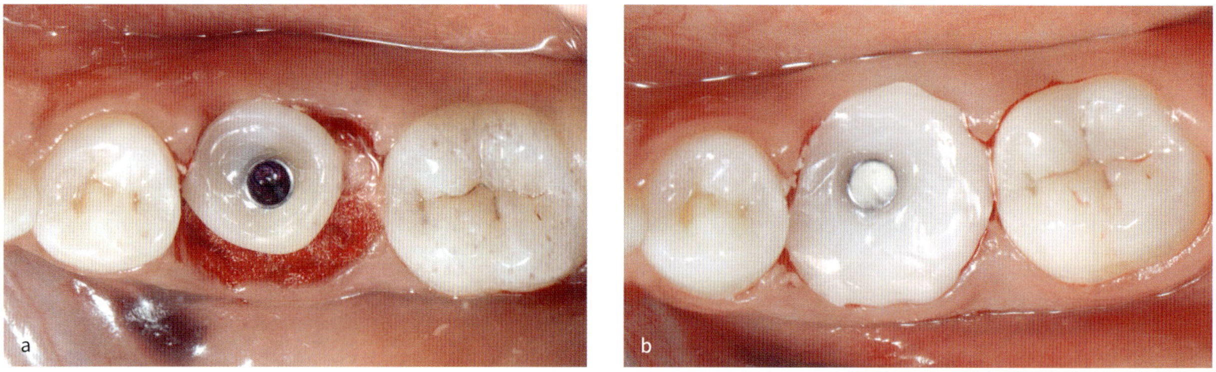

Figs 8a-b SSA in position after extraoral preparation by adding circular increments of flowable composite (a) and SSA intraoral cervical customization (b).

To obtain closure of the socket at the time of extraction, a customized sealing socket abutment was fabricated chairside and delivered immediately after implant placement. The SSA was built up with increments of conventional flowable composite following the prescribed protocol (Knafo and Finelle 2020).

SSA FABRICATION PROCESS

Use this QR code to view a highlight video of the SSA fabrication process. (Video: Courtesy of French Tooth.)

Step 1 (extraoral): Preparation. Selection of a Ti-base of the appropriate gingival height (Variobase, gingival height 2 mm: Institut Straumann AG) (Fig 7a)

Ti-base preparation: Sandblasting followed by application of a composite primer (GC, Japan)

Ti-base preparation: Circular incremental build-up of flowable composite (G-ænial Universal Flow; GC, Tokyo, Japan) around the titanium tube, located 2 to 4 mm coronal to the implant neck. The initial increments stay well within the overall alveolar contour to accommodate an average lower molar anatomy and proportion and simplify the upcoming intra oral customization phase (Fig 7b).

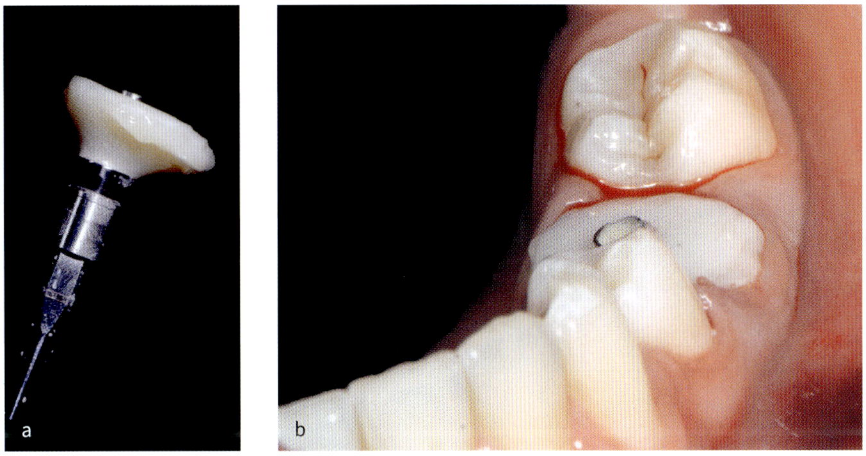

Figs 9a-b Chairside fabrication of the SSA (the customized healing abutment) using a conventional flowable composite technique. The SSA acts as a rigid barrier between the intraalveolar surgical site and the oral cavity and serves to stabilize the blood clot, to contain the biomaterials, and to support the soft tissue.

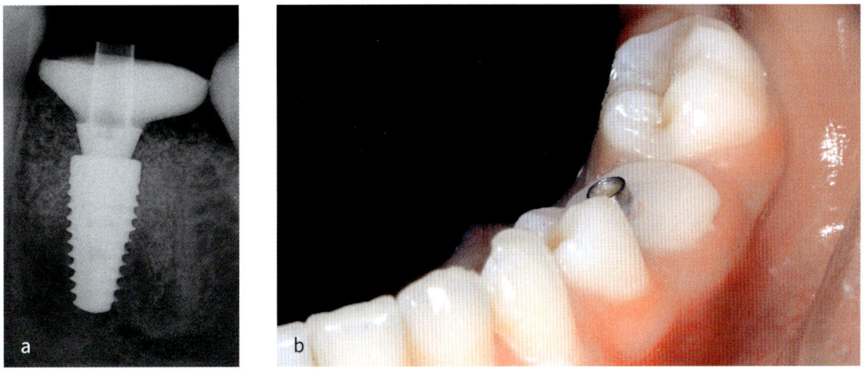

Figs 10a-b At twelve weeks. Periapical radiographs (a) and lateral view (b) showing favorable healing around the SSA.

Step 2 (intraoral): Socket outline customization. The customized abutment was connected to the implant, completing the anatomical outline from the composite base to the cervical alveolar margin (Figs 8a-b). Following this, the socket was sealed.

Step 3 (extraoral): Finalization. The transmucosal aspect was reshaped to provide a narrow concave profile close to the implant neck, becoming wider to achieve the necessary anatomical contour in the cervical emergence area (Fig 9a).

The SSA abutment was thoroughly polished and disinfected in an antiseptic solution of chlorhexidine 2%.

Step 4 (intraoral): SSA insertion. Finally, the SSA was inserted on the implant (with a manual insertion torque), in contact with the biomaterials but without a biological membrane, as defined by the dual-zone concept (Chu and coworkers 2012) (Fig 9b).

The patient was prescribed a postoperative course of antibiotics (amoxicillin 500 mg three times a day for seven days) and was advised to take paracetamol in case of pain (maximum 4 g per day) and to rinse with chlorhexidine 0.15% (three times a day) for seven days.

At the one week follow-up, the patient reported an uneventful postoperative recovery. The clinical examination at one week showed favorable soft tissue healing with minor inflammation (Figs 10a-b).

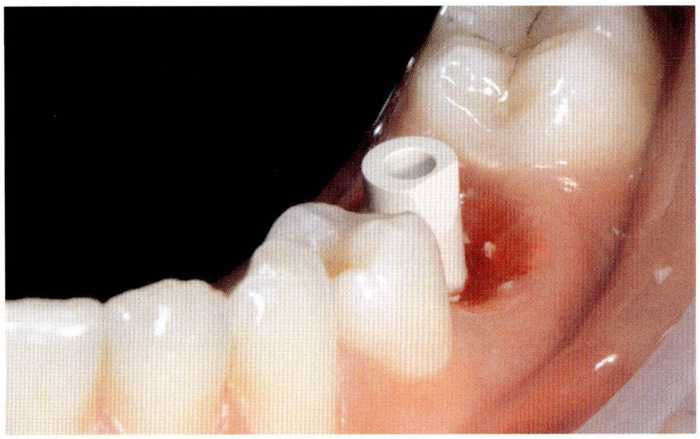

Fig 11 Lateral view at twelve weeks, after SSA removal at the time of the digital impression.

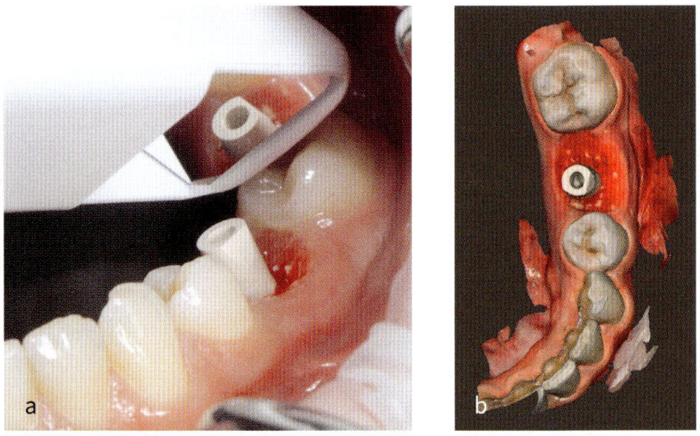

Figs 12a-b Digital implant impression using an intraoral scanner recording both the implant position and the shape of the emergence profile.

After twelve weeks of healing, the soft tissue around the SSA was healthy, and the buccal contour had been maintained (Fig 12). When the abutment was removed for the impression, a healthy and anatomical prosthetic emergence profile with a properly shaped transmucosal portion were seen (Fig 11).

A digital impression (I500; Medit, Seoul, Korea) using a digital scanbody (Straumann RC connection) was taken for an implant-supported restoration (Figs 12a-b). The digital scan provided precise information on implant positioning and the emergence profile.

The digital impression was digitally transferred to the lab (LNT; Asselin Bonichon, Paris, France) along with additional information, such as initial Standard Tessellation Language (STL) files, before extraction and shade information.

"COPY-PASTE DENTISTRY"

To reproduce the natural molar design as close as possible, the implant impression was merged with the initial diagnostic impression in the lab software (exocad, Darmstadt, Germany). A monolithic zirconia screw-retained crown was designed (Fig 13) and adapted to a Ti-base abutment (Variobase, gingival height 2 mm; Institut Straumann AG) to exactly match the coronal design of the original natural teeth and the transmucosal shape of the SSA (Fig 14a).

After milling, the implant-supported restoration was sintered, characterized by surface staining, and bonded onto the Variobase abutment (Fig 14b).

The implant crown was delivered uneventfully (Fig 14c). Minimal tissue pressure was observed at insertion. The transmucosal prosthetic contour fitted the prepared peri-implant emergence profile snugly (Figs 15a-b). The final insertion torque (35 Ncm) was applied, and the access hole was filled with a PTFE strip and covered with restorative composite (G-ænial A2; GC). A postoperative periapical radiograph was taken to verify the seating and marginal integrity after insertion (Figs 16a-b).

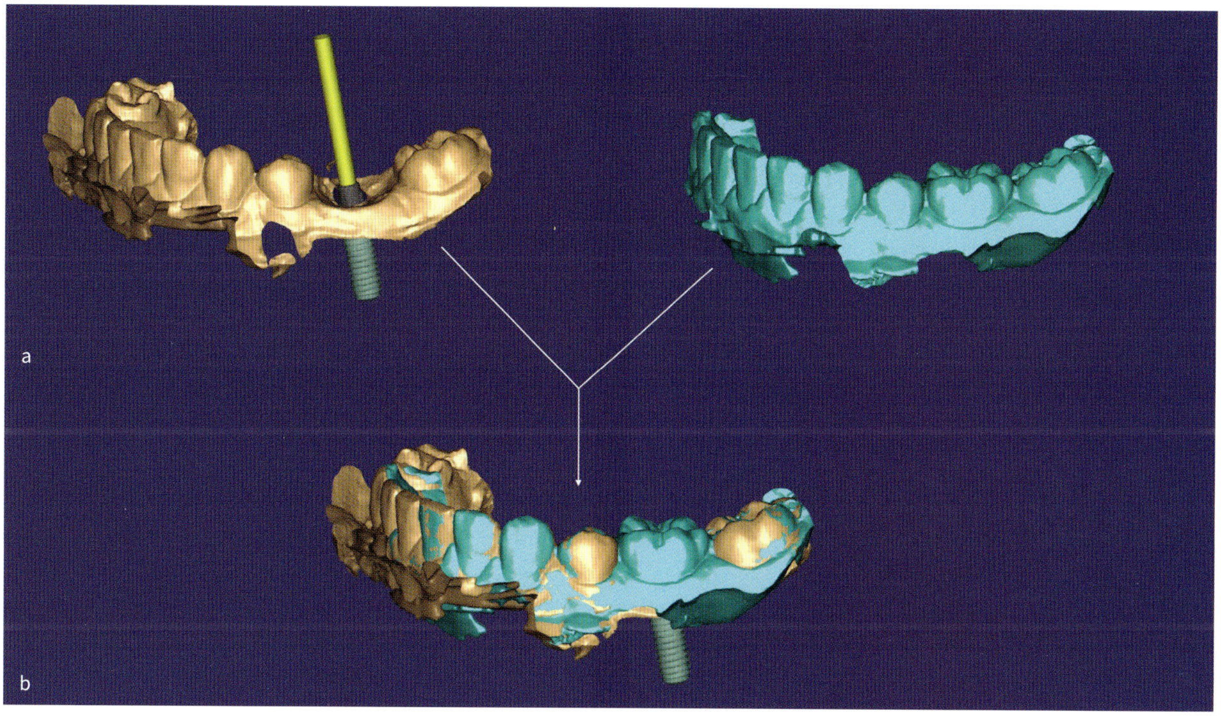

Fig 13 CAD/CAM design of the crown based on and closely guided by the shape of the emergence profile (a) and the anatomical structure of the tooth before extraction (b).

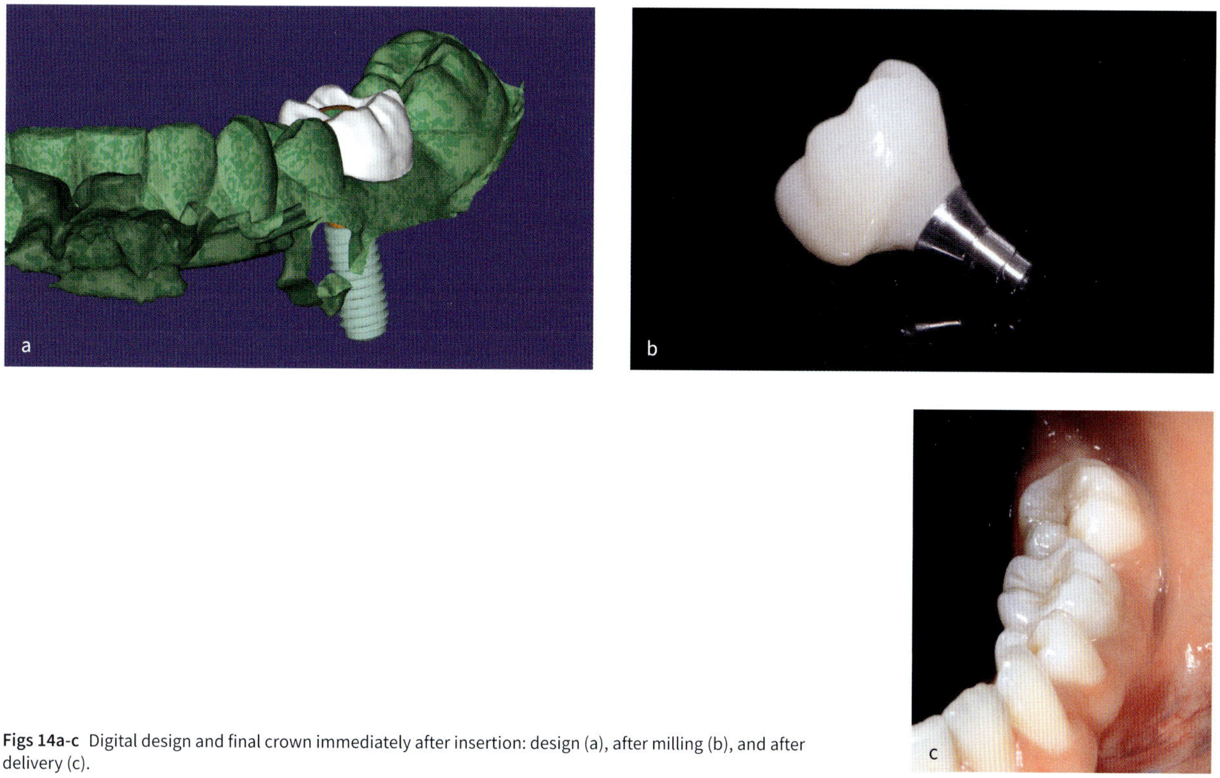

Figs 14a-c Digital design and final crown immediately after insertion: design (a), after milling (b), and after delivery (c).

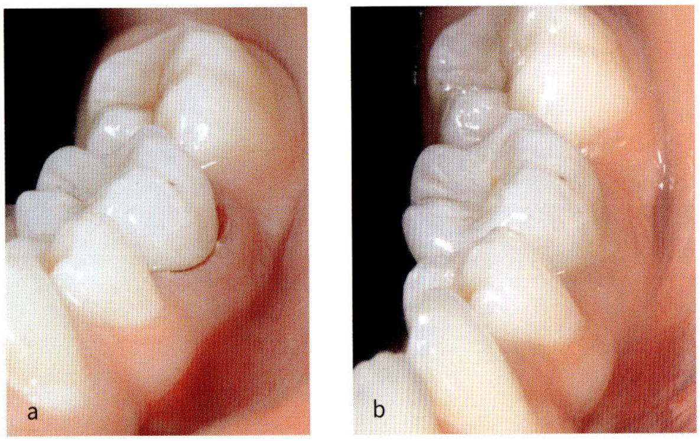

Figs 15a-b The seated screw retained implant-supported zirconia crown, before (a) and after (b) the final insertion.

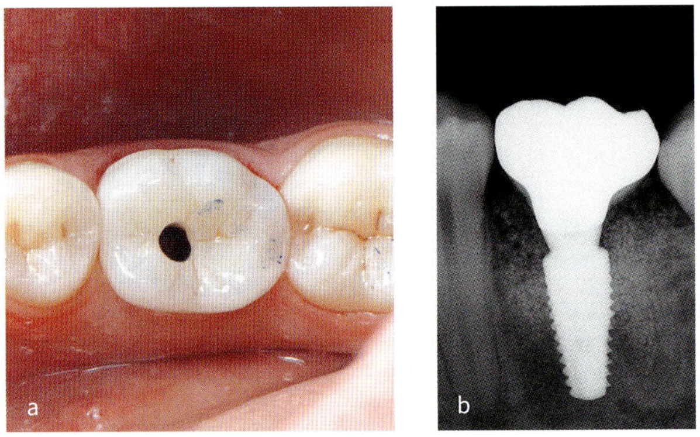

Figs 16a-b Final occlusal view (a) and final radiograph (b) immediately after crown insertion.

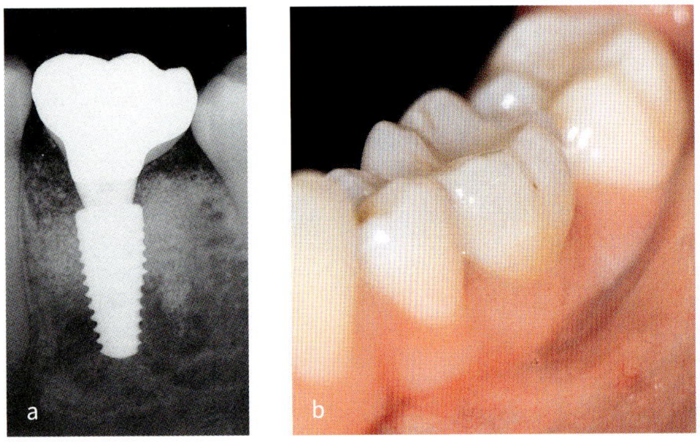

Figs 17a-b Periapical radiograph (a) and clinical lateral view (b) at the two year follow-up.

OUTCOME

At the two year follow-up, the clinical situation was stable (Figs 17a-b). No biological or technical complications were reported. The clinical assessment showed a stable position and stable soft tissue volumes (buccal contour and papillae). A CBCT was taken, as this patient was included in a recently published case series (Alexopolou and coworkers 2021) (Figs 18a-c and Figs 19a-b). At crown insertion and at the two year follow up, both the peri-implant soft tissue and the surrounding bone levels remained clinically stable in comparison to baseline situation (Alexopolou and coworkers 2021).

DISCUSSION

Immediate implant therapy at molar sites shows survival rates comparable with implants placed in healed sockets while demonstrating considerable benefits from a patient perspective.

Nevertheless, one of the major challenges during immediate implant placement in molar sites (in addition to ensuring primary stability) is the ability to obtain socket closure, given the dimension and anatomy of the molar socket.

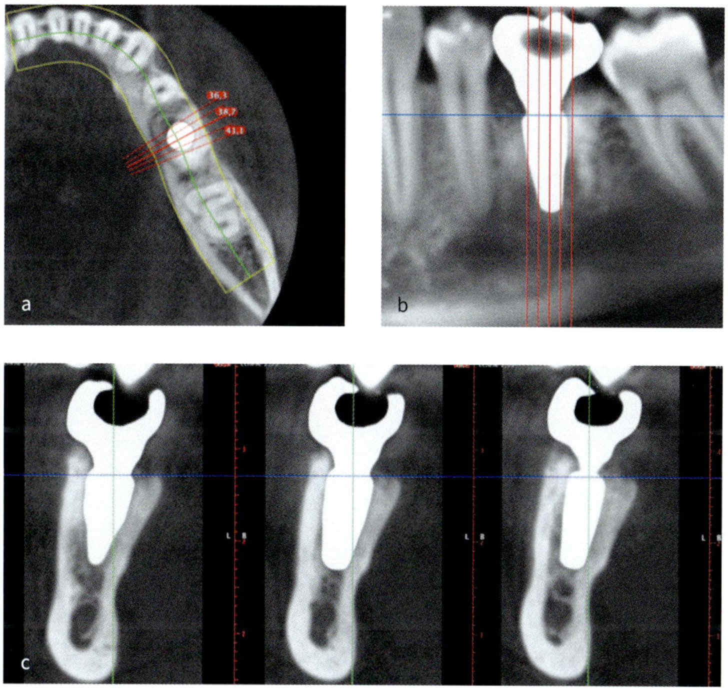

Figs 18a-c CBCT evaluation at the two year follow-up showing stable bone around the implant.

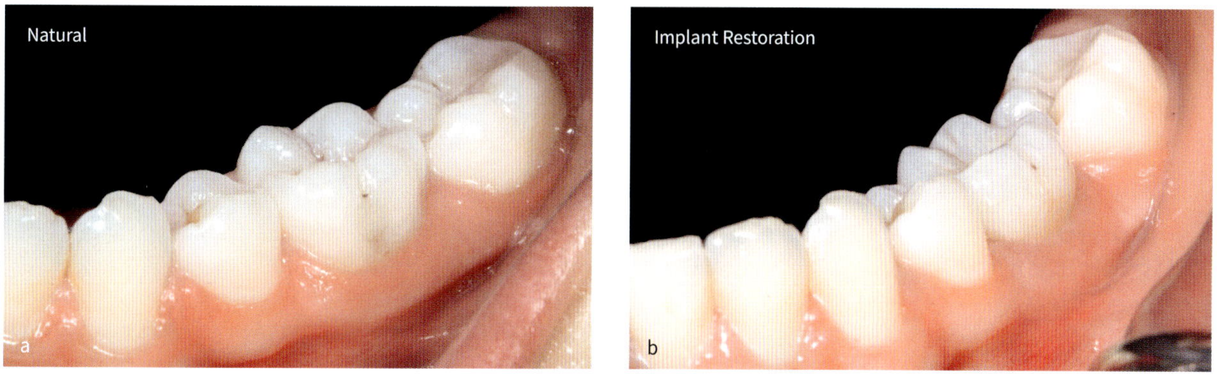

Figs 19a-b Initial preoperative situation and final outcome showing the prosthetic integration of the restoration on implant 36.

The present case report discusses a clinical protocol focusing on a minimally invasive strategy for replacing molars, combining immediate implant placement and chairside implementation of a customized sealing socket abutment technique, as reported in several previous articles (Finelle and coworkers 2016; Finelle and coworkers 2019; Ruales and coworkers 2019; Akin 2016).

While in the esthetic zone, immediate restoration appears to be a predictable strategy to guide gingival architecture and stabilize the post-extraction soft tissue (Chan and coworkers 2019), immediate provisionalization in posterior sites is also an interesting alternative to promote wound healing by supporting the peri-implant soft tissue and creating a confined bony regenerative space. Some authors have described immediate implant loading with final restorations in healed single-molar sites to guide soft tissue healing (Lambert and Mainjot 2017). Nevertheless, support for immediate loading at molar sites remains scarce and as it concerns an area highly exposed to masticatory loads during osseointegration, more evidence would be needed at this point to consider such a treatment modality on molar sites (immediate implant placement combined with immediate provisionalization, type 1A) (Gallucci and coworkers 2018).

In the present case, it was decided to proceed with an immediate placement and a delayed restoration, type 1C (Gallucci and coworkers 2018), which offers a much higher level of evidence in the lower posterior mandible than a 1A protocol (Zhou and coworkers 2021). With its customized design, the SSA protects freshly placed implants against masticatory loading while offering the biological advantages of tissue conditioning for an immediate restoration. These advantages include the following:

- Fewer appointments (combination of extraction and implant procedure)
- Less overall treatment time
- Less invasive treatment treatment (flapless procedures)
- Faster postoperative recovery
- Soft tissue support
- Fewer prosthetic manipulations

In a previous publication, SSA was described in the context of a CAD/CAM process (Finelle and coworkers 2021). This technique implies the use of chairside milling equipment, something that is not possible in most dental practices. Moreover, increased cost and long fabrication time can disrupt the workflow and make it unrealistic for routine implant procedures such as a single molar replacement.

The present case demonstrates a more autonomous, simple, and cost-efficient approach that uses conventional adhesive resin (readily available in the dental practice) at chairside immediately after surgery.

From a clinical perspective, we anticipate surgical and prosthetic benefits that directly impact wound healing at the implant site:

- Surgically, the SSA acts as a mechanical barrier, ensuring stabilization of the blood clot in the confined alveolar socket space, which favors the regenerative process. The main purpose of the SSA is to "seal" the socket, to act as a rigid "roof," isolating the alveolar bone from the oral cavity without using invasive techniques such as flaps, incisions, or sutures. As no attempt needs to be made to advance a flap to achieve primary closure, the mucogingival junction is not displaced, and the papillary architecture is maintained in its original anatomical position with minimal biological disturbance. A favorable biological response—reported in previous articles with regard to implant survival, soft tissue appearance (Lilet and coworkers 2021), and volumetric stability of the bone over time (Alexopolou and coworkers 2021)—can be seen as a direct consequence of the limited invasiveness of the surgical steps described above. It has also been observed that postoperative recovery and discomfort were well tolerated by the patient.
- From a prosthetic standpoint, the transmucosal aspect of the implant crown is designed to emerge with a cervical contour that matches the anatomy of the original natural crown, exerting a positive influence on soft tissue stability by preventing post-extraction collapse (Raj and Bhatnagar 2015). Consequently, any prosthetic manipulations at crown delivery are significantly simplified, as the tissues are already settled in their proper anatomical and prosthetic position.

CONCLUSION

By preserving alveolar structures and guiding soft tissue healing, immediate implant placement combined with SSA in molar sites might ensure predictable and safe implant procedures. While relevant evidence is currently emerging and there are promising and interesting new perspectives, further investigation using well-designed controlled clinical trials are needed.

6 Complications

F. Lambert, A. Hamilton

Immediate implant placement and immediate loading in partially edentulous patients can be a predictable treatment when planned and executed appropriately. However, complications have been reported with regard to implant esthetics, bone loss, and implant failures. While these complications are not unique to this treatment modality, careful attention should be given to minimizing any additional risks for the specific patients and tooth sites considered for treatment.

A recent systematic review and meta-analysis demonstrated that single immediate implants (type 1) had a similar survival rate, less marginal bone loss, and better pink esthetic scores than delayed implants (types 2, 3, 4) (Garcia-Sanchez and coworkers 2022). This review also revealed that immediate restoration did not influence the survival rates. However, immediate placement presented a high rate of complications (11%), with surgical and esthetic complications the most prominent examples. The authors also acknowledged that different cofounding factors may influence these outcomes such as the flap design (flap vs. flapless), the use of hard- or soft tissue grafting, the angulation and position of the implant, the position in dental arch, and the gingival phenotype.

The overall goal of this Volume 14 of the ITI Treatment Guide is to provide a structured decision-making framework for immediate implants to minimize the risk of complications, based on the literature and on the authors' clinical experience.

The first important action to decrease the risk of complications is to identify the safe indications for immediate implant placement, according to the proposed risk assessment characteristics (Chapter 6.1).

Next, the manner in which the surgical procedure is to be executed may also influence the outcome and lead to potential complications (Chapter 6.2). The ideal three-dimensional implant position remains a key aspect for the esthetic success of immediate implantation, and achieving primary implant stability in a fresh socket represents an additional challenge to adequate implant positioning. Adjunctive surgical procedures such as hard- or soft tissue grafting can assist in managing the risk of esthetic complications related to immediate implant placement. However, these adjunctive procedures increase the complexity of the treatment and may also induce additional biological or surgical complications.

Finally, immediate restoration and loading exposes the patient to mechanical complications such as abutment screw loosening, which can be detrimental to healing (Chapter 6.3).

This chapter discusses typical complications of immediate implants and provides recommendations on how these can be prevented.

6.1 Complications Related to Case Selection

6.1.1 Unfavorable Alveolar Bone Anatomy

A key factor in immediate implant placement is the requirement to place the implant in a favorable bone environment with sufficient anchorage to stabilize the implant. Beyond achieving mechanical stability, the regeneration potential of the remaining socket and the local alveolar bone anatomy are other important considerations, because post-extraction remodeling is anticipated and the regenerative potential of the socket should be respected.

Even following minimally traumatic extraction and maintenance of the alveolar bone proper, the successful integration of the grafting material placed in the gap between an immediately placed implant and the facial wall of the socket depends upon the blood supply and nutrition of the interproximal bone and periosteum. Therefore, the further the tooth root is positioned outside the alveolar bony envelope, the lower the regenerative potential of the facial bone. If the root and facial bone wall protrude outside the bony envelope, particularly when combined with a reduced facial-lingual dimension of the interproximal bone and alveolar housing, the regenerative potential of the socket is low, and immediate implants should be avoided (Figs 1a-g). In this situation, extensive resorption of the labial bone can be anticipated, resulting in dimensional changes in the alveolar contour and in esthetic complications; regeneration may fail, and a resultant lack of facial bone around the implants is more likely (Figs 2a-d and 3a-e).

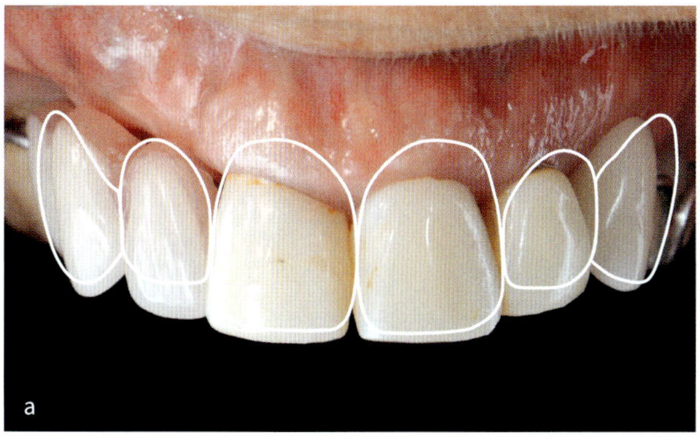

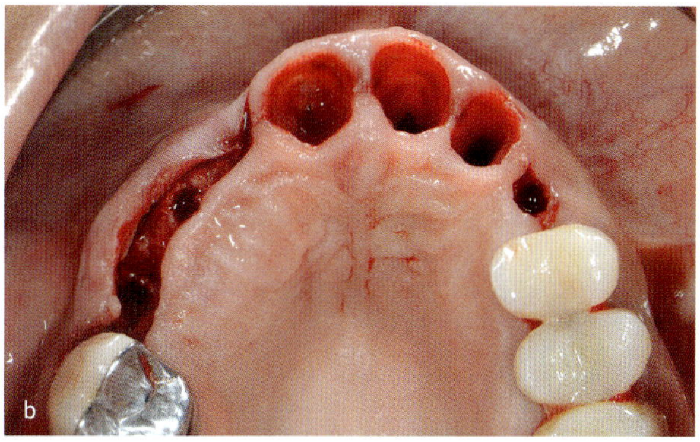

Figs 1a-g In this case, multiple implants were placed with at different time points. At sites 15 and 13, type 4 implant placement was performed nine months after a regenerative procedure. At site 23, delayed implant placement was also considered, as bone anchorage was limited by the length of the canine. But since the patient wanted a fixed provisional solution, immediate placement was planned for sites 11 and 21 with immediate loading. Comprehensive virtual implant planning was performed, but the alveolar bone at sites 11 and 21 was inappropriate for a type 1 placement. The preoperative CBCT's showed limited buccopalatal bone in the region of the implant apex, a protruded alveolar crest, and the presence of the incisal canal as anatomical characteristics that affect the indication for immediate implant placement.

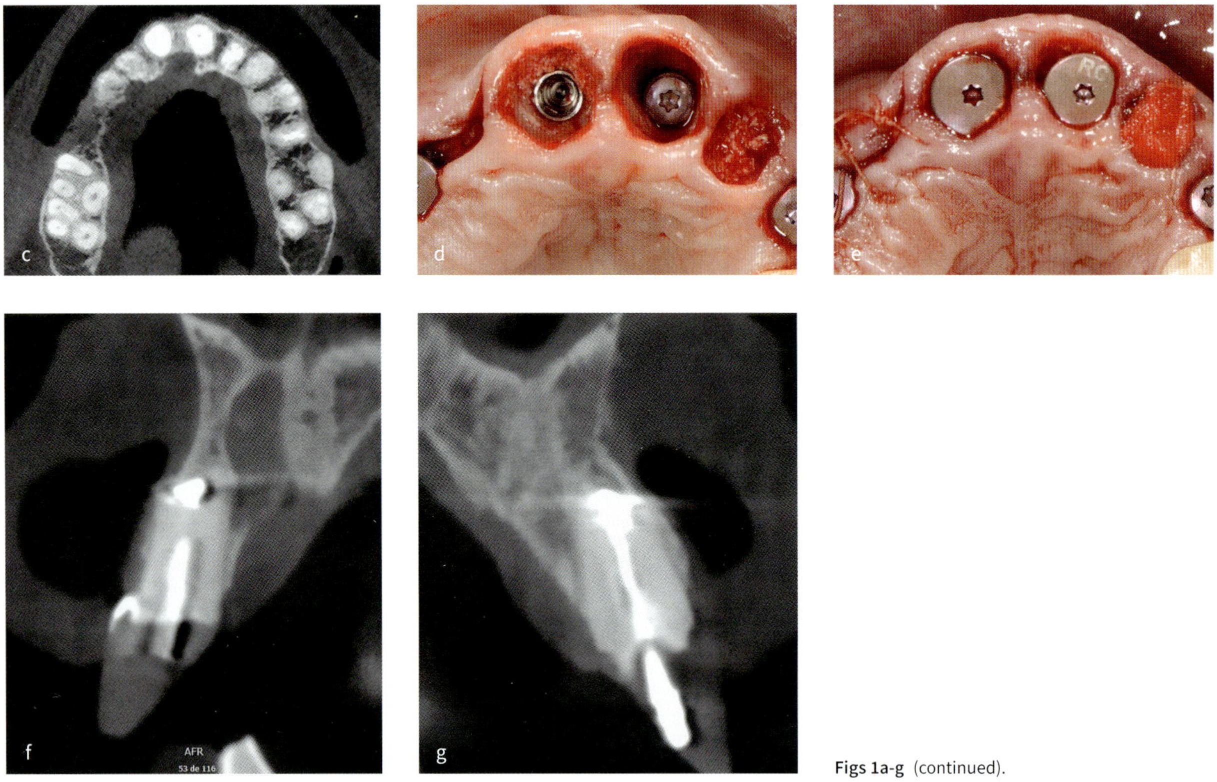

Figs 1a-g (continued).

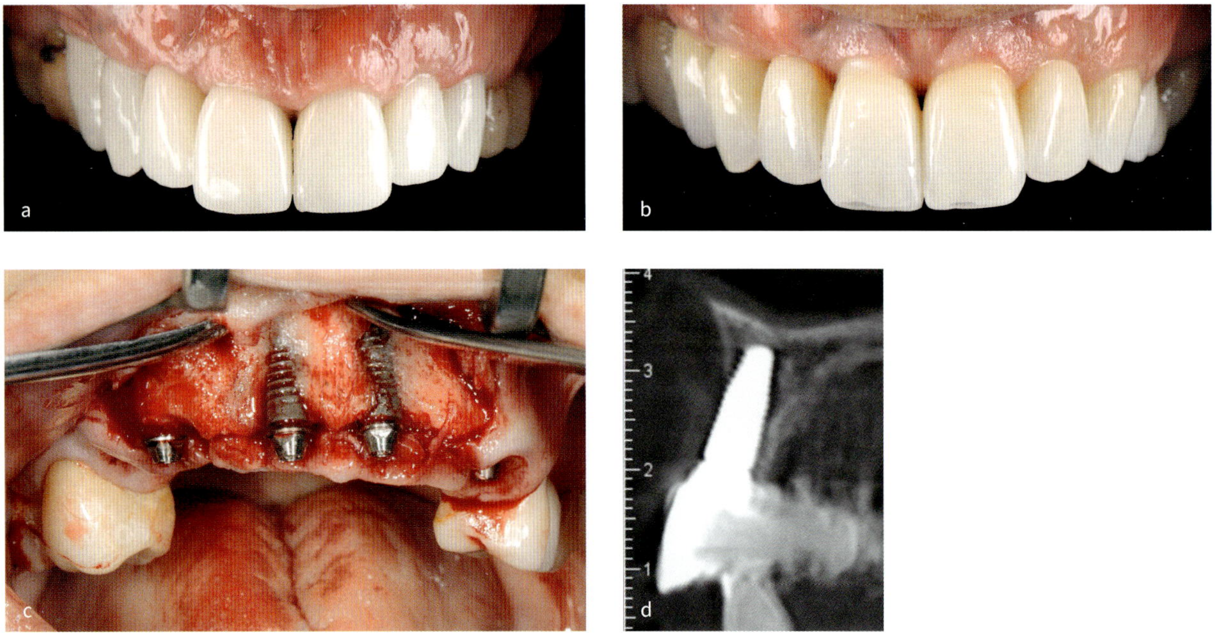

Figs 2a-d After one year, soft tissue recession was clinically identified at sites 11 and 21, and significant buccal bone resorption was observed radiographically. It was decided to perform a regenerative procedure to manage the hard tissue remodeling. A full-thickness flap was raised that confirmed the failure to regenerate bone on the labial of the immediate implants 11 and 21. By contrast, implants 13 and 24 placed at the same following a type 4 implant placement protocol had their labial bone preserved. Based on the risk assessment table in Chapter 3, these sites would have been considered "high risk," with relative contraindications for a type 1A protocol. Alternative protocols, such as early or even late placement, allowing for regenerative procedures, might have prevented these complications.

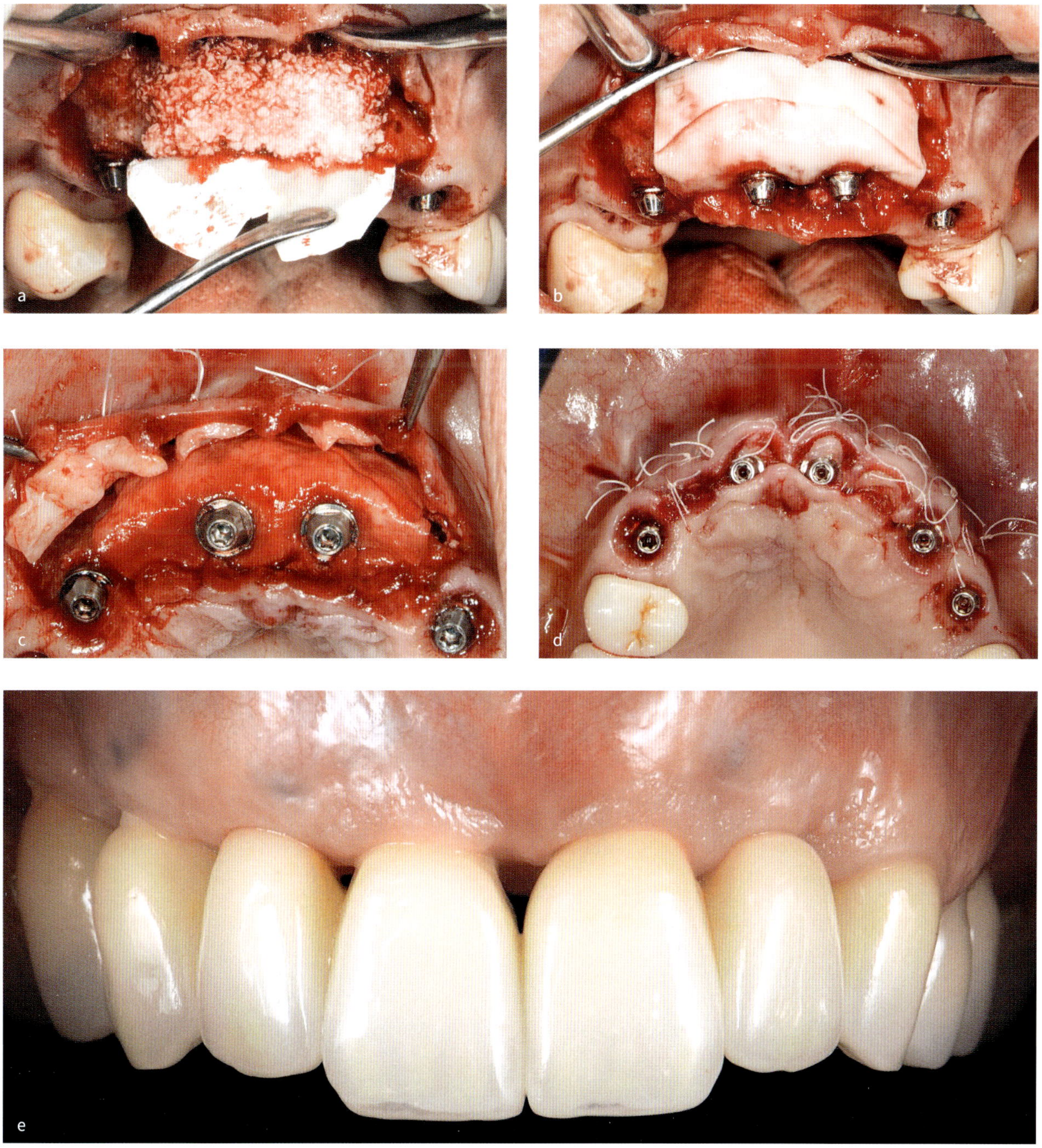

Figs 3a-e Guided bone regeneration using a demineralized bovine bone mineral and a collagen membrane was performed in combination with soft tissue grafting to manage the complication. The aim of the secondary corrective procedures was to reconstruct the facial bone wall and the contours of the alveolar ridge to minimize esthetic compromises in relation to the position of the midfacial mucosal margin and to reduce risk of implant exposure. Six months after the regenerative procedure, midfacial mucosal levels appeared to have stabilized; however, the loss of the papillae was irreversible. Early or delayed implant placement might have allowed for more predictable esthetic and biological outcomes where significant compromises were present at the local site prior to tooth extraction. (Restorative procedures: Prof. Amélie Mainjot. Laboratory procedures: Dental Team, Luc and Patrick Rutten.)

6.1.2 Unfavorable Soft Tissue Quality or Quantity

Midfacial recession is described as a common complication following immediate placement of a single implant (Kan and coworkers 2003; Kan and coworkers 2011b; Chen and Buser 2014; Yuenyongorarn and coworkers 2020) (Fig 4).

According to Cosyn and coworkers (2012), several factors contribute to these complications; the risk can be mitigated by appropriate case selection (intact buccal bone wall, thick soft tissue phenotype). The authors also emphasize the potential benefit of flapless surgery and immediate restoration.

A thin marginal gingiva is also regarded a recession risk, particularly in the esthetic zone. A recent systematic review (Seyssens and coworkers 2021) concluded that a connective tissue graft contributes to midfacial soft tissue stability following immediate implant placement and should be considered when an elevated risk for midfacial recession exists in the esthetic zone (thin gingival phenotype, less than 0.5 mm of buccal bone thickness).

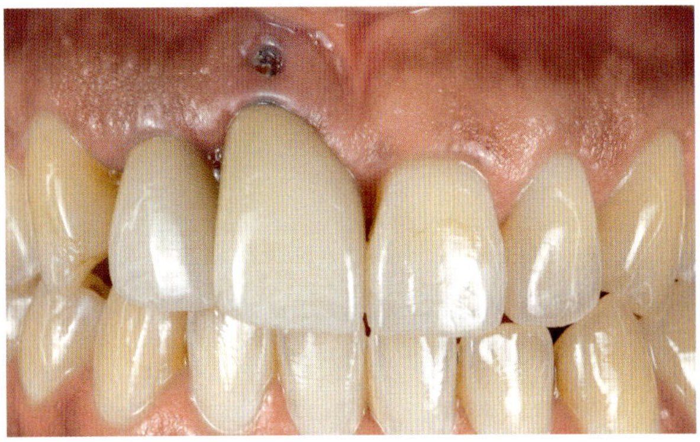

Fig 4 Midfacial recession at immediate implant 11 with loss of facial bone and soft tissue thickness.

6.2 Complications Related to Surgical Procedures

6.2.1 Implant Positioning

The ideal three-dimensional position of a dental implant plays a key role in achieving esthetic, biological, and mechanical success (Garber and Belser 1995; Buser and coworkers 2004: Grunder and coworkers 2005). Placing implants into fresh extraction sockets poses additional challenges to the surgeon's quest for an ideal implant position.

Where an osteotomy is prepared on an inclined surface, there is a tendency for the drill to be displaced, deviating from the ideal implant position. This may also occur during the implant placement itself, with the implant placed away from the inclined surface, particularly if the osteotomy has been underprepared in the hope of achieving the required insertion torque for immediate loading (Figs 5a-b). Guided implant surgery can assist in reducing the deviation; however, guided surgery systems are also subject to the same issues on inclined surfaces (El Kholy and coworkers 2019; Pimkhaokham and coworkers 2022).

To prevent this, labial displacement of the handpiece must be resisted during osteotomy preparation and implant placement. Adequate profiling of the dense palatal bone should be performed at the coronal aspect to minimize labial displacement.

Flapless surgery, recommended for type 1A implant placement, can make it challenging to visualize the surrounding alveolar bone at the implant site. This may cause inadvertent fenestration through the facial bone at the apical aspect of the implant, which may not be detected at the time of implant surgery (Figs 6a-c). Adjacent structures such as the incisive canal or neighboring teeth may also be damaged if their proximity is not assessed in detail using three-dimensional radiographic imaging. Digital planning and guided implant surgery may be advantageous in flapless placement (Figs 7a-h and Fig 8) (Romandini and coworkers 2022).

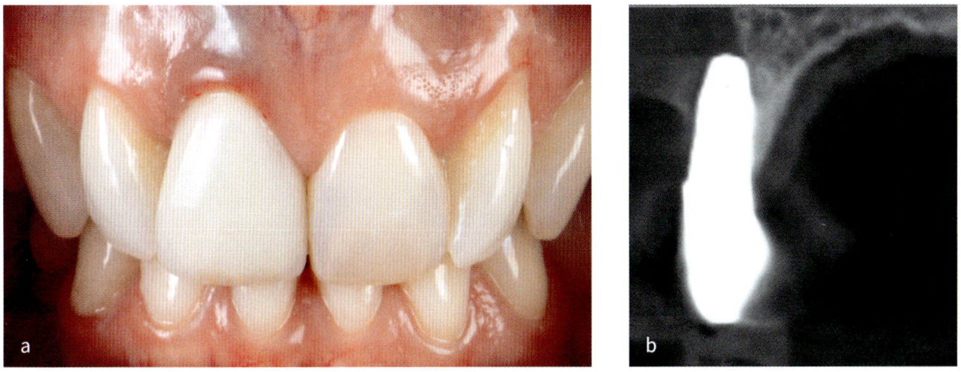

Figs 5a-b Midfacial recession, peri-implant mucositis, graying of the mucosal tissues, and significant tenderness on palpation of implant 11. A large-diameter immediate implant was facially positioned in the extraction socket and protruded through the facial bone. Subsequent remodeling of the facial bone left the implant with no surrounding facial or apical bone.

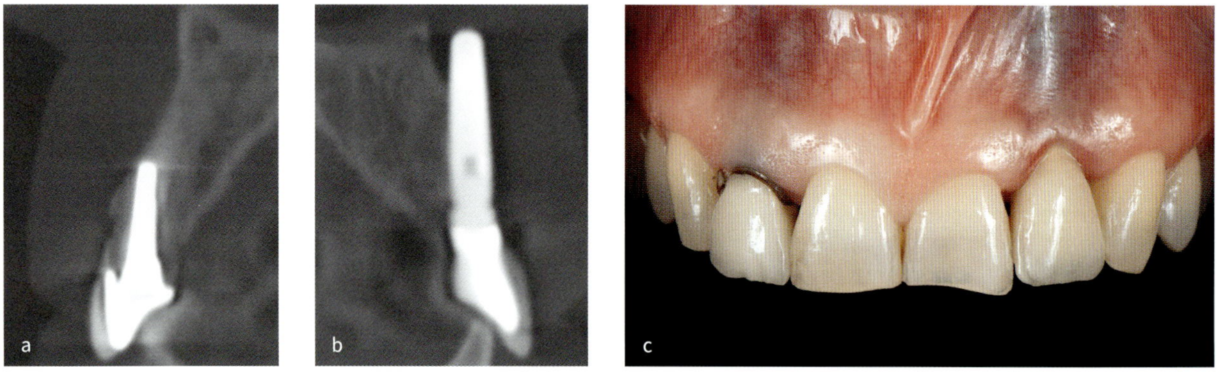

Figs 6a-c Implant 12 was immediately placed several years ago. The position of the contralateral tooth suggests that the axis of the implant was the same as that of the failing tooth, probably leading to intraoperative fenestration of the facial bone. Additional remodeling of the buccal bone has resulted in an esthetic complication after several years; the patient also reported discomfort.

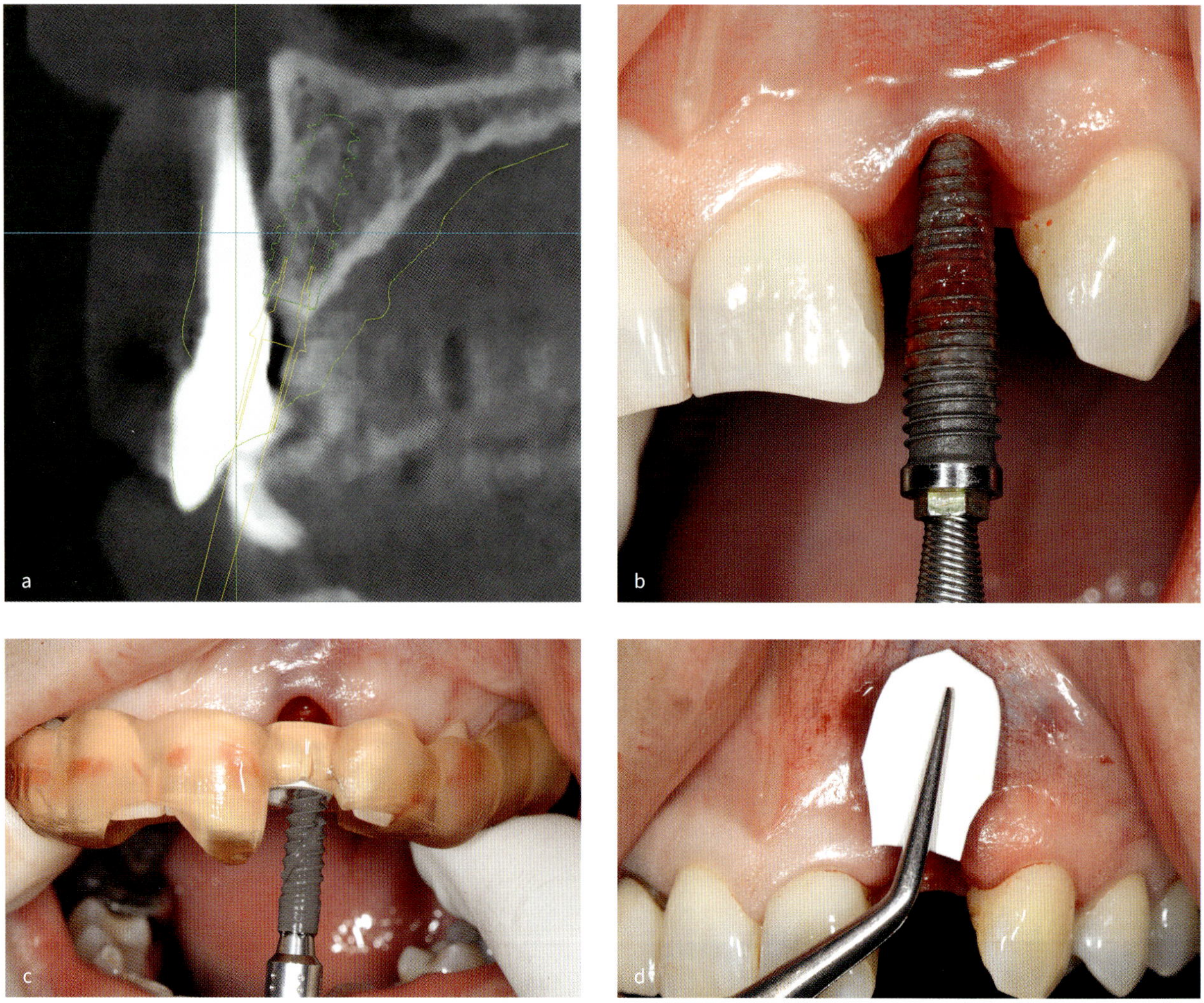

Figs 7a-h Based on digital planning (a), the implant was removed and replaced immediately in combination with simultaneous hard and soft tissue grafting. Implant removal (b), placement of a new implant immediately in a proper 3D position using a static surgical guide (c), buccal bone regeneration using a collagen membrane and xenograft (d).

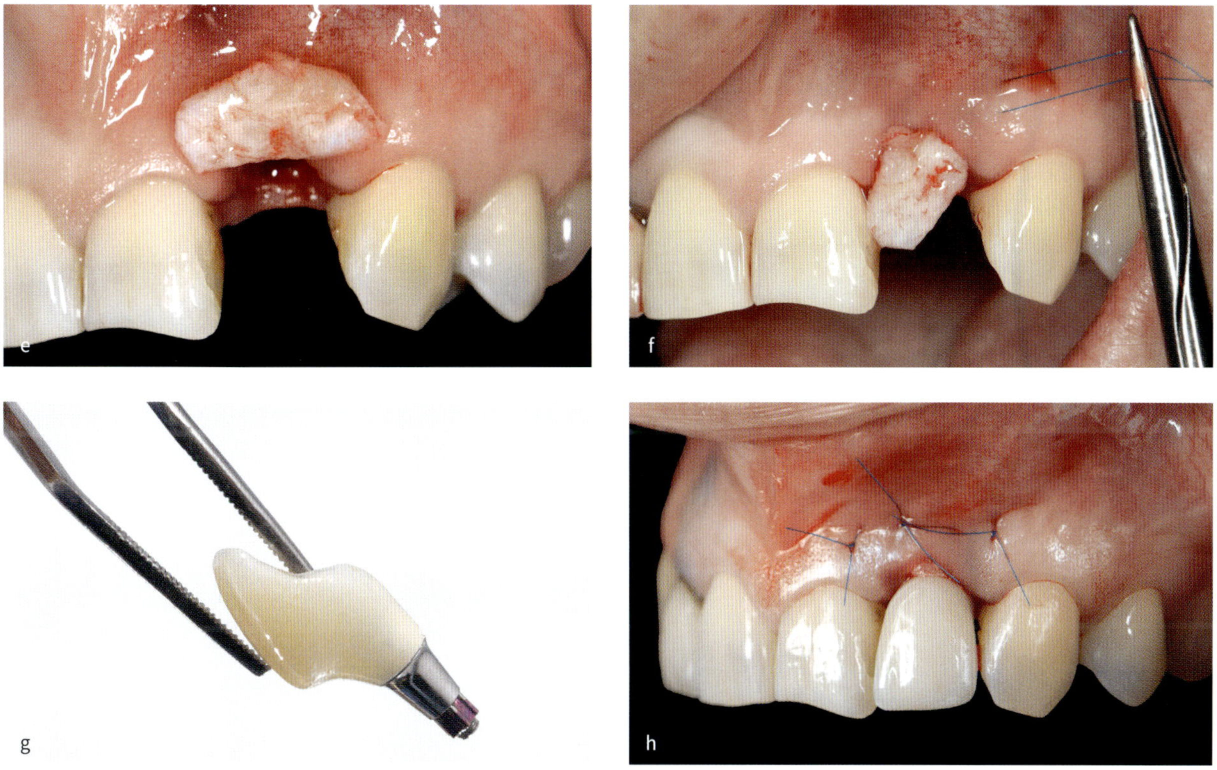

Figs 7a-h (continued) Connective tissue graft (e-f), immediate loading with a screw retained provisional fabricated prior to the surgery based on the implant digital planning (g-h).

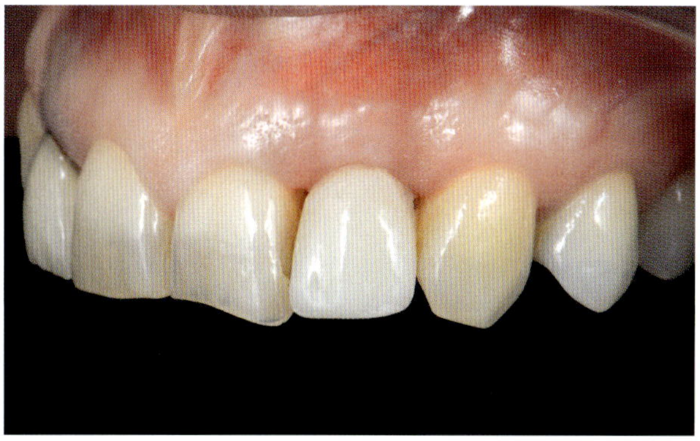

Fig 8 Provisional crown after healing. Buccal view 6 months after the implant replacement.

An excessive facial angulation of the implant may be required to achieve enough primary stability for immediate loading where palatal bone is abundant. Primary stability in type 1 implant placement may not always be achievable with an implant in the ideal position if it falls completely within the extraction socket. One might be tempted to angulate the implant apex toward the palatal aspect if there is abundant palatal bone, but this may result in a compromised facial angulation of the implant (Kan and coworkers 2021).

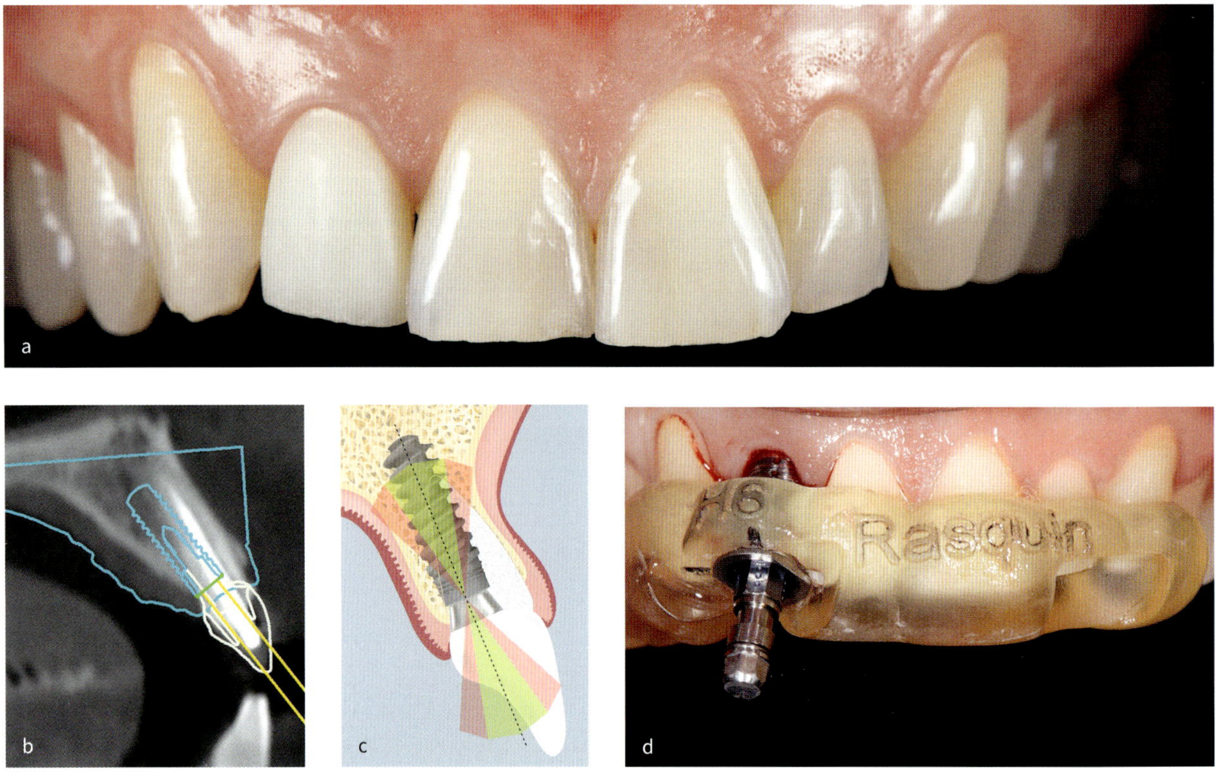

Figs 9a-d Virtual implant planning of a maxillary lateral incisor requiring extraction and replacement with an implant. The root is rather long, and the alveolar bone crest is protruded with a labial concavity toward the apex, precluding engagement of the implant with the apical bone. Engagement with the palatal bone was possible; however, this resulted in an excessive facial angulation with potential complications such as facial tissue recession.

Facial angulation of implants in the esthetic zone has been linked to an increased risk of hard and soft tissue loss with resultant midfacial recession (Figs 9a-d). It also creates restorative challenges to correct for the implant angulation. This requires angle correcting solutions, such as an angled screw channel abutment, or a cement retained restoration (Figs 10a-c). While no specific degree of facial-angulation compromise has been determined as a cut off for complications, any planned or unexpected facial inclination of the implant should be reviewed carefully preoperatively as well as at the time of implant placement surgery. If the implant is deemed to have excessive facial inclination when assessed together with additional risk factors for esthetic, biological, and mechanical complications, the implant should not be placed at the time of extraction. Alternative implant placement protocols should be considered that will allow for ideal implant positioning (Figs 11a-d).

One of the requirements for flapless immediate placement is that the implant needs to be placed slightly below the level of the labial bone crest. This provides a contained defect in which bone can regenerate to provide complete bone coverage of the implant upon healing (Clementini and coworkers 2019). With a pre-existing high-scalloped labial bone contour, or a slight vertical deficiency of labial bone, immediate placement can result in excessive implant depth. Modern implant designs with internal conical connections and platform-switching abutments are better able to maintain crestal bone levels above the implant platform when placed slightly subcrestally (Saleh and coworkers 2018; Valles and coworkers 2018; de Siqueira and coworkers 2020; Cruz and coworkers 2022).

However, favorable esthetic outcomes and a stable midfacial mucosal margin have not been demonstrated with implants placed beyond the recommended 3-4 mm from the desired facial mucosal margin. If the facial bone is vertically deficient, alternative placement protocols in which the facial bone can be regenerated in an open-flap procedure would be recommended.

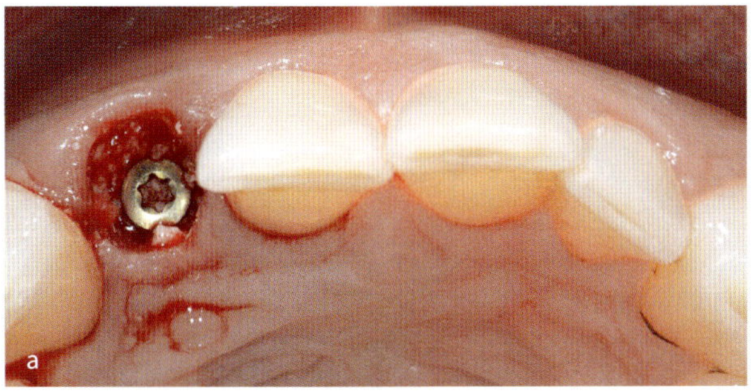

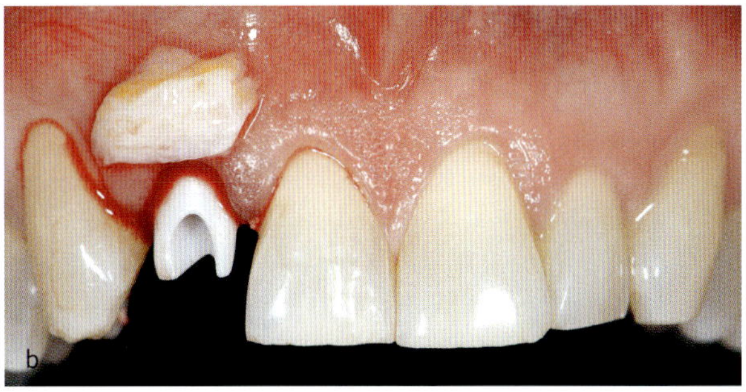

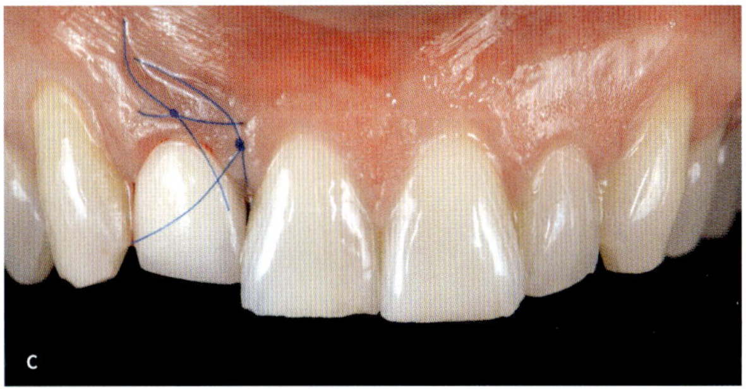

Figs 10a-c Socket grafting and a connective tissue graft were applied, creating the preconditions for immediate loading. A cemented crown was required, as the implant axis did not allow for a screw-retained restoration. The final zirconia abutment and a CAD/CAM acrylic provisional crown were fabricated prior to the surgery based on the digital planning.

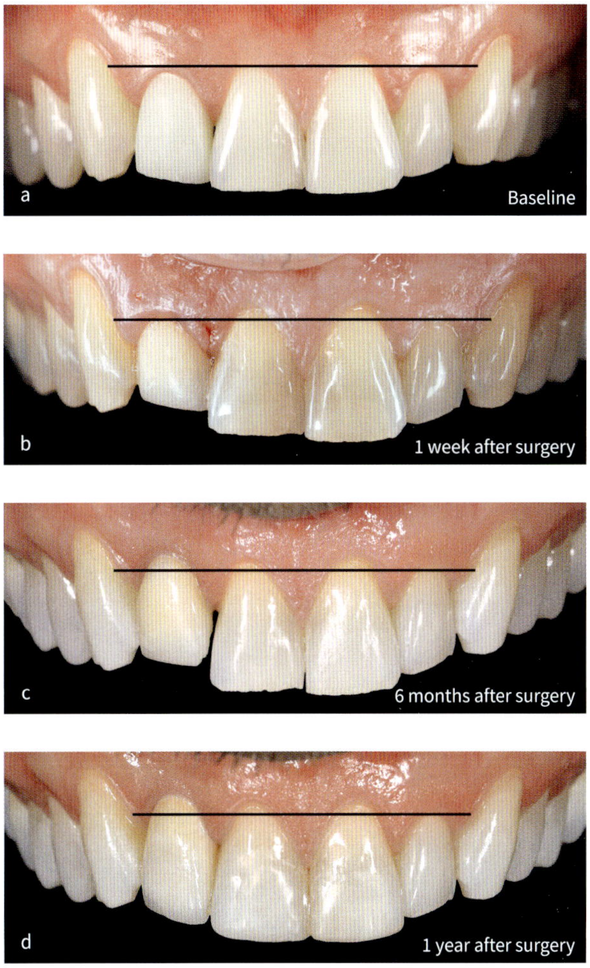

Figs 11a-d The soft tissue level was optimal after healing, but despite the hard and soft tissue management, a midfacial recession was visible after six months. Alternative placement protocols, such as early placement or late placement following socket grafting, would have permitted a more favorable axial inclination of the implant and a better esthetic outcome.

6.2.2 Complications Associated with Adjunctive Regenerative Procedures

Grafting the socket in conjunction with immediate implant placement is recommended to minimize dimensional changes in the ridge following tooth extraction (Clementini and coworkers 2019). Where favorable conditions exist for regeneration, with a contained defect within the extraction socket walls, complete bone regeneration is a predictable outcome (Clementini and coworkers 2019). Complications related to regenerative procedures have been reported for all timings of implant placement, largely related to the wound-healing capacity of the site and patient, as well to as the execution and planning of the regenerative procedures themselves (Jepsen and coworkers 2019).

With immediate implant placement, this would manifest as a potential for incomplete defect fill-in and resorption of facial bone, which has been reported in both animal and clinical studies (Gelb 1993; van Steenberghe and coworkers 2000; Chen and coworkers 2007). The clinical presentation of failed bone regeneration around an immediate implant may be indistinguishable from that of peri-implantitis, with deep probing depths, suppuration, and bone defects (Figs 12a-g to 15a-h).

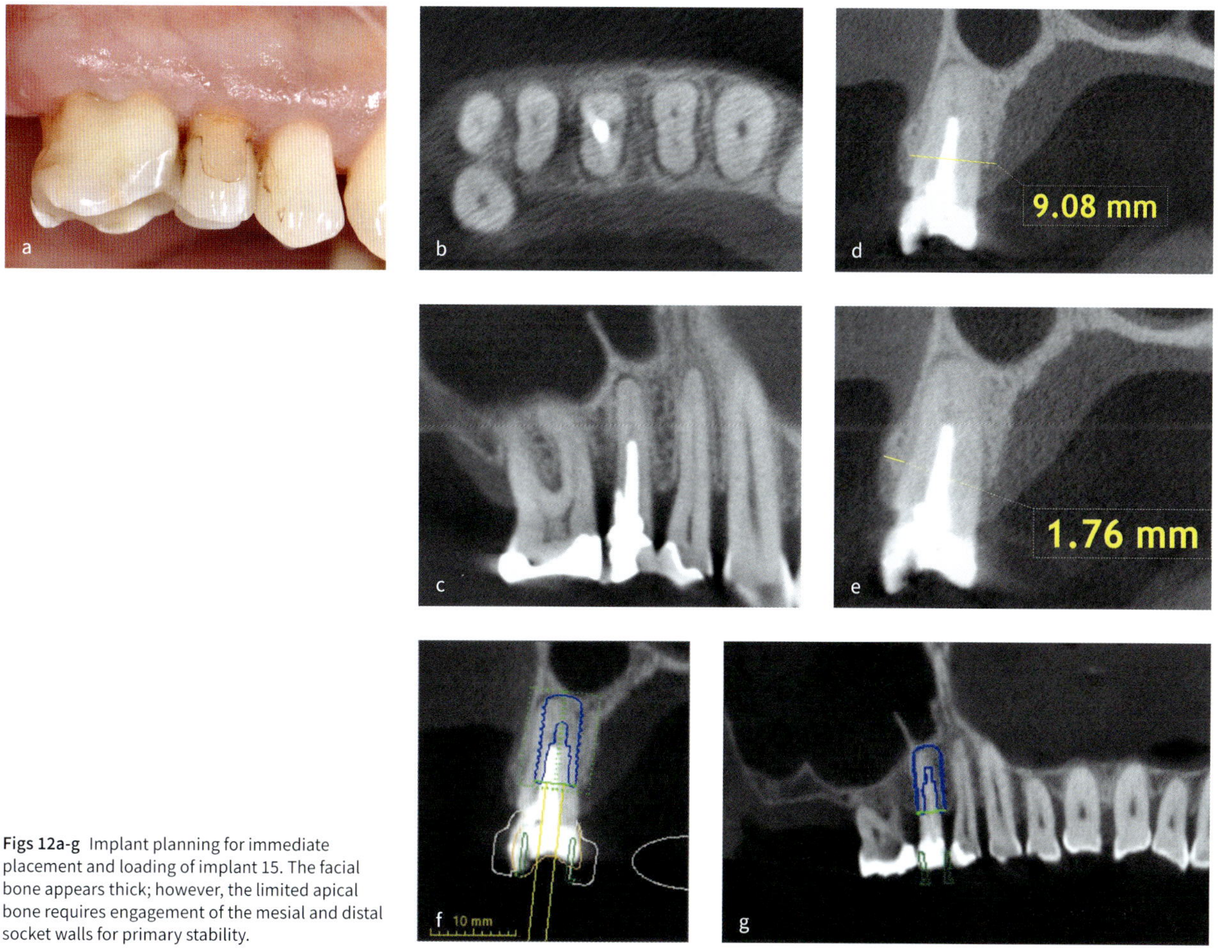

Figs 12a-g Implant planning for immediate placement and loading of implant 15. The facial bone appears thick; however, the limited apical bone requires engagement of the mesial and distal socket walls for primary stability.

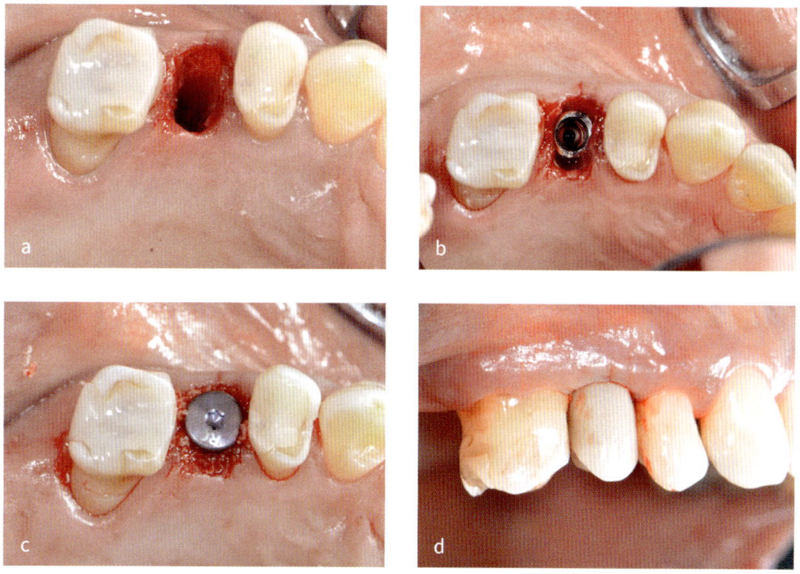

Figs 13a-d Immediate placement and loading of implant 15 with a wide-diameter bone-level implant. The small gap around the implant was grafted with deproteinized bovine bone mineral.

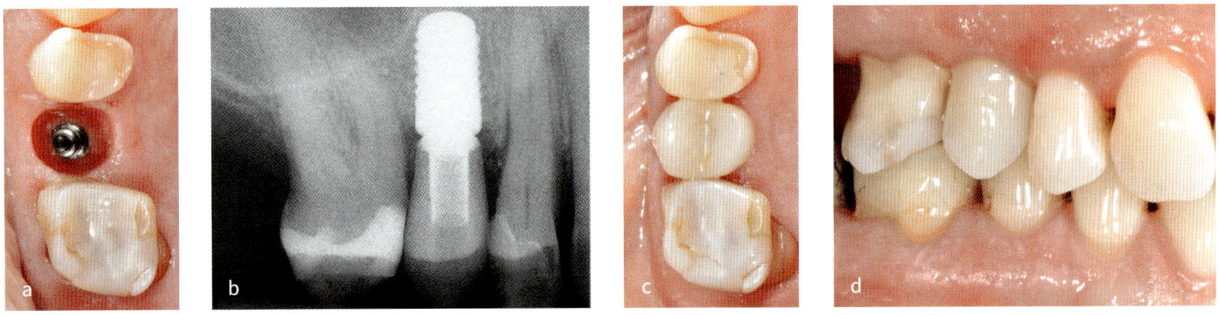

Figs 14a-d Definitive restoration delivered ten months after implant placement with excellent peri-implant soft tissue health and volume.

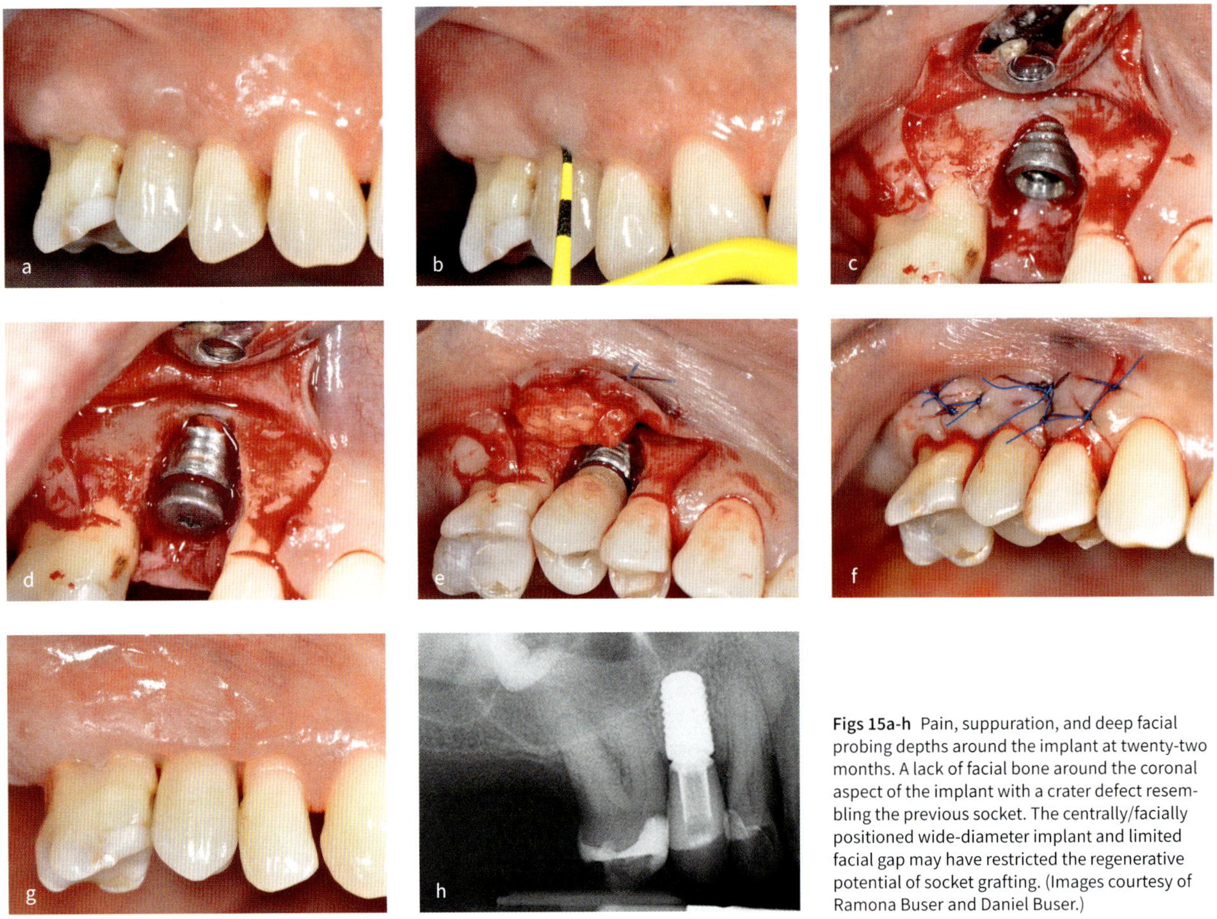

Figs 15a-h Pain, suppuration, and deep facial probing depths around the implant at twenty-two months. A lack of facial bone around the coronal aspect of the implant with a crater defect resembling the previous socket. The centrally/facially positioned wide-diameter implant and limited facial gap may have restricted the regenerative potential of socket grafting. (Images courtesy of Ramona Buser and Daniel Buser.)

When performing any placement procedure with simultaneous bone augmentation, careful consideration should be given to the regenerative potential of the site to minimize the risk of incomplete regeneration and exposure of rough implant surfaces to the peri-implant sulcus.

To minimize the risk of failed bone regeneration around an immediate implant, the following should be carefully considered:

- Selecting only healthy patients with unimpaired wound-healing capacity
- Selecting only extraction sites with a favorable socket morphology and potential implant position to provide a defect and graft with optimum biological potential for regeneration
- Providing at least 2 mm of distance between the facial bone wall and the implant surface
- Grafting the gap with a suitable biomaterial
- Closing the socket with an appropriately contoured restoration to provide stability to the graft and prosthetically guided soft tissue healing

Given the anticipated loss of facial bone following tooth extraction, soft tissue augmentation can be beneficial when used in conjunction with immediate placement protocols. This can help mitigate the anticipated minor changes in alveolar ridge dimensions following tooth extraction in conjunction with bone grafting into the facial gap. The soft tissue would be augmented facially within the coronal part of the socket above the facial bone crest; where more extensive vascularization is required to support the graft, a small split-thickness pouch can be created on the facial aspect to extend the graft slightly apical of the facial bone crest. A subepithelial connective tissue graft would then be sutured into the desired position. Early implant placement (type 2) can also be considered as an alternative, which would have the advantage of spontaneously thickening of the facial soft tissue following tooth extraction. This soft tissue can then be utilized at implant placement without with no need for concomitant soft tissue augmentation.

Potential complications reported for subepithelial connective tissue grafting are scarring or tissue hyperplasia, possibly associated with incomplete deepithelialization of the donor tissue or exposure of the graft, with epithelial downgrowth into the junction between the graft and recipient site. The differentiated esthetic appearance of the grafted tissue may also be related to specific histological differences in the donor tissue (Dellavia and coworkers 2014; Sanz-Martín and coworkers 2019). The scars may fade over time as the tissue matures; often no treatment is indicated. However, where donor tissues have a significantly different histology and gene expression at the recipient site, scars may also become more visible over time in some patients (Tavelli and coworkers 2019). If it is an esthetic concern, it can be addressed through dermal abrasion, removing the epithelium with a large round diamond bur (Figs 16a-f) or a soft tissue laser.

To prevent such complications, several aspects must be considered, such as transmucosal epithelialization, complete coverage of the graft and appropriate stabilization with sutures, and the nature of the provisional restoration. As described in Chapter 4, complete removal of the sulcular and junctional epithelium is recommended to avoid complications related to epithelial invagination; however, this is largely based on the periodontological literature on connective tissue grafting around teeth (Breault and coworkers 1997; Salhi and coworkers 2014; Cardoso and coworkers 2021; Alarcón and coworkers 2022). This removal can be performed efficiently with a high-speed handpiece and large diamond bur or with a scalpel blade, and will also improve the transmucosal vascular bed for a connective tissue graft. Scar development can be reduced by ensuring that no part of the graft is exposed beyond the sulcus and that it is adequately stabilized. The connective tissue graft should be sutured such that it does not move out of its recipient bed even under pressure of the lips or local postoperative inflammation. A provisional restoration or custom healing abutment can also contribute to the stability of the connective tissue graft by way of prosthetically guided soft tissue healing.

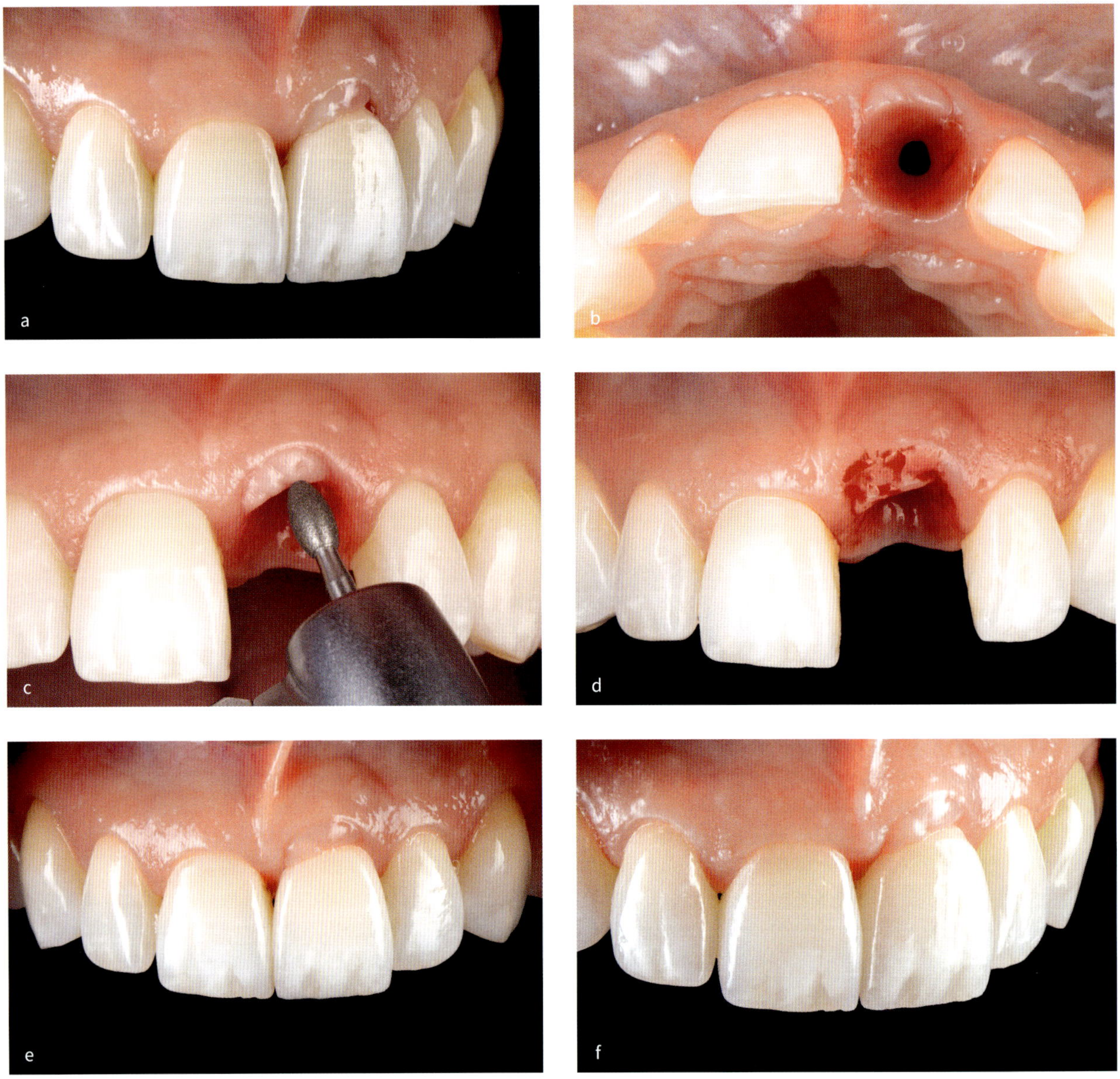

Figs 16a-f Soft tissue scar following flapless immediate implant placement and loading as a result of connective tissue grafting. The site was revised with a large round bur. The two week follow-up showed partially improved soft tissue esthetics; however, some scarring remained.

6.3 Complications Related to Loading Procedures

Abutment screws of immediately loaded provisional restorations can loosen, which can be detrimental to the healing process. The consequent micromovement will prevent the establishment of the peri-implant soft tissue. This is commonly due to contact between the abutment and adjacent bone or biomaterials, which prevents complete seating of the restoration and an adequate abutment-screw preload (Fig 17) (Schoenbaum and coworkers 2012). This can be forestalled by modifying the provisional titanium abutment to create a narrow emergence profile—not wider than the implant in the initial 2 mm of emergence (Fig 18).

Minor surgical profiling of the bone to accommodate the abutment profile can also be performed; however, maintenance of crestal bone with an appropriately contoured abutment and emergence profile is preferable. The abutment screw for provisional restorations should be tightened to the manufacturer's specifications with a torque controller to minimize the risk of screw loosening.

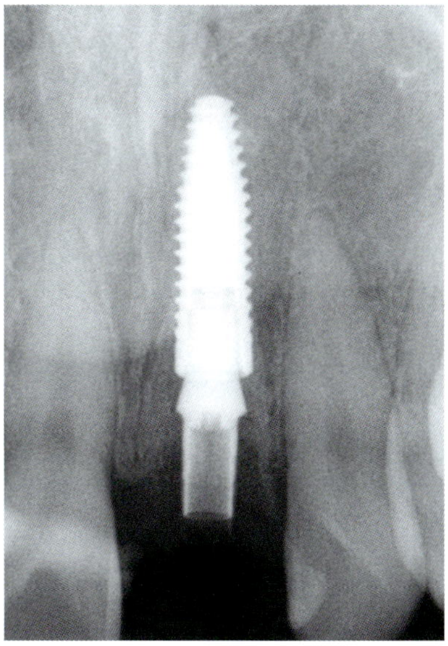

Fig 17 incomplete seating of the abutment due to contact with adjacent bone and biomaterial. This resulted in screw loosening and an associated inflammatory response, which can initiate bone remodeling.

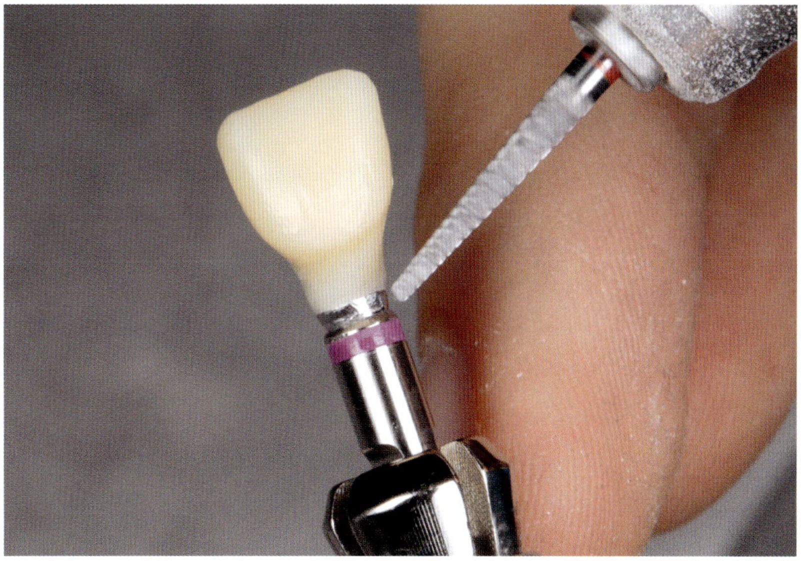

Fig 18 Modification of the abutment profile of the provisional restoration to remove contact with the adjacent bone crest. The restoration should be seated on a laboratory analog to prevent damage to the implant-abutment connection.

7 Conclusions

F. Lambert, A. Hamilton

Immediate implant placement may be indicated to reduce the overall treatment time, decrease morbidity, and maintain the peri-implant tissue architecture. Where appropriate clinical conditions and indications are present, immediate placement can be the most desirable timing—not only from a patient and time perspective, but also from an esthetic, biological, and surgical standpoint.

This Volume 14 of the ITI Treatment Guide series has provided a comprehensive update of current clinical and scientific knowledge regarding immediate implant placement and immediate loading in partially edentulous patients. The main objective has been to provide a decision-making framework that can be applied for type 1A immediate implant placement and immediate loading in a safe and reliable manner.

Understanding the biological principles of socket healing is of paramount importance in immediate implant placement. Practitioners must be aware of the dimensional changes of the alveolar tissues after tooth extraction, which will still occur when an implant is immediately inserted after extraction. Although this requires specific training, it is imperative to understand how adjunctive surgical procedures such as socket grafting or connective tissue grafting can be used and combined with immediate implant placement to limit hard and soft tissue remodeling and the resultant esthetic changes.

We think that the most important consideration in achieving success with immediate placement and loading is appropriate case selection. Careful clinical and radiographical assessment, based on prosthetic and surgical planning, permits the identification of the appropriate indications for immediacy, which minimizes the risks of complications.

Immediate placement should be selected for replacing teeth with optimal bone and soft tissue conditions. Adjunctive measures such as socket grafting with biomaterials or connective tissue grafting should be considered to compensate the expected post-extraction tissue shrinkage, following a diligent risk assessment. In sites with insufficient bone anchorage, soft tissues discrepancies, acute infections, or alveolar or buccal bone-plate defects, an alternative timing of implant placement should be considered. Additionally, one of the key aspects of successful immediate implant placement is based on the possibility to anchor and stabilize the implant within the fresh extraction socket. However, correct three-dimensional implant positioning should never be compromised in order to obtain primary implant stability.

Immediate loading (restoration) can be combined with immediate placement if indicated. Alternatively, conventional loading can always be considered if the risk assessment shows this to be the more suitable choice. If conventional loading is performed, a custom healing abutment can be considered for an immediate implant to provide prosthetically guided soft tissue healing. Immediate loading requires a thorough analysis of the occlusal scheme, together with optimal anchorage and stability of the implant, and is usually not recommended in the molar region.

Although complications related to immediate implant procedures may still occur, a careful case selection and an appropriate application of the surgical and prosthetic principles described in this volume will assist in managing the risk of these cases.

Finally, immediate placement and loading are operator-sensitive techniques and should be reserved for clinicians with an appropriate level of experience and training.

8 References

References have been listed in the order of (1) the first or only author's last name and (2) the year of publication. Identical short references are distinguished in the text by lowercase letters, which if used are given in parentheses at the end of the respective entry in this list of references.

Digital Object Identifier (DOI) names have been added to the individual references wherever they were available with reasonable effort, to allow readers to check the respective references quickly. For more information, refer to https://www.doi.org. When entering a DOI name in the search field on that site, make sure not to enter the leading "doi:" or the trailing period. You may also access a reference by pointing your browser to https://doi.org/<DOI name>, where <DOI name> should be replaced with the actual DOI name without the leading "doi:" or the trailing period (e.g., "10.1000/xyz123").

Abrahamsson I, Berglundh T, Lindhe J. Soft tissue response to plaque formation at different implant systems. A comparative study in the dog. Clin Oral Implants Res. **1998** Apr; 9(2): 73–79. doi: 10.1034/j.1600-0501.1998.090202.x.

Adell R, Lekholm U, Rockler B, Brånemark PI. A 15-year study of osseointegrated implants in the treatment of the edentulous jaw. Int J Oral Surg. **1981** Dec; 10(6): 387–416. doi: 10.1016/s0300-9785(81)80077-4.

Ainamo J, Bay I. Problems and proposals for recording gingivitis and plaque. Int Dent J. **1975** Dec; 25(4): 229–235.

Akagawa Y, Ichikawa Y, Nikai H, Tsuru H. Interface histology of unloaded and early loaded partially stabilized zirconia endosseous implant in initial bone healing. J Prosthet Dent. **1993** Jun; 69(6): 599–604. doi: 10.1016/0022-3913(93)90289-z.

Akin R. A new concept in maintaining the emergence profile in immediate posterior implant placement: the anatomic harmony abutment. J Oral Maxillofac Surg. **2016** Dec; 74(12): 2385–2392. doi: 10.1016/j.joms.2016.06.184.

Alarcón MA, Moses AX, Palma D, García-Roncero H, de Carvalho PFM. Unusual complications at the recipient site following periodontal plastic surgery procedures: a systematic review. Clin Oral Investig. **2022** Sep; 26(9): 5595–5609. doi: 10.1007/s00784-022-04596-6.

Al-Askar M, O'Neill R, Stark PC, Griffin T, Javed F, Al-Hezaimi K. Effect of single and contiguous teeth extractions on alveolar bone remodeling: a study in dogs. Clin Implant Dent Relat Res. **2013** Aug; 15(4): 569–575. doi: 10.1111/j.1708-8208.2011.00403.x.

Albrektsson T, Zarb GA. Current interpretations of the osseointegrated response: clinical significance. Int J Prosthodont. **1993** Mar–Apr; 6(2): 95–105.

Albrektsson T, Brånemark PI, Hansson HA, Lindström J. Osseointegrated titanium implants. Requirements for ensuring a long-lasting, direct bone-to-implant anchorage in man. Acta Orthop Scand. **1981**; 52(2): 155–170. doi: 10.3109/17453678108991776.

Alexopoulou M, Lambert F, Knafo B, Popelut A, Vandenberghe B, Finelle G. Immediate implant in the posterior region combined with alveolar ridge preservation and sealing socket abutment: a retrospective 3D radiographic analysis. Clin Implant Dent Relat Res. **2021** Feb; 23(1): 61–72. doi: 10.1111/cid.12974.

Al-Harbi SA, Edgin WA. Preservation of soft tissue contours with immediate screw-retained provisional implant crown. J Prosthet Dent. **2007** Oct; 98(4): 329–332. doi: 10.1016/S0022-3913(07)60107-3.

Alqutaibi AY. Cement- and screw-retained implant-supported restorations showed comparable marginal bone loss and implant survival rate. J Evid Based Dent Pract. **2017** Jun; 17(2): 107–109. doi: 10.1016/j.jebdp.2017.03.009.

Alves D, Faria-Almeida R, Azevedo Á, Liñares A, Muñoz F, Blanco-Carrion J. Immediate one-piece zirconia implants with/without xenograft in the buccal gap: a 6-month pre-clinical study. Clin Oral Implants Res. **2021** May; 32(5): 629–640. doi: 10.1111/clr.13735

Andreiotelli M, Kohal RJ. Fracture strength of zirconia implants after artificial aging. Clin Implant Dent Relat Res. **2009** Jun; 11(2): 158–166. doi: 10.1111/j.1708-8208.2008.00105.x.

Araújo MG, Lindhe J. Dimensional ridge alterations following tooth extraction. An experimental study in the dog. J Clin Periodontol. **2005** Feb; 32(2): 212–218. doi: 10.1111/j.1600-051X.2005.00642.x.

Araújo MG, Sukekava F, Wennström JL, Lindhe J. Ridge alterations following implant placement in fresh extraction sockets: an experimental study in the dog. J Clin Periodontol. **2005** Jun; 32(6): 645–652. doi: 10.1111/j.1600-051X.2005.00726.x.

Araújo MG, Sukekava F, Wennström JL, Lindhe J. Tissue modeling following implant placement in fresh extraction sockets. Clin Oral Implants Res. **2006** Dec; 17(6): 615–624. doi: 10.1111/j.1600-0501.2006.01317.x. (**a**)

Araújo MG, Wennström JL, Lindhe J. Modeling of the buccal and lingual bone walls of fresh extraction sites following implant installation. Clin Oral Implants Res. **2006** Dec; 17(6): 606–614. doi: 10.1111/j.1600-0501.2006.01315.x. (**b**)

Araújo MG, Linder E, Lindhe J. Bio-Oss collagen in the buccal gap at immediate implants: a 6-month study in the dog. Clin Oral Implants Res. **2011** Jan; 22(1): 1–8. doi: 10.1111/j.1600-0501.2010.01920.x.

Araújo MG, Silva CO, Misawa M, Sukekava F. Alveolar socket healing: what can we learn? Periodontol 2000. **2015** Jun; 68(1): 122–134. doi: 10.1111/prd.12082.

Araújo MG, Silva CO, Souza AB, Sukekava F. Socket healing with and without immediate implant placement. Periodontol 2000. **2019** Feb; 79(1): 168–177. doi: 10.1111/prd.12252

Arcuri C, Barlattani A Jr, Mazzetti V, Carosi P, Ferrigno N, Ferrigno N. Immediate restoration of a single upper central integrating digital workflow and a novel dental implant: a case report. J Biol Regul Homeost Agents. **2019** Nov–Dec; 33 (6 Suppl. 2): 171–177.

Atieh MA, Payne AG, Duncan WJ, de Silva RK, Cullinan MP. Immediate placement or immediate restoration/loading of single implants for molar tooth replacement: a systematic review and meta-analysis. Int J Oral Maxillofac Implants. **2010** Mar–Apr; 25(2): 401–415.

Atieh MA, Alsabeeha NH, Payne AG, Duncan W, Faggion CM, Esposito M. Interventions for replacing missing teeth: alveolar ridge preservation techniques for dental implant site development. Cochrane Database Syst Rev. **2015** May 28; 2015(5): CD010176. doi: 10.1002/14651858.CD010176.pub2. Update in: Cochrane Database Syst Rev. **2021** Apr 26; 4: CD010176.

Atwood DA. Reduction of residual ridges: a major oral disease entity. J Prosthet Dent. **1971** Sep; 26(3): 266–279. doi: 10.1016/0022-3913(71)90069-2.

Avila G, Galindo P, Rios H, Wang HL. Immediate implant loading: current status from available literature. Implant Dent. **2007** Sep; 16(3): 235–245. doi: 10.1097/ID.0b013e3180de4ec5.

Avila-Ortiz G, Elangovan S, Kramer KW, Blanchette D, Dawson DV. Effect of alveolar ridge preservation after tooth extraction: a systematic review and meta-analysis. J Dent Res. **2014** Oct; 93(10): 950–968. doi: 10.1177/0022034514541127.

Avila-Ortiz G, Chambrone L, Vignoletti F. Effect of alveolar ridge preservation interventions following tooth extraction: A systematic review and meta-analysis. J Clin Periodontol. **2019** Jun; 46 Suppl 21: 195–223. doi: 10.1111/jcpe.13057.

Babbush CA, Kent JN, Misiek DJ. Titanium plasma-sprayed (TPS) screw implants for the reconstruction of the edentulous mandible. J Oral Maxillofac Surg. **1986** Apr; 44(4): 274–282. doi: 10.1016/0278-2391(86)90078-9.

Bakshi M, Tarnow D, Bittner N. Changes in ridge dimension with pontics immediately placed at extraction sites: a pilot study. Int J Periodontics Restorative Dent. **2018** Jul–Aug; 38(4): 541–547. doi: 10.11607/prd.3496.

Balmer M, Spies BC, Kohal RJ, Hämmerle CH, Vach K, Jung RE. Zirconia implants restored with single crowns or fixed dental prostheses: 5-year results of a prospective cohort investigation. Clin Oral Implants Res. **2020** May; 31(5): 452–462. doi: 10.1111/clr.13581.

Barzilay I, Graser GN, Iranpour B, Caton J, Schenkle G. Immediate implantation of pure titanium implants into extraction sockets [abstract 234]. J Dent Res. **1988**; 67 (special issue): 142.

Barzilay I, Graser GN, Iranpour B, Natiella JR. Immediate implantation of a pure titanium implant into an extraction socket: report of a pilot procedure. Int J Oral Maxillofac Implants. **1991** Fall; 6(3): 277–284.

Bäumer D, Zuhr O, Rebele S, Hürzeler M. Socket Shield Technique for immediate implant placement—clinical, radiographic and volumetric data after 5 years. Clin Oral Implants Res. **2017** Nov; 28(11): 1450–1458. doi: 10.1111/clr.13012.

Becker W, Becker BE. Guided tissue regeneration for implants placed into extraction sockets and for implant dehiscences: surgical techniques and case report. Int J Periodontics Restorative Dent. **1990**; 10(5): 376–391.

Behneke A, Burwinkel M, Behneke N. Factors influencing transfer accuracy of cone beam CT-derived template-based implant placement. Clin Oral Implants Res. **2012** Apr; 23(4): 416–423. doi: 10.1111/j.1600-0501.2011.02337.x.

Bell CL, Diehl D, Bell BM, Bell RE. The immediate placement of dental implants into extraction sites with periapical lesions: a retrospective chart review. J Oral Maxillofac Surg. **2011** Jun; 69(6): 1623–1627. doi: 10.1016/j.joms.2011.01.022.

Belser UC, Grütter L, Vailati F, Bornstein MM, Weber HP, Buser D. Outcome evaluation of early placed maxillary anterior single-tooth implants using objective esthetic criteria: a cross-sectional, retrospective study in 45 patients with a 2- to 4-year follow-up using pink and white esthetic scores. J Periodontol. **2009** Jan; 80(1): 140–151. doi: 10.1902/jop.2009.080435.

Bernabeu-Mira JC, Soto-Peñaloza D, Peñarrocha-Diago M, Camacho-Alonso F, Rivas-Ballester R, Peñarrocha-Oltra D. Low-speed drilling without irrigation versus conventional drilling for dental implant osteotomy preparation: a systematic review. Clin Oral Investig. **2021** Jul; 25(7): 4251-4267. doi: 10.1007/s00784-021-03939-z.

Bethke A, Pieralli S, Kohal RJ, Burkhardt F, von Stein-Lausnitz M, Vach K, Spies BC. Fracture resistance of zirconia oral implants in vitro: a systematic review and meta-analysis. Materials (Basel). **2020** Jan 24; 13(3): 562. doi: 10.3390/ma13030562.

Bianchi AE, Sanfilippo F. Single-tooth replacement by immediate implant and connective tissue graft: a 1–9-year clinical evaluation. Clin Oral Implants Res. **2004** Jun; 15(3): 269–277. doi: 10.1111/j.1600-0501.2004.01020.x.

Bittner N, Schulze-Späte U, Silva C, Da Silva JD, Kim DM, Tarnow D, et al. Changes of the alveolar ridge dimension and gingival recession associated with implant position and tissue phenotype with immediate implant placement: a randomised controlled clinical trial. Int J Oral Implantol (Berl). **2019**; 12(4): 469–480.

Blaschke C, Schwass DR. The socket-shield technique: a critical literature review. Int J Implant Dent. **2020** Sep 7; 6(1): 52. doi: 10.1186/s40729-020-00246-2.

Block MS, Mercante DE, Lirette D, Mohamed W, Ryser M, Castellon P. Prospective evaluation of immediate and delayed provisional single tooth restorations. J Oral Maxillofac Surg. **2009** Nov; 67(11 Suppl): 89–107. doi: 10.1016/j.joms.2009.07.009.

Blus C, Szmukler-Moncler S. Atraumatic tooth extraction and immediate implant placement with Piezosurgery: evaluation of 40 sites after at least 1 year of loading. Int J Periodontics Restorative Dent. **2010** Aug; 30(4): 355–363.

Boardman N, Darby I, Chen S. A retrospective evaluation of aesthetic outcomes for single-tooth implants in the anterior maxilla. Clin Oral Implants Res. **2016** Apr; 27(4): 443–451. doi: 10.1111/clr.12593.

Borges H, Correia ARM, Castilho RM, de Oliveira Fernandes GV. Zirconia implants and marginal bone loss: a systematic review and meta-analysis of clinical studies. Int J Oral Maxillofac Implants. **2020** Jul–Aug; 35(4): 707–720. doi: 10.11607/jomi.8097.

Bormann KH, Gellrich NC, Kniha H, Schild S, Weingart D, Gahlert M. A prospective clinical study to evaluate the performance of zirconium dioxide dental implants in single-tooth edentulous area: 3-year follow-up. BMC Oral Health. **2018** Nov 1; 18(1): 181. doi: 10.1186/s12903-018-0636-x.

Bornstein MM, Cionca N, Mombelli A. Systemic conditions and treatments as risks for implant therapy. Int J Oral Maxillofac Implants. **2009**; 24 Suppl: 12-27.

Bornstein MM, Horner K, Jacobs R. Use of cone beam computed tomography in implant dentistry: current concepts, indications and limitations for clinical practice and research. Periodontol 2000. **2017** Feb; 73(1): 51-72. doi: 10.1111/prd.12161.

Bosshardt DD, Chappuis V, Buser D. Osseointegration of titanium, titanium alloy and zirconia dental implants: current knowledge and open questions. Periodontol 2000. **2017** Feb; 73(1): 22-40. doi: 10.1111/prd.12179.

Botelho SV, Perussolo J, Misawa MY, Zadeh HH, Araújo MG. the basal bone and alveolar process in the maxillary anterior region in humans: a cone beam computed tomographic study. Int J Periodontics Restorative Dent. **2020** Nov–Dec; 40(6): 907–914. doi: 10.11607/prd.4571.

Botilde G, Colin PE, González-Martín O, Lecloux G, Rompen E, Lambert F. Hard and soft tissue analysis of alveolar ridge preservation in esthetic zone using deproteinized bovine bone mineral and a saddle connective tissue graft: A long-term prospective case series. Clin Implant Dent Relat Res. **2020** Jun; 22(3): 387–396. doi: 10.1111/cid.12899.

Botticelli D, Berglundh T, Buser D, Lindhe J. The jumping distance revisited: An experimental study in the dog. Clin Oral Implants Res. **2003** Feb; 14(1):35–42. doi: 10.1034/j.1600-0501.2003.140105.x.

Botticelli D, Berglundh T, Lindhe J. Hard tissue alterations following immediate implant placement in extraction sites. J Clin Periodontol. **2004** Oct; 31(10): 820–828. doi: 10.1111/j.1600-051X.2004.00565.x.

Bramanti E, Norcia A, Cicciù M, Matacena G, Cervino G, Troiano G, et al. Postextraction dental implant in the aesthetic zone, socket shield technique versus conventional protocol. J Craniofac Surg. **2018** Jun; 29(4): 1037–1041. doi: 10.1097/SCS.0000000000004419.

Brånemark PI, Adell R, Breine U, Hansson BO, Lindström J, Ohlsson A. Intra-osseous anchorage of dental prostheses. I. Experimental studies. Scand J Plast Reconstr Surg. **1969**; 3(2): 81–100. doi: 10.3109/02844316909036699.

Brånemark PI, Hansson BO, Adell R, Breine U, Lindström J, Hallén O, Ohman A. Osseointegrated implants in the treatment of the edentulous jaw. Experience from a 10-year period. Scand J Plast Reconstr Surg Suppl. **1977**; 16: 1–132.

Braut V, Bornstein MM, Belser U, Buser D. Thickness of the anterior maxillary facial bone wall—a retrospective radiographic study using cone beam computed tomography. Int J Periodontics Restorative Dent. **2011** Apr; 31(2): 125–131.

Braut V, Bornstein MM, Lauber R, Buser D. Bone dimensions in the posterior mandible: a retrospective radiographic study using cone beam computed tomography. Part 1—analysis of dentate sites. Int J Periodontics Restorative Dent. **2012** Apr; 32(2): 175–184.

Breault LG, Billman MA, Lewis DM. Report of a gingival "surgical cyst" developing secondarily to a subepithelial connective tissue graft. J Periodontol. **1997** Apr; 68(4): 392–395. doi: 10.1902/jop.1997.68.4.392.

Bressan E, Grusovin MG, D'Avenia F, Neumann K, Sbricoli L, Luongo G, et al. The influence of repeated abutment changes on peri-implant tissue stability: 3-year post-loading results from a multicentre randomised controlled trial. Eur J Oral Implantol. **2017**; 10(4): 373–390.

Buser D, von Arx T, ten Bruggenkate C, Weingart D. Basic surgical principles with ITI implants. Clin Oral Implants Res. **2000**; 11 Suppl 1: 59–68. doi: 10.1034/j.1600-0501.2000.011s1059.x.

Buser D, Martin W, Belser UC. Optimizing esthetics for implant restorations in the anterior maxilla: anatomic and surgical considerations. Int J Oral Maxillofac Implants. **2004**; 19 Suppl: 43–61.

Buser D, Chappuis V, Belser UC, Chen S. Implant placement post extraction in esthetic single tooth sites: when immediate, when early, when late? Periodontol 2000. **2017** Feb; 73(1): 84–102. doi: 10.1111/prd.12170.

Buser D, Chappuis V, Belser UC, Chen S. Implant placement post extraction in esthetic single tooth sites: when immediate, when early, when late? Periodontol 2000. **2017** Feb; 73(1): 84–102. doi: 10.1111/prd.12170.

Buser D, Chen S, Wismeijer D. Implant therapy in the esthetic zone: current modalities and materials for single-tooth replacments. Berlin: Quintessence Publishing, **2017**. ISBN 978-3-86867-343-2.

Cai H, Chen J, Li C, Wang J, Wan Q, Liang X. Quantitative discoloration assessment of peri-implant soft tissue around zirconia and other abutments with different colours: A systematic review and meta-analysis. J Dent. **2018** Mar; 70: 110–117. doi: 10.1016/j.jdent.2018.01.003.

Cairo F, Barbato L, Tonelli P, Batalocco G, Pagavino G, Nieri M. Xenogeneic collagen matrix versus connective tissue graft for buccal soft tissue augmentation at implant site. A randomized, controlled clinical trial. J Clin Periodontol. **2017** Jul; 44(7): 769–776. doi: 10.1111/jcpe.12750.

Calvo-Guirado JL, Aguilar-Salvatierra A, Gomez-Moreno G, Guardia J, Delgado-Ruiz RA, Mate-Sanchez de Val JE. Histological, radiological and histomorphometric evaluation of immediate vs. non-immediate loading of a zirconia implant with surface treatment in a dog model. Clin Oral Implants Res. **2014** Jul; 25(7): 826–830. doi: 10.1111/clr.12145.

Caneva M, Salata LA, de Souza SS, Baffone G, Lang NP, Botticelli D. Influence of implant positioning in extraction sockets on osseointegration: histomorphometric analyses in dogs. Clin Oral Implants Res. **2010** Jan; 21(1): 43–49. doi: 10.1111/j.1600-0501.2009.01842.x.

Caneva M, Botticelli D, Viganò P, Morelli F, Rea M, Lang NP. Connective tissue grafts in conjunction with implants installed immediately into extraction sockets. An experimental study in dogs. Clin Oral Implants Res. **2013** Jan; 24(1): 50–56. doi: 10.1111/j.1600-0501.2012.02450.x.

Canullo L, Pesce P, Penarrocha D. One abutment—one time approach to maximize peri-implant tissue expression in the aesthetic area. Clin Oral Impl Res. **2018 Oct**; 20: 80. doi: 10.1111/clr.37_13356.

Cardaropoli G, Araújo M, Lindhe J. Dynamics of bone tissue formation in tooth extraction sites. An experimental study in dogs. J Clin Periodontol. **2003** Sep; 30(9): 809–818. doi: 10.1034/j.1600-051x.2003.00366.x.

Cardoni A, MacBeath A, Lucas M. Methods for reducing cutting temperature in ultrasonic cutting of bone. Ultrasonics. **2006** Dec 22; 44 Suppl 1: e37–e42. doi: 10.1016/j.ultras.2006.06.046.

Cardoso MV, Lara VS, Sant'Ana ACP, Damante CA, Ragghianti Zangrando MS. Late complications after root coverage with two types of subepithelial connective tissue grafts, clinical and histopathological evaluation: A prospective cohort study. J Clin Periodontol. **2021** Mar; 48(3):431–440. doi: 10.1111/jcpe.13413.

Cawood JI, Howell RA. A classification of the edentulous jaws. Int J Oral Maxillofac Surg. **1988** Aug; 17(4): 232-6. doi: 10.1016/s0901-5027(88)80047-x.

Chackartchi T, Romanos GE, Sculean A. Soft tissue-related complications and management around dental implants. Periodontol 2000. **2019** Oct; 81(1): 124–138. doi: 10.1111/prd.12287.

Chan HL, George F, Wang IC, Suárez López Del Amo F, Kinney J, Wang HL. A randomized controlled trial to compare aesthetic outcomes of immediately placed implants with and without immediate provisionalization. J Clin Periodontol. **2019** Oct; 46(10): 1061–1069. doi: 10.1111/jcpe.13171.

Chang PC, Lang NP, Giannobile WV. Evaluation of functional dynamics during osseointegration and regeneration associated with oral implants. Clin Oral Implants Res. **2010** Jan; 21(1): 1–12. doi: 10.1111/j.1600-0501.2009.01826.x.

Chappuis V, Engel O, Reyes M, Shahim K, Nolte LP, Buser D. Ridge alterations post-extraction in the esthetic zone: a 3D analysis with CBCT. J Dent Res. **2013** Dec; 92(12 Suppl): 195S–201S. doi: 10.1177/0022034513506713.

Chappuis V, Engel O, Shahim K, Reyes M, Katsaros C, Buser D. Soft tissue alterations in esthetic postextraction sites: a 3-dimensional analysis. J Dent Res. **2015** Sep; 94(9 Suppl): 187S–193S. doi: 10.1177/0022034515592869.

Chappuis V, Araújo MG, Buser D. Clinical relevance of dimensional bone and soft tissue alterations post-extraction in esthetic sites. Periodontol 2000. **2017** Feb; 73(1): 73–83. doi: 10.1111/prd.12167.

Chen ST, Buser D. Advantages and disadvantages of treatment options for implant placement and post-extraction sites. In: Buser D, Wismeijer D, Belser U (eds). ITI Treatment Guide, Volume 3: Implant placement in post-extraction sites—treatment options. Berlin: Quintessence Publishing, **2008**. ISBN: 978-3-938947-14-2. 29–37.

Chen ST, Buser D. Clinical and esthetic outcomes of implants placed in postextraction sites. Int J Oral Maxillofac Implants. **2009**; 24 Suppl: 186–217.

Chen ST, Buser D. Esthetic outcomes following immediate and early implant placement in the anterior maxilla—a systematic review. Int J Oral Maxillofac Implants. **2014**; 29 Suppl: 186–215. doi: 10.11607/jomi.2014suppl.g3.3.

Chen ST, Wilson TG Jr, Hämmerle CH. Immediate or early placement of implants following tooth extraction: review of biologic basis, clinical procedures, and outcomes. Int J Oral Maxillofac Implants. **2004**; 19 Suppl: 12–25.

Chen ST, Darby IB, Reynolds EC. A prospective clinical study of non-submerged immediate implants: clinical outcomes and esthetic results. Clin Oral Implants Res. **2007** Oct; 18(5): 552–562. doi: 10.1111/j.1600-0501.2007.01388.x.

Chen ST, Darby IB, Reynolds EC, Clement JG. Immediate implant placement postextraction without flap elevation. J Periodontol. **2009** Jan; 80(1): 163–172. doi: 10.1902/jop.2009.080243.

Chen MH, Lyons KM, Tawse-Smith A, Ma S. Clinical significance of the use of resonance frequency analysis in assessing implant stability: a systematic review. Int J Prosthodont. **2019** Jan/Feb; 32(1): 51–58. doi: 10.11607/ijp.6048.

Chen YW, Finkelman M, Papaspirisdakos P, César-Neto JB, Weber HP, de Souza AB. Comparative analysis of dimensional alterations following extraction of maxillary molars using three-dimensional images' superimposition: a CBCT study. Odontology. **2021** Apr; 109(2): 514–523. doi: 10.1007/s10266-020-00568-y.

Chrcanovic BR, Martins MD, Wennerberg A. Immediate placement of implants into infected sites: a systematic review. Clin Implant Dent Relat Res. **2015** Jan; 17 Suppl 1: e1–e16. doi: 10.1111/cid.12098.

Christel P, Meunier A, Heller M, Torre JP, Peille CN. Mechanical properties and short-term in-vivo evaluation of yttrium-oxide-partially-stabilized zirconia. J Biomed Mater Res. **1989** Jan; 23(1): 45–61. doi: 10.1002/jbm.820230105.

Chu SJ, Salama MA, Salama H, Garber DA, Saito H, Sarnachiaro GO, Tarnow DP. The dual-zone therapeutic concept of managing immediate implant placement and provisional restoration in anterior extraction sockets. Compend Contin Educ Dent. **2012** Jul–Aug; 33(7): 524–532, 534.

Chu SJ, Salama MA, Garber DA, Salama H, Sarnachiaro GO, Sarnachiaro E, et al. Flapless postextraction socket implant placement, Part 2: The effects of bone grafting and provisional restoration on peri-implant soft tissue height and thickness—a retrospective study. Int J Periodontics Restorative Dent. **2015** Nov–Dec; 35(6): 803–809. doi: 10.11607/prd.2178.

Cionca N, Hashim D, Cancela J, Giannopoulou C, Mombelli A. Pro-inflammatory cytokines at zirconia implants and teeth. A cross-sectional assessment. Clin Oral Investig. **2016** Nov; 20(8): 2285–2291. doi: 10.1007/s00784-016-1729-z.

Clementini M, Agostinelli A, Castelluzzo W, Cugnata F, Vignoletti F, De Sanctis M. The effect of immediate implant placement on alveolar ridge preservation compared to spontaneous healing after tooth extraction: Radiographic results of a randomized controlled clinical trial. J Clin Periodontol. **2019** Jul; 46(7): 776–786. doi: 10.1111/jcpe.13125.

Coachman C, Paravina RD. Digitally enhanced esthetic dentistry—from treatment planning to quality control. J Esthet Restor Dent. **2016** Mar; 28 Suppl 1: S3–4. doi: 10.1111/jerd.12205.

Cochran DL, Morton D, Weber HP. Consensus statements and recommended clinical procedures regarding loading protocols for endosseous dental implants. Int J Oral Maxillofac Implants. **2004**; 19 Suppl: 109–113.

Cordaro L, Torsello F, Roccuzzo M. Clinical outcome of submerged vs. non-submerged implants placed in fresh extraction sockets. Clin Oral Implants Res. **2009** Dec; 20(12): 1307–1313. doi: 10.1111/j.1600-0501.2009.01724.x.

Cosyn J, Hooghe N, De Bruyn H. A systematic review on the frequency of advanced recession following single immediate implant treatment. J Clin Periodontol. **2012** Jun; 39(6): 582–589. doi: 10.1111/j.1600-051X.2012.01888.x.

Cosyn J, Eghbali A, Hermans A, Vervaeke S, De Bruyn H, Cleymaet R. A 5-year prospective study on single immediate implants in the aesthetic zone. J Clin Periodontol. **2016** Aug; 43(8): 702–709. doi: 10.1111/jcpe.12571.

Crespi R, Capparè P, Gherlone E. Immediate loading of dental implants placed in periodontally infected and non-infected sites: a 4-year follow-up clinical study. J Periodontol. **2010** Aug; 81(8): 1140–1146. doi: 10.1902/jop.2010.090666.

Cruz RS, Lemos CAA, de Luna Gomes JM, Fernandes E Oliveira HF, Pellizzer EP, Verri FR. Clinical comparison between crestal and subcrestal dental implants: a systematic review and meta-analysis. J Prosthet Dent. **2022** Mar; 127(3): 408–417. doi: 10.1016/j.prosdent.2020.11.003.

Dada K, Pariente L, Valois J. A new method of conclusively creating and transferring the emergence profile on single tooth immediate implant restorations: the E-merge protocol. Int J Comput Dent. 2021 Dec 21; 24(4): 457–477. doi: 10.3290/j.ijcd.b2382983.

Dahlin C, Linde A, Gottlow J, Nyman S. Healing of bone defects by guided tissue regeneration. Plast Reconstr Surg. **1988** May; 81(5): 672–676. doi: 10.1097/00006534-198805000-00004.

Dahlin C, Sennerby L, Lekholm U, Linde A, Nyman S. Generation of new bone around titanium implants using a membrane technique: an experimental study in rabbits. Int J Oral Maxillofac Implants. **1989** Spring; 4(1): 19–25.

Darby I, Chen ST, Buser D. Ridge preservation techniques for implant therapy. Int J Oral Maxillofac Implants. **2009**; 24 Suppl: 260–271.

Dawson A, Martin WC, Polido W (eds). The SAC Classification in Implant Dentistry. 2nd edn. Berlin: Quintessence Publishing, **2021**. ISBN 978-1-78698-110-3.

de Carvalho Barbara JG, Luz D, Vianna K, Porto Barboza E. The influence of abutment disconnections on peri-implant marginal bone: a systematic review. Int J Oral Implantol (Berl). **2019**; 12(3): 283–296.

De Carvalho B, Rompen E, Lecloux G, Schupbach P, Dory E, Art JF, Lambert F. Effect of sintering on in vivo biological performance of chemically deproteinized bovine hydroxyapatite. Materials (Basel). **2019** Nov 28; 12(23): 3946. doi: 10.3390/ma12233946.

De Rouck T, Eghbali R, Collys K, De Bruyn H, Cosyn J. The gingival biotype revisited: transparency of the periodontal probe through the gingival margin as a method to discriminate thin from thick gingiva. J Clin Periodontol. **2009** May; 36(5): 428–433. doi: 10.1111/j.1600-051X.2009.01398.x.

de Siqueira RAC, Savaget Gonçalves Junior R, Dos Santos PGF, de Mattias Sartori IA, Wang HL, Fontão FNGK. Effect of different implant placement depths on crestal bone levels and soft tissue behavior: A 5-year randomized clinical trial. Clin Oral Implants Res. **2020** Mar; 31(3): 282–293. doi: 10.1111/clr.13569.

de Sousa Gomes P, Daugela P, Poskevicius L, Mariano L, Fernandes MH. Molecular and cellular aspects of socket healing in the absence and presence of graft materials and autologous platelet concentrates: a focused review. J Oral Maxillofac Res. **2019** Sep 5; 10(3): e2. doi: 10.5037/jomr.2019.10302.

Dellavia C, Ricci G, Pettinari L, Allievi C, Grizzi F, Gagliano N. Human palatal and tuberosity mucosa as donor sites for ridge augmentation. Int J Periodontics Restorative Dent. **2014** Mar–Apr; 34(2): 179–186. doi: 10.11607/prd.1929.

Denissen HW, Kalk W, Veldhuis HA, van Waas MA. Anatomic consideration for preventive implantation. Int J Oral Maxillofac Implants. **1993**; 8(2): 191–196.

Derks J, Tomasi C. Peri-implant health and disease. A systematic review of current epidemiology. J Clin Periodontol. **2015** Apr; 42 Suppl 16: S158–S171. doi: 10.1111/jcpe.12334.

El Kholy K, Lazarin R, Janner SFM, Faerber K, Buser R, Buser D. Influence of surgical guide support and implant site location on accuracy of static computer-assisted implant surgery. Clin Oral Implants Res. **2019** Nov; 30(11): 1067–1075. doi: 10.1111/clr.13520.

Elian N, Cho SC, Froum S, Smith RB, Tarnow DP. A simplified socket classification and repair technique. Pract Proced Aesthet Dent. **2007** Mar; 19(2): 99–104.

Eriksson AR, Albrektsson T. Temperature threshold levels for heat-induced bone tissue injury: a vital-microscopic study in the rabbit. J Prosthet Dent. **1983** Jul; 50(1): 101–107. doi: 10.1016/0022-3913(83)90174-9.

Esposito M, Grusovin MG, Polyzos IP, Felice P, Worthington HV. Timing of implant placement after tooth extraction: immediate, immediate-delayed or delayed implants? A Cochrane systematic review. Eur J Oral Implantol. **2010** Autumn; 3(3): 189–205.

Evans CD, Chen ST. Esthetic outcomes of immediate implant placements. Clin Oral Implants Res. **2008** Jan; 19(1): 73–80. doi: 10.1111/j.1600-0501.2007.01413.x.

Fabbri G, Fradeani M, Dellificorelli G, De Lorenzi M, Zarone F, Sorrentino R. Clinical evaluation of the influence of connection type and restoration height on the reliability of zirconia abutments: a retrospective study on 965 abutments with a mean 6-year follow-up. Int J Periodontics Restorative Dent. **2017** Jan–Feb; 37(1): 19–31. doi: 10.11607/prd.2974.

Falco A, Berardini M, Trisi P. Correlation between implant geometry, implant surface, insertion torque, and primary stability: in vitro biomechanical analysis. Int J Oral Maxillofac Implants. **2018** Jul–Aug; 33(4): 824–830.

Ferrus J, Cecchinato D, Pjetursson EB, Lang NP, Sanz M, Lindhe J. Factors influencing ridge alterations following immediate implant placement into extraction sockets. Clin Oral Implants Res. **2010** Jan; 21(1): 22–29. doi: 10.1111/j.1600-0501.2009.01825.x.

Fickl S, Kebschull M, Schupbach P, Zuhr O, Schlagenhauf U, Hürzeler MB. Bone loss after full-thickness and partial-thickness flap elevation. J Clin Periodontol. **2011** Feb; 38(2): 157–162. doi: 10.1111/j.1600-051X.2010.01658.x.

Finelle G, Lee SJ. Guided immediate implant placement with wound closure by computer-aided design/computer-assisted manufacture sealing socket abutment: case report. Int J Oral Maxillofac Implants. **2017** Mar–Apr; 32(2) :e63–e67. doi: 10.11607/jomi.4770.

Finelle G, Papadimitriou DEV, Souza AB, Katebi N, Gallucci GO, Araújo MG. Peri-implant soft tissue and marginal bone adaptation on implant with non-matching healing abutments: micro-CT analysis. Clin Oral Implants Res. **2015** Apr; 26(4): e42–e46. doi: 10.1111/clr.12328.

Finelle G, Sanz-Martín I, Knafo B, Figué M, Popelut A. Digitalized CAD/CAM protocol for the fabrication of customized sealing socket healing abutments in immediate implants in molar sites. Int J Comput Dent. **2019**; 22(2): 187–204.

Finelle G, Popelut A, Knafo B, Martín IS. Sealing socket abutments (SSAs) in molar immediate implants with a digitalized CAD/CAM protocol: soft tissue contour changes and radiographic outcomes after 2 years. Int J Periodontics Restorative Dent. **2021** Mar–Apr; 41(2): 235–244. doi: 10.11607/prd.4579..

Fischer KR, Testori T, Wachtel H, Mühlemann S, Happe A, Del Fabbro M. Soft tissue augmentation applying a collagenated porcine dermal matrix during second stage surgery: a prospective multicenter case series. Clin Implant Dent Relat Res. **2019** Oct; 21(5): 923–930. doi: 10.1111/cid.12817.

Frizzera F, de Freitas RM, Muñoz-Chávez OF, Cabral G, Shibli JA, Marcantonio E Jr. Impact of soft tissue grafts to reduce peri-implant alterations after immediate implant placement and provisionalization in compromised sockets. Int J Periodontics Restorative Dent. **2019** May–June; 39(3): 381–389. doi: 10.11607/prd.3224.

Fürhauser R, Florescu D, Benesch T, Haas R, Mailath G, Watzek G. Evaluation of soft tissue around single-tooth implant crowns: the pink esthetic score. Clin Oral Implants Res. **2005** Dec; 16(6): 639–644. doi: 10.1111/j.1600-0501.2005.01193.x.

Gahlert M, Röhling S, Wieland M, Sprecher CM, Kniha H, Milz S. Osseointegration of zirconia and titanium dental implants: a histological and histomorphometrical study in the maxilla of pigs. Clin Oral Implants Res. **2009** Nov; 20(11): 1247–1253. doi: 10.1111/j.1600-0501.2009.01734.x

Gallucci GO, Benic GI, Eckert SE, Papaspyridakos P, Schimmel M, Schrott A, Weber HP. Consensus statements and clinical recommendations for implant loading protocols. Int J Oral Maxillofac Implants. **2014**; 29 Suppl: 287–290. doi: 10.11607/jomi.2013.g4.

Gallucci GO, Khoynezhad S, Yansane AI, Taylor J, Buser D, Friedland B. Influence of the posterior mandible ridge morphology on virtual implant planning. Int J Oral Maxillofac Implants. **2017** Jul/Aug; 32(4): 801–806. doi: 10.11607/jomi.5546.

Gallucci GO, Hamilton A, Zhou W, Buser D, Chen S. Implant placement and loading protocols in partially edentulous patients: a systematic review. Clin Oral Implants Res. **2018** Oct; 29 Suppl 16: 106–134. doi: 10.1111/clr.13276.

Garber DA, Belser UC. Restoration-driven implant placement with restoration-generated site development. Compend Contin Educ Dent. **1995** Aug; 16(8): 796, 798–802, 804.

Garcia-Sanchez R, Dopico J, Kalemaj Z, Buti J, Pardo Zamora G, Mardas N. Comparison of clinical outcomes of immediate versus delayed placement of dental implants: A systematic review and meta-analysis. Clin Oral Implants Res. **2022** Mar; 33(3): 231–277. doi: 10.1111/clr.13892.

Gelb DA. Immediate implant surgery: three-year retrospective evaluation of 50 consecutive cases. Int J Oral Maxillofac Implants. **1993**; 8(4): 388–399.

Ghiasi MS, Chen J, Vaziri A, Rodriguez EK, Nazarian A. Bone fracture healing in mechanobiological modeling: a review of principles and methods. Bone Rep. **2017** Mar 16; 6: 87–100. doi: 10.1016/j.bonr.2017.03.002.

Gluckman H, Salama M, Du Toit J. A retrospective evaluation of 128 socket-shield cases in the esthetic zone and posterior sites: Partial extraction therapy with up to 4 years follow-up. Clin Implant Dent Relat Res. **2018** Apr; 20(2): 122–129. doi: 10.1111/cid.12554.

González-Martín O, Lee EA, Veltri M. CBCT fractal dimension changes at the apex of immediate implants placed using undersized drilling. Clin Oral Implants Res. **2012** Aug; 23(8): 954–957. doi: 10.1111/j.1600-0501.2011.02246.x.

González-Martín O, Lee E, Weisgold A, Veltri M, Su H. Contour management of implant restorations for optimal emergence profiles: guidelines for immediate and delayed provisional restorations. Int J Periodontics Restorative Dent. **2020** Jan–Feb; 40(1): 61–70. doi: 10.11607/prd.4422.

Grassi FR, Capogreco M, Consonni D, Bilardi G, Buti J, Kalemaj Z. Immediate occlusal loading of one-piece zirconia implants: five-year radiographic and clinical evaluation. Int J Oral Maxillofac Implants. **2015** May–Jun; 30(3): 671–680. doi: 10.11607/jomi.3831.

Grenade C, De Pauw-Gillet MC, Gailly P, Vanheusden A, Mainjot A. Biocompatibility of polymer-infiltrated-ceramic-network (PICN) materials with Human Gingival Fibroblasts (HGFs). Dent Mater. **2016** Sep; 32(9): 1152–1164. doi: 10.1016/j.dental.2016.06.020.

Grenade C, De Pauw-Gillet MC, Pirard C, Bertrand V, Charlier C, Vanheusden A, Mainjot A. Biocompatibility of polymer-infiltrated-ceramic-network (PICN) materials with Human Gingival Keratinocytes (HGKs). Dent Mater. **2017** Mar; 33(3): 333–343. doi: 10.1016/j.dental.2017.01.001.

Grunder U. Crestal ridge width changes when placing implants at the time of tooth extraction with and without soft tissue augmentation after a healing period of 6 months: report of 24 consecutive cases. Int J Periodontics Restorative Dent. **2011** Feb; 31(1): 9-17.

Grunder U, Gracis S, Capelli M. Influence of the 3-D bone-to-implant relationship on esthetics. Int J Periodontics Restorative Dent. **2005** Apr; 25(2): 113–119.

Gupta SK. Intention-to-treat concept: A review. Perspect Clin Res. **2011** Jul; 2(3): 109–112. doi: 10.4103/2229-3485.83221.

Hamilton A, Gonzaga L, Amorim K, Wittneben JG, Martig L, Morton D, et al. Selection criteria for immediate implant placement and immediate loading for single tooth replacement in the maxillary esthetic zone: a systematic review and meta-analysis. Clin Oral Implants Res. **2023**; 34 [forthcoming].

Hamilton A, Obermaier B, Doliveux S, Negreiros WM, Al-nasser M, Gallucci GO. Digitally fabricated provisional implant restorations prior to implant placement: a clinical case series. Int J Prosthodont. **2022** Jan–Feb; 35(1): 94–108. doi: 10.11607/ijp.7623.

Hamilton A, Vazouras K, Friedland B, Gallucci GO, De Souza A. Influence of implant diameter and taper on virtual implant placement in the maxillary central incisor position: a CBCT analysis. Int J Oral Maxillofac Implants. **2022** May–Jun;37(3):525-532. doi: 10.11607/jomi.9367.

Hämmerle CH, Chen ST, Wilson TG Jr. Consensus statements and recommended clinical procedures regarding the placement of implants in extraction sockets. Int J Oral Maxillofac Implants. **2004**; 19 Suppl: 26–28.

Happe A, Röling N, Schäfer A, Rothamel D. Effects of different polishing protocols on the surface roughness of Y-TZP surfaces used for custom-made implant abutments: a controlled morphologic SEM and profilometric pilot study. J Prosthet Dent. **2015** May; 113(5): 440–447. doi: 10.1016/j.prosdent.2014.12.005.

Happe A, Fehmer V, Herklotz I, Nickenig HJ, Sailer I. Possibilities and limitations of computer-assisted implant planning and guided surgery in the anterior region. Int J Comput Dent. **2018**; 21(2): 147–162.

Happe A, Schmidt, Fehmer, V, Neugebauer, J. immediate implant placement in conjunction with xenogeneic acellular dermal matrix or connective tissue graft. a randomized controlled clinical volumetric study. Int J Periodontics Restorative Dent. **2021** (accepted for publication).

Happe A, Debring L, Schmidt A, Fehmer V, Neugebauer J. Immediate implant placement in conjunction with acellular dermal matrix or connective tissue graft: a randomized controlled clinical volumetric study. Int J Periodontics Restorative Dent. **2022** May–Jun; 42(3): 381–390. doi: 10.11607/prd.5632.

Happe A, Schmidt A, Neugebauer J. Peri-implant soft tissue esthetic outcome after immediate implant placement in conjunction with xenogeneic acellular dermal matrix or connective tissue graft: A randomized controlled clinical study. J Esthet Restor Dent. **2022** Jan; 34(1): 215–225. doi: 10.1111/jerd.12866.

Haro Adánez M, Nishihara H, Att W. A systematic review and meta-analysis on the clinical outcome of zirconia implant-restoration complex. J Prosthodont Res. **2018** Oct; 62(4): 397–406. doi: 10.1016/j.jpor.2018.04.007.

Harvey BV. Optimizing the esthetic potential of implant restorations through the use of immediate implants with immediate provisionals. J Periodontol. **2007** Apr; 78(4): 770–776. doi: 10.1902/jop.2007.060278.

Heithersay GS. Management of tooth resorption. Aust Dent J. **2007** Mar; 52(1 Suppl): S105–121. doi: 10.1111/j.1834-7819.2007.tb00519.x.

Heitz-Mayfield LJ, Darby I, Heitz F, Chen S. Preservation of crestal bone by implant design. A comparative study in minipigs. Clin Oral Implants Res. **2013** Mar; 24(3): 243-9. doi: 10.1111/j.1600-0501.2012.02513.x.

Heritier SR, Gebski VJ, Keech AC. Inclusion of patients in clinical trial analysis: the intention-to-treat principle. Med J Aust. **2003** Oct 20; 179(8): 438–440. doi: 10.5694/j.1326-5377.2003.tb05627.x.

Hürzeler MB, Zuhr O, Schupbach P, Rebele SF, Emmanouilidis N, Fickl S. The socket-shield technique: a proof-of-principle report. J Clin Periodontol. **2010** Sep; 37(9): 855–862. doi: 10.1111/j.1600-051X.2010.01595.x.

Ikar M, Grobecker-Karl T, Karl M, Steiner C. Mechanical stress during implant surgery and its effects on marginal bone: a literature review. Quintessence Int. **2020**; 51(2): 142–150. doi: 10.3290/j.qi.a43664.

Janner SFM, Gahlert M, Bosshardt DD, Röhling S, Milz S, Higginbottom F, Buser D, Cochran DL. Bone response to functionally loaded, two-piece zirconia implants: A preclinical histometric study. Clin Oral Implants Res. **2018** Mar; 29(3): 277–289. doi: 10.1111/clr.13112.

Januário AL, Barriviera M, Duarte WR. Soft tissue cone-beam computed tomography: a novel method for the measurement of gingival tissue and the dimensions of the dentogingival unit. J Esthet Restor Dent. **2008**; 20(6): 366–373; discussion 374. doi: 10.1111/j.1708-8240.2008.00210.x.

Januário AL, Barriviera M, Duarte WR. Soft tissue cone-beam computed tomography: a novel method for the measurement of gingival tissue and the dimensions of the dentogingival unit. J Esthet Restor Dent. **2008**; 20(6): 366–373. doi: 10.1111/j.1708-8240.2008.00210.x.

Januário AL, Duarte WR, Barriviera M, Mesti JC, Araújo MG, Lindhe J. Dimension of the facial bone wall in the anterior maxilla: a cone-beam computed tomography study. Clin Oral Implants Res. **2011** Oct; 22(10): 1168–1171. doi: 10.1111/j.1600-0501.2010.02086.x.

Javed F, Romanos GE. The role of primary stability for successful immediate loading of dental implants. A literature review. J Dent. **2010** Aug; 38(8): 612–620. doi: 10.1016/j.jdent.2010.05.013.

Javed F, Ahmed HB, Crespi R, Romanos GE. Role of primary stability for successful osseointegration of dental implants: factors of influence and evaluation. Interv Med Appl Sci. **2013** Dec; 5(4): 162–167. doi: 10.1556/IMAS.5.2013.4.3.

Jepsen S, Caton JG, Albandar JM, Bissada NF, Bouchard P, Cortellini P, et al. Periodontal manifestations of systemic diseases and developmental and acquired conditions: Consensus report of workgroup 3 of the 2017 World Workshop on the Classification of Periodontal and Peri-Implant Diseases and Conditions. J Periodontol. **2018** Jun; 89 Suppl 1: S237–S248. doi: 10.1002/JPER.17-0733.

Jepsen S, Schwarz F, Cordaro L, Derks J, Hämmerle CHF, Heitz-Mayfield LJ, et al. Regeneration of alveolar ridge defects. Consensus report of group 4 of the 15th European Workshop on Periodontology on Bone Regeneration. J Clin Periodontol. **2019** Jun; 46 Suppl 21: 277–286. doi: 10.1111/jcpe.13121.

Johnson K. A study of the dimensional changes occurring in the maxilla following tooth extraction. Aust Dent J. **1969** Aug; 14(4): 241–244. doi: 10.1111/j.1834-7819.1969.tb06001.x.

Jung RE, Zaugg B, Philipp AO, Truninger TC, Siegenthaler DW, Hämmerle CH. A prospective, controlled clinical trial evaluating the clinical radiological and aesthetic outcome after 5 years of immediately placed implants in sockets exhibiting periapical pathology. Clin Oral Implants Res. **2013** Aug; 24(8): 839–846. doi: 10.1111/j.1600-0501.2012.02491.x.

Jung RE, Al-Nawas B, Araújo M, Avila-Ortiz G, Barter S, Brodala N, et al. Group 1 ITI Consensus Report: The influence of implant length and design and medications on clinical and patient-reported outcomes. Clin Oral Implants Res. **2018** Oct; 29 Suppl 16: 69–77. doi: 10.1111/clr.13342.

Jung RE, Becker K, Bienz SP, Dahlin C, Donos N, Hammächer C, et al. Effect of peri-implant mucosal thickness on esthetic outcomes and the efficacy of soft tissue augmentation procedures: Consensus report of group 2 of the SEPA/DGI/OF workshop. Clin Oral Implants Res. **2022** Jun; 33 Suppl 23(Suppl 23): 100–108. doi: 10.1111/clr.13955.

Juodzbalys G, Wang HL. Soft and hard tissue assessment of immediate implant placement: a case series. Clin Oral Implants Res. **2007** Apr; 18(2): 237–243. doi: 10.1111/j.1600-0501.2006.01312.x.

Kan JY, Rungcharassaeng K, Kois JC. Removable ovate pontic for peri-implant architecture preservation during immediate implant placement. Pract Proced Aesthet Dent. **2001** Nov–Dec; 13(9): 711–715.

Kan JYK, Rungcharassaeng K, Deflorian M, Weinstein T, Wang HL, Testori T. Immediate implant placement and provisionalization of maxillary anterior single implants. Periodontol 2000. **2018** Jun; 77(1): 197–212. doi: 10.1111/prd.12212.

Kan JY, Rungcharassaeng K, Lozada JL. Bilaminar subepithelial connective tissue grafts for immediate implant placement and provisionalization in the esthetic zone. J Calif Dent Assoc. **2005** Nov; 33(11): 865-71.

Kan JY, Rungcharassaeng K, Sclar A, Lozada JL. Effects of the facial osseous defect morphology on gingival dynamics after immediate tooth replacement and guided bone regeneration: 1-year results. J Oral Maxillofac Surg. **2007** Jul; 65 (7 Suppl 1): 13–19. doi: 10.1016/j.joms.2007.04.006.

Kan JY, Rungcharassaeng K, Morimoto T, Lozada J. Facial gingival tissue stability after connective tissue graft with single immediate tooth replacement in the esthetic zone: consecutive case report. J Oral Maxillofac Surg. **2009** Nov; 67(11 Suppl): 40–48. doi: 10.1016/j.joms.2009.07.004.

Kan JY, Roe P, Rungcharassaeng K, Patel RD, Waki T, Lozada JL, Zimmerman G. Classification of sagittal root position in relation to the anterior maxillary osseous housing for immediate implant placement: a cone beam computed tomography study. Int J Oral Maxillofac Implants. **2011** Jul–Aug; 26(4): 873–876. (**a**)

Kan JY, Rungcharassaeng K, Lozada JL, Zimmerman G. Facial gingival tissue stability following immediate placement and provisionalization of maxillary anterior single implants: a 2- to 8-year follow-up. Int J Oral Maxillofac Implants. **2011** Jan–Feb; 26(1): 179–187. (**b**)

Kan JYK, Rungcharassaeng K, Deflorian M, Weinstein T, Wang HL, Testori T. Immediate implant placement and provisionalization of maxillary anterior single implants. Periodontol 2000. **2018** Jun; 77(1): 197q212. doi: 10.1111/prd.12212.

Kan JY, Rungcharassaeng K, Lin GH, Zucchelli G, Kamolroongwarakul P, Matsuda H, Lozada J. Incidence of straight-channel screw-retained single crown following immediate implant placement and provisionalization in the esthetic zone: A CBCT study. Int J Oral Maxillofac Implants. **2021** Jul–Aug; 36(4): 793–798. doi: 10.11607/jomi.8887.

Ketabi M, Deporter D, Atenafu EG. A systematic review of outcomes following immediate molar iplant placement based on recently published studies. Clin Implant Dent Relat Res. **2016** Dec; 18(6): 1084–1094. doi: 10.1111/cid.12390.

Khoury G, Chamieh F, Fromentin O. One-by-one immediate dental implants: A papillae preservation concept for adjacent implants in a compromised periodontal case. Clin Case Rep. **2020** Aug 20; 8(12): 2664–2672. doi: 10.1002/ccr3.2929.

Kleinheinz J, Büchter A, Kruse-Lösler B, Weingart D, Joos U. Incision design in implant dentistry based on vascularization of the mucosa. Clin Oral Implants Res. **2005** Oct; 16(5): 518–523. doi: 10.1111/j.1600-0501.2005.01158.x.

Knafo B, Finelle G. 2020 Procédés de fabrication des piliers de cicatrisation anatomique SSA. Titane. **2018**: 17(2): 55–60.

Kniha K, Gahlert M, Hicklin S, Brägger U, Kniha H, Milz S. Evaluation of hard and soft tissue dimensions around zirconium oxide implant-supported crowns: a 1-year retrospective study. J Periodontol. **2016** May; 87(5): 511–528. doi: 10.1902/jop.2015.150441.

Kniha K, Kniha H, Möhlhenrich SC, Milz S, Hölzle F, Modabber A. Papilla and alveolar crest levels in immediate versus delayed single-tooth zirconia implants. Int J Oral Maxillofac Surg. **2017** Aug; 46(8): 1039–1044. doi: 10.1016/j.ijom.2017.02.007.

Koenig V, Vanheusden AJ, Le Goff SO, Mainjot AK. Clinical risk factors related to failures with zirconia-based restorations: an up to 9-year retrospective study. J Dent. **2013** Dec; 41(12): 1164–1174. doi: 10.1016/j.jdent.2013.10.009.

Koutouzis T, Gholami F, Reynolds J, Lundgren T, Kotsakis GA. Abutment disconnection/reconnection affects peri-implant marginal bone levels: a meta-analysis. Int J Oral Maxillofac Implants. 2017 May–June; 32(3): 575–581. doi: 10.11607/jomi.5367.

Koyano K, Esaki D. Occlusion on oral implants: current clinical guidelines. J Oral Rehabil. **2015** Feb; 42(2): 153–161. doi: 10.1111/joor.12239.

Kuchler U, Chappuis V, Gruber R, Lang NP, Salvi GE. Immediate implant placement with simultaneous guided bone regeneration in the esthetic zone: 10-year clinical and radiographic outcomes. Clin Oral Implants Res. **2016** Feb; 27(2): 253–257. doi: 10.1111/clr.12586.

Lajolo C, Valente NA, Romandini WG, Petruzzi M, Verdugo F, D'Addona A. Bone heat generated using conventional implant drills versus piezosurgery unit during apical cortical plate perforation. J Periodontol. **2018** Jun; 89(6): 661–668. doi: 10.1002/JPER.17-0502.

Lambert F, Mainjot A. One-Tooth One-Time (1T1T): A straightforward approach to reeplace missing teeth in the posterior region. J Oral Implantol. **2017** Oct; 43(5): 371–377. doi: 10.1563/aaid-joi-D-17-00136.

Lambert F, Vincent K, Vanhoutte V, Seidel L, Lecloux G, Rompen E. A methodological approach to assessing alveolar ridge preservation procedures in humans: hard tissue profile. J Clin Periodontol. **2012** Sep; 39(9): 887–894. doi: 10.1111/j.1600-051X.2012.01900.x.

Lambert F, Baćević M, Layrolle P, Schüpbach P, Drion P, Rompen E. Impact of biomaterial microtopography on bone regeneration: comparison of three hydroxyapatites. Clin Oral Implants Res. **2017** Oct; 28(10): e201–e207. doi: 10.1111/clr.12986.

Lang NP, Brägger U, Hämmerle CH, Sutter F. Immediate transmucosal implants using the principle of guided tissue regeneration. I. Rationale, clinical procedures and 30-month results. Clin Oral Implants Res. **1994** Sep; 5(3): 154–163. doi: 10.1034/j.1600-0501.1994.050306.x.

Lang NP, Salvi GE, Huynh-Ba G, Ivanovski S, Donos N, Bosshardt DD. Early osseointegration to hydrophilic and hydrophobic implant surfaces in humans. Clin Oral Implants Res. **2011** Apr; 22(4): 349–356. doi: 10.1111/j.1600-0501.2011.02172.x.

Langer B. Spontaneous in situ gingival augmentation. Int J Periodontics Restorative Dent. **1994** Dec; 14(6): 524–535.

Lanis A, Álvarez Del Canto O. The combination of digital surface scanners and cone beam computed tomography technology for guided implant surgery using 3Shape implant studio software: a case history report. Int J Prosthodont. **2015** Mar–Apr; 28(2): 169–178. doi: 10.11607/ijp.4148.

Lanis A, Llorens P, Álvarez Del Canto O. Selecting the appropriate digital planning pathway for computer-guided implant surgery. Int J Comput Dent. **2017**; 20(1): 75–85.

Lazzara RJ. Immediate implant placement into extraction sites: surgical and restorative advantages. Int J Periodontics Restorative Dent. **1989**; 9(5): 332–343.

Ledermann P. Stegprothetische Versorgung des zahnlosen Unterkiefers mit Hilfe von plasmabeschichteten Titanschraubenimplantaten [Bar-prosthetic management of the edentulous mandible by means of plasma-coated implantation with titanium screws]. Dtsch Zahnärztl Z. **1979** Dec; 34(12): 907–911. German.

Lee, EA, Su H, Gonzalez-Martin O. Modified drilling sequence for immediate loading of non-conical single implants placed in extraction sockets. J Pract Proced Aesthet Dent. **2009** Jan; 21: 207–214.

Lemos CA, de Souza Batista VE, Almeida DA, Santiago Júnior JF, Verri FR, Pellizzer EP. Evaluation of cement-retained versus screw-retained implant-supported restorations for marginal bone loss: A systematic review and meta-analysis. J Prosthet Dent. **2016** Apr; 115(4): 419–427. doi: 10.1016/j.prosdent.2015.08.026.

Levine RA, Huynh-Ba G, Cochran DL. Soft tissue augmentation procedures for mucogingival defects in esthetic sites. Int J Oral Maxillofac Implants. **2014**; 29 Suppl: 155–185. doi: 10.11607/jomi.2014suppl.g3.2.

Levine RA, Ganeles J, Gonzaga L, Kan JK, Randel H, Evans CD, Chen ST. 10 keys for successful esthetic-zone single immediate implants. Compend Contin Educ Dent. **2017** Apr; 38(4): 248–260.

Levine RA, Dias DR, Wang P, Araújo MG. Effect of the buccal gap width following immediate implant placement on the buccal bone wall: A retrospective cone-beam computed tomography analysis. Clin Implant Dent Relat Res. **2022** Aug; 24(4): 403–413. doi: 10.1111/cid.13095.

Li P, Zhu H, Huang D. Autogenous DDM versus Bio-Oss granules in GBR for immediate implantation in periodontal postextraction sites: a prospective clinical study. Clin Implant Dent Relat Res. **2018** Dec; 20(6): 923–928. doi: 10.1111/cid.12667.

Lilet R, Desiron M, Finelle G, Lecloux G, Seidel L, Lambert F. Immediate implant placement combining socket seal abutment and peri-implant socket filling: a prospective case series. Clin Oral Implants Res. **2022** Jan; 33(1): 33–44. doi: 10.1111/clr.13852.

Lilet R, Desiron M, Finelle G, Lecloux G, Seidel L, Lambert F. Immediate implant placement combining socket seal abutment and peri-implant socket filling: a prospective case series. Clin Oral Implants Res. **2022** Jan; 33(1): 33–44. doi: 10.1111/clr.13852.

Liñares A, Muñoz F, Permuy M, Dard M, Blanco J. Soft tissue histomorphology at implants with a transmucosal modified surface. A study in minipigs. Clin Oral Implants Res. **2015** Sep; 26(9): 996–1005. doi: 10.1111/clr.12417.

Linkevicius T, Apse P. Influence of abutment material on stability of peri-implant tissues: a systematic review. Int J Oral Maxillofac Implants. **2008** May–Jun; 23(3): 449–456.

Linkevicius T, Vaitelis J. The effect of zirconia or titanium as abutment material on soft peri-implant tissues: a systematic review and meta-analysis. Clin Oral Implants Res. **2015** Sep; 26 Suppl 11: 139–147. doi: 10.1111/clr.12631.

Lioubavina-Hack N, Lang NP, Karring T. Significance of primary stability for osseointegration of dental implants. Clin Oral Implants Res. **2006** Jun; 17(3): 244–250. doi: 10.1111/j.1600-0501.2005.01201.x.

Lissek M, Boeker M, Happe A. How thick is the oral mucosa around implants after augmentation with different materials: a systematic review of the effectiveness of substitute matrices in comparison to connective tissue grafts. Int J Mol Sci. **2020** Jul 17; 21(14): 5043. doi: 10.3390/ijms21145043.

Listgarten MA, Lang NP, Schroeder HE, Schroeder A. Periodontal tissues and their counterparts around endosseous implants. [corrected and republished with original paging, article originally printed in Clin Oral Implants Res **1991** Jan–Mar; 2(1): 1–19]. Clin Oral Implants Res. **1991** Jul–Sep; 2(3): 1–19. doi: 10.1034/j.1600-0501.1991.020309.x.

Lopez-Píriz R, Fernández A, Goyos-Ball L, Rivera S, Díaz LA, Fernández-Domínguez M, Prado C, Moya JS, Torrecillas R. Performance of a new Al_2O_3/Ce-TZP ceramic nanocomposite dental implant: a pilot study in dogs. Materials (Basel). **2017** Jun 3; 10(6): 614. doi: 10.3390/ma10060614.

Magne P, Magne M, Belser U. The diagnostic template: a key element to the comprehensive esthetic treatment concept. Int J Periodontics Restorative Dent. **1996** Dec; 16(6): 560–569.

Mainjot AK, Schajer GS, Vanheusden AJ, Sadoun MJ. Influence of veneer thickness on residual stress profile in veneering ceramic: measurement by hole-drilling. Dent Mater. **2012** Feb; 28(2): 160–177. doi: 10.1016/j.dental.2011.11.008. (**a**)

Mainjot AK, Schajer GS, Vanheusden AJ, Sadoun MJ. Influence of zirconia framework thickness on residual stress profile in veneering ceramic: measurement by hole-drilling. Dent Mater. **2012** Apr; 28(4): 378–384. doi: 10.1016/j.dental.2011.11.009. (**b**)

Mankoo T. Single-tooth implant restorations in the esthetic zone—contemporary concepts for optimization and maintenance of soft tissue esthetics in the replacement of failing teeth in compromised sites. Eur J Esthet Dent. **2007** Autumn; 2(3): 274–295.

Margeas RC. Predictable periimplant gingival esthetics: use of the natural tooth as a provisional following implant placement. J Esthet Restor Dent. **2006**; 18(1): 5–12. doi: 10.2310/6130.2006.00006.

Marsell R, Einhorn TA. The biology of fracture healing. Injury. **2011** Jun; 42(6): 551–555. doi: 10.1016/j.injury.2011.03.031.

Martin W, Chappuis V, Morton D, Buser D. Esthetic Risk Assessment. In: Buser D, Chen S, Wismeijer D (eds). ITI Treatment Guide Vol. 10: Implant therapy in the esthetic zone: current treatment modalities and materials for single-tooth replacements. Berlin: Quintessence Publishing, **2017**. ISBN 978-3-86867-343-2.

Matta RE, Bergauer B, Adler W, Wichmann M, Nickenig HJ. The impact of the fabrication method on the three-dimensional accuracy of an implant surgery template. J Craniomaxillofac Surg. **2017** Jun; 45(6): 804–808. doi: 10.1016/j.jcms.2017.02.015.

Mayfield LJA. Immediate, delayed and late submerged and transmucosal implants. In: Lang NP, Karring T, Lindhe J (ed). Proceedings of the 3rd European Workshop on Periodontology: Implant Dentistry. Berlin: Quintessence Publishing, **1999**. ISBN 10: 3-87652-306-0.

Meredith N, Alleyne D, Cawley P. Quantitative determination of the stability of the implant-tissue interface using resonance frequency analysis. Clin Oral Implants Res. **1996** Sep; 7(3): 261–267. doi: 10.1034/j.1600-0501.1996.070308.x.

Merheb J, Vercruyssen M, Coucke W, Beckers L, Teughels W, Quirynen M. The fate of buccal bone around dental implants. A 12-month postloading follow-up study. Clin Oral Implants Res. **2017** Jan; 28(1): 103–108. doi: 10.1111/clr.12767.

Miani C, Piconi C, Piselli D. <Untitled>. Italian J Osseoint. **1993**; 69, 599–604.

Miyamoto Y, Obama T. Dental cone beam computed tomography analyses of postoperative labial bone thickness in maxillary anterior implants: comparing immediate and delayed implant placement. Int J Periodontics Restorative Dent. **2011** Jun; 31(3): 215–225.

Miyazaki T, Nakamura T, Matsumura H, Ban S, Kobayashi T. Current status of zirconia restoration. J Prosthodont Res. **2013** Oct; 57(4): 236–261. doi: 10.1016/j.jpor.2013.09.001.

Möhlhenrich SC, Modabber A, Steiner T, Mitchell DA, Hölzle F. Heat generation and drill wear during dental implant site preparation: systematic review. Br J Oral Maxillofac Surg. **2015** Oct; 53(8): 679–689. doi: 10.1016/j.bjoms.2015.05.004.

Monje A, Ravidà A, Wang HL, Helms JA, Brunski JB. Relationship between primary/mechanical and secondary/biological implant stability. Int J Oral Maxillofac Implants. **2019** Suppl; 34: s7–s23. doi: 10.11607/jomi.19suppl.g1.

Monzavi M, Zhang F, Meille S, Douillard T, Adrien J, Noumbissi S, et al. Influence of artificial aging on mechanical properties of commercially and non-commercially available zirconia dental implants. J Mech Behav Biomed Mater. **2020** Jan; 101: 103423. doi: 10.1016/j.jmbbm.2019.103423.

Moore PA, Hersh EV. Combining ibuprofen and acetaminophen for acute pain management after third-molar extractions: translating clinical research to dental practice. J Am Dent Assoc. **2013** Aug; 144(8): 898–908. doi: 10.14219/jada.archive.2013.0207.

Morton D, Chen ST, Martin WC, Levine RA, Buser D. Consensus statements and recommended clinical procedures regarding optimizing esthetic outcomes in implant dentistry. Int J Oral Maxillofac Implants. **2014**; 29 Suppl: 216–220. doi: 10.11607/jomi.2013.g3.

Morton D, Gallucci G, Lin WS, et al. Group 2 ITI Consensus Report: Prosthodontics and implant dentistry. Clin Oral Implants Res. **2018** Oct; 29 Suppl 16: 215–223. doi: 10.1111/clr.13298.

Morton D, Wismeijer D, Chen S, Hamilton A, Wittneben JG, Casentini P, et al. Group 5 ITI Consensus Report: Implant placement and loading protocols. Clin Oral Implants Res. **2023**; 34 [forthcoming].

Newell DJ. Intention-to-treat analysis: implications for quantitative and qualitative research. Int J Epidemiol. **1992** Oct; 21(5): 837–841. doi: 10.1093/ije/21.5.837.

Noelken R, Moergel M, Pausch T, Kunkel M, Wagner W. Clinical and esthetic outcome with immediate insertion and provisionalization with or without connective tissue grafting in presence of mucogingival recessions: a retrospective analysis with follow-up between 1 and 8 years. Clin Implant Dent Relat Res. **2018** Jun; 20(3): 285–293. doi: 10.1111/cid.12595.

Norton MR. The influence of insertion torque on the survival of immediately placed and restored single-tooth implants. Int J Oral Maxillofac Implants. **2011** Nov–Dec; 26(6): 1333–1343.

Norton M. Primary stability versus viable constraint—a need to redefine. Int J Oral Maxillofac Implants. **2013** Jan–Feb; 28(1): 19–21.

Novaes AB Jr, Vidigal Júnior GM, Novaes AB, Grisi MF, Polloni S, Rosa A. Immediate implants placed into infected sites: a histomorphometric study in dogs. Int J Oral Maxillofac Implants. **1998** May–Jun; 13(3): 422–427.

Oates TW, Valderrama P, Bischof M, Nedir R, Jones A, Simpson J, et al. Enhanced implant stability with a chemically modified SLA surface: a randomized pilot study. Int J Oral Maxillofac Implants. **2007** Sep–Oct; 22(5): 755–760.

Ogawa T, Sitalaksmi RM, Miyashita M, Maekawa K, Ryu M, Kimura-Ono A, et al. Effectiveness of the socket shield technique in dental implant: a systematic review. J Prosthodont Res. **2022** Jan 11; 66(1): 12–18. doi: 10.2186/jpr.JPR_D_20_00054.

Ok E, Güngör E, Colak M, Altunsoy M, Nur BG, Ağlarci OS. Evaluation of the relationship between the maxillary posterior teeth and the sinus floor using cone-beam computed tomography. Surg Radiol Anat. **2014** Nov; 36(9): 907–914. doi: 10.1007/s00276-014-1317-3.

Osman RB, Ma S, Duncan W, De Silva RK, Siddiqi A, Swain MV. Fractured zirconia implants and related implant designs: scanning electron microscopy analysis. Clin Oral Implants Res. **2013** May; 24(5): 592–597. doi: 10.1111/j.1600-0501.2011.02411.x.

Ottoni JM, Oliveira ZF, Mansini R, Cabral AM. Correlation between placement torque and survival of single-tooth implants. Int J Oral Maxillofac Implants. **2005** Sep–Oct; 20(5): 769–776.

Paolantonio M, Dolci M, Scarano A, d'Archivio D, di Placido G, Tumini V, et al. Immediate implantation in fresh extraction sockets. A controlled clinical and histological study in man. J Periodontol. **2001** Nov; 72(11): 1560–1571. doi: 10.1902/jop.2001.72.11.1560.

Papageorgiou SN, Eliades T, Hämmerle CHF. Frequency of infraposition and missing contact points in implant-supported restorations within natural dentitions over time: a systematic review with meta-analysis. Clin Oral Implants Res. **2018** Oct; 29 Suppl 18: 309–325. doi: 10.1111/clr.13291.

Papaspyridakos P, Chen CJ, Chuang SK, Weber HP. Implant loading protocols for edentulous patients with fixed prostheses: a systematic review and meta-analysis. Int J Oral Maxillofac Implants. **2014**; 29 Suppl: 256–270. doi: 10.11607/jomi.2014suppl.g4.3.

Payer M, Arnetzl V, Kirmeier R, Koller M, Arnetzl G, Jakse N. Immediate provisional restoration of single-piece zirconia implants: a prospective case series—results after 24 months of clinical function. Clin Oral Implants Res. **2013** May; 24(5): 569–575. doi: 10.1111/j.1600-0501.2012.02425.x.

Payer M, Heschl A, Koller M, Arnetzl G, Lorenzoni M, Jakse N. All-ceramic restoration of zirconia two-piece implants—a randomized controlled clinical trial. Clin Oral Implants Res. **2015** Apr; 26(4): 371–376. doi: 10.1111/clr.12342.

Pellegrino G, Ferri A, Del Fabbro M, Prati C, Gandolfi MG, Marchetti C. Dynamic navigation in implant dentistry: a systematic review and meta-analysis. Int J Oral Maxillofac Implants. **2021** Sep–Oct; 36(5): e121–e140. doi: 10.11607/jomi.8770.

Perez A, Caiazzo A, Valente NA, Toti P, Alfonsi F, Barone A. Standard vs customized healing abutments with simultaneous bone grafting for tissue changes around immediate implants. 1-year outcomes from a randomized clinical trial. Clin Implant Dent Relat Res. **2020** Feb; 22(1): 42–53. doi: 10.1111/cid.12871.

Pieralli S, Kohal RJ, Jung RE, Vach K, Spies BC. Clinical outcomes of zirconia dental implants: a systematic review. J Dent Res. **2017** Jan; 96(1): 38–46. doi: 10.1177/0022034516664043.

Pietrokovski J, Massler M. Alveolar ridge resorption following tooth extraction. J Prosthet Dent. **1967** Jan; 17(1): 21–27. doi: 10.1016/0022-3913(67)90046-7.

Pimkhaokham A, Jiaranuchart S, Kaboosaya B, Arunjaroensuk S, Subbalekha K, Mattheos N. Can computer-assisted implant surgery improve clinical outcomes and reduce the frequency and intensity of complications in implant dentistry? A critical review. Periodontol 2000. **2022** Oct; 90(1): 197–223. doi: 10.1111/prd.12458.

Pitta J, Zarauz C, Pjetursson B, Sailer I, Liu X, Pradies G. A systematic review and meta-analysis of the influence of abutment material on peri-implant soft tissue color measured using spectrophotometry. Int J Prosthodont. **2020** Jan–Feb; 33(1): 39–47. doi: 10.11607/ijp.6393.

Raghavendra S, Wood MC, Taylor TD. Early wound healing around endosseous implants: a review of the literature. Int J Oral Maxillofac Implants. **2005** May–Jun; 20(3): 425–431.

Ragucci GM, Elnayef B, Criado-Cámara E, Del Amo FS, Hernández-Alfaro F. Immediate implant placement in molar extraction sockets: a systematic review and meta-analysis. Int J Implant Dent. **2020** Oct 13; 6(1): 40. doi: 10.1186/s40729-020-00235-5.

Raj A, Bhatnagar A. Preservation of optimal gingival architecture through customised healing abutment in immediate implant placement: a clinical report. Int J Adv Res. **2015** Nov; 3(11): 156–160.

Rashad A, Sadr-Eshkevari P, Heiland M, Smeets R, Hanken H, Gröbe A, et al. Intraosseous heat generation during sonic, ultrasonic and conventional osteotomy. J Craniomaxillofac Surg. **2015** Sep; 43(7): 1072–1077. doi: 10.1016/j.jcms.2015.05.018.

Rilo B, da Silva JL, Mora MJ, Santana U. Guidelines for occlusion strategy in implant-borne prostheses. A review. Int Dent J. **2008** Jun; 58(3): 139–145. doi: 10.1111/j.1875-595x.2008.tb00189.x.

Röhling S, Astasov-Frauenhoffer M, Hauser-Gerspach I, Braissant O, Wölfler H, Waltimo T, et al. In vitro biofilm formation on titanium and zirconia implant surfaces. J Periodontol. **2017** Mar; 88(3): 298–307. doi: 10.1902/jop.2016.160245.

Röhling S, Schlegel KA, Wölfler H, Gahlert M. Performance and outcome of zirconia dental implants in clinical studies: a meta-analysis. Clin Oral Implants Res. **2018** Oct; 29 Suppl 16: 135–153. doi: 10.1111/clr.13352.

Röhling S, Gahlert M, Janner S, Meng B, Wölfler H, Cochran DL. Ligature-induced peri-implant bone loss around loaded zirconia and titanium implants. Int J Oral Maxillofac Implants. **2019** Mar–Apr; 34(2): 357–365. doi: 10.11607/jomi.7015.

Röhling S, Schlegel KA, Wölfler H, Gahlert M. Zirconia compared to titanium dental implants in preclinical studies—a systematic review and meta-analysis. Clin Oral Implants Res. **2019** May; 30(5): 365–395. doi: 10.1111/clr.13425.

Romandini M, Pedrinaci I, Lima C, Soldini MC, Araoz A, Sanz M. Prevalence and risk/protective indicators of buccal soft tissue dehiscence around dental implants. J Clin Periodontol. **2021** Mar; 48(3): 455–463. doi: 10.1111/jcpe.13417.

Romandini M, Ruales-Carrera E, Sadilina S, Hämmerle CHF, Sanz M. Minimal invasiveness at dental implant placement: A systematic review with meta-analyses on flapless fully guided surgery. Periodontol 2000. **2022** Jul 30. [Epub ahead of print.] doi: 10.1111/prd.12440.

Romanos GE, Ciornei G, Jucan A, Malmstrom H, Gupta B. In vitro assessment of primary stability of Straumann implant designs. Clin Implant Dent Relat Res. **2014** Feb; 16(1): 89–95. doi: 10.1111/j.1708-8208.2012.00464.x.

Romanos GE, Delgado-Ruiz R, Sculean A. Concepts for prevention of complications in implant therapy. Periodontol 2000. **2019** Oct; 81(1): 7–17. doi: 10.1111/prd.12278.

Ruales-Carrera E, Pauletto P, Apaza-Bedoya K, Volpato CAM, Özcan M, Benfatti CAM. Peri-implant tissue management after immediate implant placement using a customized healing abutment. J Esthet Restor Dent. **2019** Nov; 31(6): 533–541. doi: 10.1111/jerd.12512.

Sailer I, Philipp A, Zembic A, Pjetursson BE, Hämmerle CH, Zwahlen M. A systematic review of the performance of ceramic and metal implant abutments supporting fixed implant reconstructions. Clin Oral Implants Res. **2009** Sep; 20 Suppl 4: 4–31. doi: 10.1111/j.1600-0501.2009.01787.x.

Sailer I, Mühlemann S, Zwahlen M, Hämmerle CH, Schneider D. Cemented and screw-retained implant reconstructions: a systematic review of the survival and complication rates. Clin Oral Implants Res. **2012** Oct; 23 Suppl 6: 163–201. doi: 10.1111/j.1600-0501.2012.02538.x.

Saito H, Chu SJ, Reynolds MA, Tarnow DP. Provisional restorations used in immediate implant placement provide a platform to promote peri-implant soft tissue healing: a pilot study. Int J Periodontics Restorative Dent. **2016** Jan–Feb; 36(1): 47–52. doi: 10.11607/prd.1945.

Saleh MHA, Ravidà A, Suárez-López Del Amo F, Lin GH, Asa'ad F, et al. The effect of implant-abutment junction position on crestal bone loss: A systematic review and meta-analysis. Clin Implant Dent Relat Res. **2018** Aug; 20(4): 617–633. doi: 10.1111/cid.12600.

Salhi L, Lecloux G, Seidel L, Rompen E, Lambert F. Coronally advanced flap versus the pouch technique combined with a connective tissue graft to treat Miller's class I gingival recession: a randomized controlled trial. J Clin Periodontol. **2014** Apr; 41(4): 387–395. doi: 10.1111/jcpe.12207.

Salvi GE, Bosshardt DD, Lang NP, Abrahamsson I, Berglundh T, Lindhe J, et al. Temporal sequence of hard and soft tissue healing around titanium dental implants. Periodontol 2000. **2015** Jun; 68(1): 135–152. doi: 10.1111/prd.12054.

Sanz M, Ivanoff CJ, Weingart D, Wiltfang J, Gahlert M, Cordaro L, et al. Clinical and radiologic outcomes after submerged and transmucosal implant placement with two-piece implants in the anterior maxilla and mandible: 3-year results of a randomized controlled clinical trial. Clin Implant Dent Relat Res. **2015** Apr; 17(2): 234–246. doi: 10.1111/cid.12107.

Sanz M, Lindhe J, Alcaraz J, Sanz-Sanchez I, Cecchinato D. The effect of placing a bone replacement graft in the gap at immediately placed implants: a randomized clinical trial. Clin Oral Implants Res. **2017** Aug; 28(8): 902–910. doi: 10.1111/clr.12896.

Sanz-Martín I, Rojo E, Maldonado E, Stroppa G, Nart J, Sanz M. Structural and histological differences between connective tissue grafts harvested from the lateral palatal mucosa or from the tuberosity area. Clin Oral Investig. **2019** Feb; 23(2): 957–964. doi: 10.1007/s00784-018-2516-9.

Sanz-Martín I, Regidor E, Cosyn J, Wiedemeier DB, Thoma DS. Buccal soft tissue dehiscence defects at dental implants–associated factors and frequency of occurrence: A systematic review and meta-analysis. Clin Oral Implants Res. **2022** Jun; 33 Suppl 23: 109–124. doi: 10.1111/clr.13888.

Sanz-Sánchez I, Sanz-Martín I, Figuero E, Sanz M. Clinical efficacy of immediate implant loading protocols compared to conventional loading depending on the type of the restoration: a systematic review. Clin Oral Implants Res. **2015** Aug; 26(8): 964–982. doi: 10.1111/clr.12428.

Schneider D, Marquardt P, Zwahlen M, Jung RE. A systematic review on the accuracy and the clinical outcome of computer-guided template-based implant dentistry. Clin Oral Implants Res. **2009** Sep; 20 Suppl 4: 73–86. doi: 10.1111/j.1600-0501.2009.01788.x.

Schnitman PA, Wohrle PS, Rubenstein JE. Immediate fixed interim prostheses supported by two-stage threaded implants: methodology and results. J Oral Implantol. **1990**; 16(2): 96–105.

Schnutenhaus S, Edelmann C, Rudolph H, Dreyhaupt J, Luthardt RG. 3D accuracy of implant positions in template-guided implant placement as a function of the remaining teeth and the surgical procedure: a retrospective study. Clin Oral Investig. **2018** Jul; 22(6): 2363–2372. doi: 10.1007/s00784-018-2339-8.

Schoenbaum TR, Chang YY, Klokkevold PR, Snowden JS. Abutment emergence modification for immediate implant provisional restorations. J Esthet Restor Dent. **2013** Apr; 25(2): 103–107. doi: 10.1111/jerd.12007.

Schroeder A, Pohler O, Sutter F. Gewebsreaktion auf ein Titan-Hohlzylinderimplantat mit Titan-Spritzschichtoberfläche [Tissue reaction to an implant of a titanium hollow cylinder with a titanium surface spray layer]. SSO Schweiz Monatsschr Zahnheilkd. **1976** Jul; 86(7): 713–727. German.

Schroeder A, van der Zypen E, Stich H, Sutter F. The reactions of bone, connective tissue, and epithelium to endosteal implants with titanium-sprayed surfaces. J Maxillofac Surg. **1981** Feb; 9(1): 15–25. doi: 10.1016/s0301-0503(81)80007-0.

Schropp L, Wenzel A, Kostopoulos L, Karring T. Bone healing and soft tissue contour changes following single-tooth extraction: a clinical and radiographic 12-month prospective study. Int J Periodontics Restorative Dent. **2003** Aug; 23(4): 313–323.

Schubert O, Beuer F, Schweiger J, Güth J. Digital tissue preservation concept: a workflow for guided immediate implant placement and restoration. J Prosthodont. **2019** Jul; 28(6): 613–617. doi: 10.1111/jopr.13089.

Schulte W, Kleineikenscheidt H, Lindner K, Schareyka R. Das Tübinger Sofortimplantat in der klinischen Prüfung [The Tübingen immediate implant in clinical studies]. Dtsch Zahnärztl Z. **1978** May; 33(5): 348–359. German.

Schütz S, Egger J, Kühl S, Filippi A, Lambrecht JT. Intraosseous temperature changes during the use of piezosurgical inserts in vitro. Int J Oral Maxillofac Surg. **2012** Nov; 41(11): 1338–1343. doi: 10.1016/j.ijom.2012.06.007.

Schwartz-Arad D, Chaushu G. The ways and wherefores of immediate placement of implants into Fresh extraction sites: a literature review. J Periodontol. **1997** Oct; 68(10): 915–923. doi: 10.1902/jop.1997.68.10.915.

Schwarz F, Herten M, Sager M, Wieland M, Dard M, Becker J. Bone regeneration in dehiscence-type defects at chemically modified (SLActive) and conventional SLA titanium implants: a pilot study in dogs. J Clin Periodontol. **2007** Jan; 34(1): 78–86. doi: 10.1111/j.1600-051X.2006.01008.x.

Schwimer C, Pette GA, Gluckman H, Salama M, Du Toit J. Human histologic evidence of new bone formation and osseointegration between root dentin (unplanned socket-shield) and dental implant: case report. Int J Oral Maxillofac Implants. **2018** Jan–Feb; 33(1): e19–e23. doi: 10.11607/jomi.6215.

Seyssens L, Eghbali A, Cosyn J. A 10-year prospective study on single immediate implants. J Clin Periodontol. **2020** Oct; 47(10): 1248–1258. doi: 10.1111/jcpe.13352.

Seyssens L, De Lat L, Cosyn J. Immediate implant placement with or without connective tissue graft: A systematic review and meta-analysis. J Clin Periodontol. **2021** Feb; 48(2): 284–301. doi: 10.1111/jcpe.13397.

Seyssens L, Eeckhout C, Cosyn J. Immediate implant placement with or without socket grafting: a systematic review and meta-analysis. Clin Implant Dent Relat Res. **2022** Jun; 24(3): 339–351. doi: 10.1111/cid.13079.

Shahramian K, Gasik M, Kangasniemi I, Walboomers XF, Willberg J, Abdulmajeed A, Närhi T. Zirconia implants with improved attachment to the gingival tissue. J Periodontol. **2020** Sep; 91(9): 1213–1224. doi: 10.1002/JPER.19-0323.

Silva NR, Coelho PG, Fernandes CA, Navarro JM, Dias RA, Thompson VP. Reliability of one-piece ceramic implant. J Biomed Mater Res B Appl Biomater. **2009** Feb; 88(2): 419–426. doi: 10.1002/jbm.b.31113.

Smith RB, Tarnow DP. Classification of molar extraction sites for immediate dental implant placement: technical note. Int J Oral Maxillofac Implants. 2013 May–Jun; 28(3): 911–916. doi: 10.11607/jomi.2627.

Song SJ, Tao G, Shariff J, Tarnow DP, Bittner N. Evaluation of dimensional changes and ridge contour around ovate pontics inserted immediately after extraction with alveolar ridge preservation in the esthetic zone. Int J Periodontics Restorative Dent. **2022** Jan–Feb; 42(1): 83–91. doi: 10.11607/prd.5352.

Souza AB, Tormena M, Matarazzo F, Araújo MG. The influence of peri-implant keratinized mucosa on brushing discomfort and peri-implant tissue health. Clin Oral Implants Res. **2016** Jun; 27(6): 650–655. doi: 10.1111/clr.12703.

Souza AB, Alshihri A, Kämmerer PW, Araújo MG, Gallucci GO. Histological and micro-CT analysis of peri-implant soft and hard tissue healing on implants with different healing abutments configurations. Clin Oral Implants Res. **2018** Oct; 29(10): 1007–1015. doi: 10.1111/clr.13367.

Spies BC, Balmer M, Patzelt SB, Vach K, Kohal RJ. Clinical and patient-reported outcomes of a zirconia oral iImplant: three-year results of a prospective cohort investigation. J Dent Res. **2015** Oct; 94(10): 1385–1391. doi: 10.1177/0022034515598962.

Staehler P, Abraha SM, Bastos J, Zuhr O, Hürzeler M. The socket-shield technique: a step-by-step protocol after 12 years of experience. Int J Esthet Dent. **2020**; 15(3): 288–305.

Staubli N, Walter C, Schmidt JC, Weiger R, Zitzmann NU. Excess cement and the risk of peri-implant disease—a systematic review. Clin Oral Implants Res. **2017** Oct; 28(10): 1278–1290. doi: 10.1111/clr.12954.

Stavropoulos A, Cochran D, Obrecht M, Pippenger BE, Dard M. Effect of osteotomy preparation on osseointegration of immediately loaded, tapered dental implants. Adv Dent Res. **2016** Mar; 28(1): 34–41. doi: 10.1177/0022034515624446.

Steigmann M, Cooke J, Wang HL. Use of the natural tooth for soft tissue development: a case series. Int J Periodontics Restorative Dent. **2007** Dec; 27(6): 603–608.

Su H, Gonzalez-Martin O, Weisgold A, Lee E. Considerations of implant abutment and crown contour: critical contour and subcritical contour. Int J Periodontics Restorative Dent. **2010** Aug; 30(4): 335–343.

Tahmaseb A, Wismeijer D, Coucke W, Derksen W. Computer technology applications in surgical implant dentistry: a systematic review. Int J Oral Maxillofac Implants. **2014**; 29 Suppl: 25–42. doi: 10.11607/jomi.2014suppl.g1.2.

Tahmaseb A, Wu V, Wismeijer D, Coucke W, Evans C. The accuracy of static computer-aided implant surgery: a systematic review and meta-analysis. Clin Oral Implants Res. **2018** Oct; 29 Suppl 16: 416–435. doi: 10.1111/clr.13346.

Tan WL, Wong TL, Wong MC, Lang NP. A systematic review of post-extractional alveolar hard and soft tissue dimensional changes in humans. Clin Oral Implants Res. **2012** Feb; 23 Suppl 5: 1–21. doi: 10.1111/j.1600-0501.2011.02375.x.

Tarnow DP, Cho SC, Wallace SS. The effect of inter-implant distance on the height of inter-implant bone crest. J Periodontol. **2000** Apr; 71(4): 546–549. doi: 10.1902/jop.2000.71.4.546.

Tarnow DP, Chu SJ. Human histologic verification of osseointegration of an immediate implant placed into a fresh extraction socket with excessive gap distance without primary flap closure, graft, or membrane: a case report. Int J Periodontics Restorative Dent. **2011** Sep–Oct; 31(5): 515–521.

Tarnow DP, Chu SJ, Salama MA, Stappert CF, Salama H, Garber DA, et al. Flapless postextraction socket implant placement in the esthetic zone. Part 1: The effect of bone grafting and/or provisional restoration on facial-palatal ridge dimensional change–a retrospective cohort study. Int J Periodontics Restorative Dent. 2014 May–Jun; 34(3): 323–331. doi: 10.11607/prd.1821.

Tavelli L, Barootchi S, Greenwell H, Wang HL. Is a soft tissue graft harvested from the maxillary tuberosity the approach of choice in an isolated site? J Periodontol. **2019** Aug; 90(8): 821–825. doi: 10.1002/JPER.18-0615.

Tavelli L, Barootchi S, Avila-Ortiz G, Urban IA, Giannobile WV, Wang HL. Peri-implant soft tissue phenotype modification and its impact on peri-implant health: A systematic review and network meta-analysis. J Periodontol. **2021** Jan; 92(1): 21–44. doi: 10.1002/JPER.19-0716.

Testori T, Weinstein T, Scutellà F, Wang HL, Zucchelli G. Implant placement in the esthetic area: criteria for positioning single and multiple implants. Periodontol 2000. **2018** Jun; 77(1): 176–196. doi: 10.1111/prd.12211.

Thoma DS, Ioannidis A, Cathomen E, Hämmerle CH, Hüsler J, Jung RE. Discoloration of the peri-implant mucosa caused by zirconia and titanium implants. Int J Periodontics Restorative Dent. **2016** Jan–Feb; 36(1): 39–45. doi: 10.11607/prd.2663.

Thoma DS, Naenni N, Benic GI, Hämmerle CH, Jung RE. Soft tissue volume augmentation at dental implant sites using a volume stable three-dimensional collagen matrix—histological outcomes of a preclinical study. J Clin Periodontol. **2017** Feb; 44(2): 185–194. doi: 10.1111/jcpe.12635.

Thoma DS, Naenni N, Figuero E, Hämmerle CHF, Schwarz F, Jung RE, Sanz-Sánchez I. Effects of soft tissue augmentation procedures on peri-implant health or disease: a systematic review and meta-analysis. Clin Oral Implants Res. **2018** Mar; 29 Suppl 15: 32–49. doi: 10.1111/clr.13114.

Tian XM, Qian L, Xin XZ, Wei B, Gong Y. An analysis of the proximity of maxillary posterior teeth to the maxillary sinus using cone-beam computed tomography. J Endod. **2016** Mar; 42(3): 371–377. doi: 10.1016/j.joen.2015.10.017.

Tomasi C, Sanz M, Cecchinato D, Pjetursson B, Ferrus J, Lang NP, Lindhe J. Bone dimensional variations at implants placed in fresh extraction sockets: a multilevel multivariate analysis. Clin Oral Implants Res. **2010** Jan; 21(1): 30–36. doi: 10.1111/j.1600-0501.2009.01848.x.

Tonetti MS, Cortellini P, Graziani F, Cairo F, Lang NP, Abundo R, et al. Immediate versus delayed implant placement after anterior single tooth extraction: the timing randomized controlled clinical trial. J Clin Periodontol. **2017** Feb; 44(2): 215–224. doi: 10.1111/jcpe.12666.

Tonetti MS, Jung RE, Avila-Ortiz G, Blanco J, Cosyn J, Fickl S, et al. Management of the extraction socket and timing of implant placement: Consensus report and clinical recommendations of group 3 of the XV European Workshop in Periodontology. J Clin Periodontol. **2019** Jun; 46 Suppl 21: 183–194. doi: 10.1111/jcpe.13131.

Trimpou G, Weigl P, Krebs M, Parvini P, Nentwig GH. Rationale for esthetic tissue preservation of a fresh extraction socket by an implant treatment concept simulating a tooth replantation. Dent Traumatol. **2010** Feb; 26(1): 105–111. doi: 10.1111/j.1600-9657.2009.00831.x

Truninger TC, Philipp AO, Siegenthaler DW, Roos M, Hämmerle CH, Jung RE. A prospective, controlled clinical trial evaluating the clinical and radiological outcome after 3 years of immediately placed implants in sockets exhibiting periapical pathology. Clin Oral Implants Res. **2011** Jan; 22(1): 20–27. doi: 10.1111/j.1600-0501.2010.01973.x.

Tsuda H, Rungcharassaeng K, Kan JY, Roe P, Lozada JL, Zimmerman G. Peri-implant tissue response following connective tissue and bone grafting in conjunction with immediate single-tooth replacement in the esthetic zone: a case series. Int J Oral Maxillofac Implants. **2011** Mar–Apr; 26(2): 427–436.

Valles C, Rodríguez-Ciurana X, Clementini M, Baglivo M, Paniagua B, Nart J. Influence of subcrestal implant placement compared with equicrestal position on the peri-implant hard and soft tissues around platform-switched implants: a systematic review and meta-analysis. Clin Oral Investig. **2018** Mar; 22(2): 555–570. doi: 10.1007/s00784-017-2301-1.

Valles C, Vilarrasa J, Barallat L, Pascual A, Nart J. Efficacy of soft tissue augmentation procedures on tissue thickening around dental implants: A systematic review and meta-analysis. Clin Oral Implants Res. **2022** Jun; 33 Suppl 23: 72–99. doi: 10.1111/clr.13920.

van Nimwegen WG, Raghoebar GM, Zuiderveld EG, Jung RE, Meijer HJA, Mühlemann S. Immediate placement and provisionalization of implants in the aesthetic zone with or without a connective tissue graft: a 1-year randomized controlled trial and volumetric study. Clin Oral Implants Res. **2018** Jul; 29(7): 671–678. doi: 10.1111/clr.13258.

van Steenberghe D, Callens A, Geers L, Jacobs R. The clinical use of deproteinized bovine bone mineral on bone regeneration in conjunction with immediate implant installation. Clin Oral Implants Res. **2000** Jun; 11(3): 210–216. doi: 10.1034/j.1600-0501.2000.011003210.x.

Vanhoutte V, Rompen E, Lecloux G, Rues S, Schmitter M, Lambert F. A methodological approach to assessing alveolar ridge preservation procedures in humans: soft tissue profile. Clin Oral Implants Res. **2014** Mar; 25(3): 304–309. doi: 10.1111/clr.12144.

Vera C, De Kok IJ, Chen W, Reside G, Tyndall D, Cooper LF. Evaluation of post-implant buccal bone resorption using cone beam computed tomography: a clinical pilot study. Int J Oral Maxillofac Implants. **2012** Sep–Oct; 27(5): 1249–1257.

Wang IC, Chan HL, Kinney J, Wang HL. Volumetric facial contour changes of immediately placed implants with and without immediate provisionalization. J Periodontol. **2020** Jul; 91(7): 906–916. doi: 10.1002/JPER.19-0308.

Welander M, Abrahamsson I, Berglundh T. The mucosal barrier at implant abutments of different materials. Clin Oral Implants Res. **2008** Jul; 19(7): 635–641. doi: 10.1111/j.1600-0501.2008.01543.x.

Wilson TG Jr, Miller RJ, Trushkowsky R, Dard M. Tapered implants in dentistry: revitalizing concepts with technology: a review. Adv Dent Res. **2016** Mar; 28(1): 4–9. doi: 10.1177/0022034516628868.

Wittneben JG, Molinero-Mourelle P, Hamilton A, Alnasser M, Obermaier B, Morton D, et al. Clinical performance of immediately loaded single implants in the esthetic zone. A systematic review and meta-analysis. Clin Oral Implants Res. **2023**; 34 [forthcoming].

Wöhrle PS. Single-tooth replacement in the aesthetic zone with immediate provisionalization: fourteen consecutive case reports. Pract Periodontics Aesthet Dent. **1998** Nov–Dec; 10(9): 1107–1114.

Yamaguchi Y, Shiota M, Munakata M, Kasugai S, Ozeki M. Effect of implant design on primary stability using torque-time curves in artificial bone. Int J Implant Dent. **2015** Dec; 1(1): 21. doi: 10.1186/s40729.015-0024-0.

Yuenyongorarn P, Kan JYK, Rungcharassaeng K, Matsuda H, Roe P, Lozada JL, Caruso J. Facial gingival changes with and without socket gap grafting following single maxillary anterior immediate tooth replacement: one-year results. J Oral Implantol. **2020** Oct 1; 46(5): 496–505. doi: 10.1563/aaid-joi-D-19-00187.

Zhang YQ, Yan XB, Meng Y, Zhao YN, Liu DG. Morphologic analysis of maxillary sinus floor and its correlation to molar roots using cone beam computed tomography. Chin J Dent Res. **2019**; 22(1): 29–36. doi: 10.3290/j.cjdr.a41772.

Zhou W, Gallucci GO, Chen S, Buser D, Hamilton A. Placement and loading protocols for single implants in different locations: a systematic review. Int J Oral Maxillofac Implants. **2021** Jul–Aug; 36(4): e72–e89. doi: 10.11607/jomi.8750.